Terminal Care Strategies for Managing Elderly Patients

Adil Hamad Alharthi
https://orcid.org/0000-0001-6124-5907
King Fahad Armed Forces Hospital, Saudi Arabia

Marwa Mohammed Eleawa
https://orcid.org/0000-0003-1666-2167
Beni-Suef University, Egypt

IGI Global
Scientific Publishing
Publishing Tomorrow's Research Today

Vice President of Editorial	Melissa Wagner
Director of Acquisitions	Mikaela Felty
Director of Book Development	Jocelynn Hessler
Production Manager	Mike Brehm
Cover Design	Jose Rosado

Published in the United States of America by
IGI Global Scientific Publishing
701 East Chocolate Avenue
Hershey, PA, 17033, USA
Tel: 717-533-8845 | Fax: 717-533-7115
Website: https://www.igi-global.com E-mail: cust@igi-global.com

Library of Congress Cataloging-in-Publication Data

LCCN: 2025945280 (CIP Data Pending)
ISBN13: 979-8-3373-4099-9
Isbn13Softcover: 979-8-3373-4100-2
EISBN13: 979-8-3373-4101-9
British Cataloguing in Publication Data
A Cataloguing in Publication record for this book is available from the British Library.

Table of Contents

Detailed Table of Contents

Current trends in geriatric palliative care require expert team engagement with acknowledgement of challenges and opportunities for improvement. The unique requirements of elderly patients across different societal settings need practical consideration. As such, models for delivery of geriatric palliative care services should be feasible, with consideration of the population demographics. Healthcare disparities still affect geriatric palliative care. Training and the need for global standardization of geriatric palliative care is also discussed.

Quality of life (QoL) in terminal care for elderly patients is a multifaceted concept that includes not only physical symptoms but also psychological, social, and spiritual aspects of well-being. With the global aging population and rising rates of chronic,

Elderly patients often face advanced chronic illnesses, emphasizing the urgent need for timely access to palliative care (PC). Loss of function is among the most distressing symptoms for patients nearing end of life (EOL). In such contexts, rehabilitation becomes essential for adapting care to changing needs and improving patients' quality of life. The World Health Organization's Rehabilitation initiative and its PC policy framework advocate for the integration of rehabilitation into PC systems globally. These initiatives support functional independence, enabling individuals with incurable conditions to remain socially engaged and self-sufficient despite limited life expectancy. Physical therapy (PT) plays a pivotal role in preserving dignity and independence, and supports emotional well-being through patient education, movement restoration, and interdisciplinary collaboration. This chapter concludes by emphasizing the essential role of PT in palliative and EOL care across a range of serious conditions affecting elderly patients

Pressure ulcers (PUs) pose a significant health concern, especially among frail older adults. Effective management of PUs necessitates a coordinated, multidisciplinary approach. Despite significant advancements in medical technology, a universally effective, accessible, and adaptable treatment option that addresses the varied needs of individuals with PUs remains elusive. This persistent gap has led researchers to explore novel and unconventional therapeutic avenues, including those rooted in the field of physical therapy. Within this collaborative framework, physiotherapeutic modalities present promising opportunities as integral components of comprehensive, interprofessional wound care strategies. This chapter presents in brief the surgical management of PUs in the elderly, in addition to a cohesive framework for integrating physiotherapy-based interventions with conventional medical management to optimise healing outcomes. It underscores the pivotal role of caregiver education and the implementation of individualised preventive strategies tailored to each patient's unique needs.

The increase in population of elderly people across the world is presenting a dauting challenge for palliative cares because elderly people are often encountered health challenges and other chronic diseases. This chapter delves into integration of artificial intelligence (AI)-powered wearable devices into elderly palliative cares. These advanced technologies allow proper monitoring of patient vital signs, track symptoms and adopt predictive analysis to prove patient's outcome. (AI)-powered wearable can monitor disease progression, allow remote monitoring which promote patient autonomy especially at home or hospices settings. We presented a comprehensive framework that include diagnostic and therapeutic advantages, case studies and other ethical issues such data privacy and informed consent. This chapter also present challenges such users' acceptability, we also mentioned other real-world applications such as CardioMEMS, Control-IQ, Sepsis Watch and the rest. We conclude the chapter by providing guidelines and recommendation to sharpen future research

Home care has emerged as a cornerstone of contemporary health systems, driven by demographic aging, escalating chronic disease prevalence, and imperatives for cost-effective, patient-centric models of care. This chapter critically interrogates the evolving landscape of home care delivery, foregrounding its most pressing challenges and strategic responses through the lenses of workforce deficits, technological discontinuities, regulatory disarticulation, and entrenched social inequities. Drawing on robust empirical evidence, it delineates pathways to fortify workforce capacity, harness digital health innovations, enhance care integration, and galvanize policy reform. It further explores transformative trends, including artificial intelligence, precision medicine, and pandemic preparedness, that increasingly intersect with domiciliary care. Bridging these systemic gaps holds the potential to reimagine home health care as an equitable, resilient, and high-quality alternative to institutional modalities.

Caring for terminally ill elderly individuals imposes profound psychological, emotional, and physical stress on caregivers, often resulting in anxiety, depression, and anticipatory grief that diminish well-being and end-of-life care quality. Mindfulness-Based Interventions (MBIs), rooted in Buddhist contemplative practice and supported by clinical research, offer an evidence-based means to reduce distress and enhance resilience and compassion. This chapter outlines the theoretical foundations and empirical evidence of MBIs in geriatric palliative care, presenting a practical "Mindfulness Care Pathway" featuring formal and brief practices adaptable for busy caregivers. Cultural adaptation, ethical concerns, and implementation strategies are discussed, alongside outcome measures such as caregiver burden and quality of life. Mindfulness emerges as a compassionate, scalable, and cost-effective approach to sustain caregiver wellness and deliver dignified end-of-life care.

End-of-life care in multicultural societies requires sensitivity to diverse cultural, religious, and trauma-informed perspectives. This work explores how beliefs rooted in Islam, Christianity, Buddhism, Confucianism, and African traditions shape dying experiences, family roles, and clinical decisions. It highlights tensions between Western individualism and communal values, emphasizing the need for cultural safety, humility, and trust. Trauma histories further complicate care, especially among

Preface

The global demographic shift towards an aging population presents one of the most significant challenges and opportunities for modern healthcare systems. As life expectancy increases, so does the prevalence of chronic, end-stage diseases, making the need for effective, compassionate, and specialized terminal care for the elderly more urgent than ever. This phase of life demands a nuanced approach that moves beyond curative intent to a model that prioritizes quality of life, manages complex symptom burdens, and honors the holistic needs of the individual emotional, psychological, and spiritual support.

Terminal Care Strategies for Managing Elderly Patients is dedicated to exploring this critical frontier, offering a comprehensive examination of the strategies that ensure care for the elderly is not only medically sound but also deeply humanistic and respectful.

The subject of terminal care in geriatrics occupies a vital and expanding space in today's world, intersecting with fields like gerontology, palliative medicine, ethics, health management, and digital health. It responds to a growing imperative within healthcare to provide care that aligns with patient values, especially when curing a disease is no longer possible. This book situates itself at this confluence, addressing the gap between generalized medical care and the specialized needs of the terminally ill elderly. It delves into the practical, clinical, and systemic innovations required to navigate the complexities of multimorbidity, functional decline, and the profound psychosocial transitions at the end of life.

This volume is designed as an essential resource for a broad spectrum of healthcare professionals. Practicing physicians, nurses, physical therapists, and home health care providers will find evidence-based clinical guidance. Non-palliative specialists, who often form the first line of management for elderly patients, will gain crucial insights into symptom control and palliative principles. Furthermore, healthcare administrators, policymakers, and technology developers working in the geriatric care space will benefit from the discussions on systemic challenges, AI integration, and novel care models.

The strength of this book lies in the specific and timely contributions of its chapters. Each chapter submission addresses a critical facet of the terminal care ecosystem:

CHAPTER OVERVIEW

Chapter 1: Holistic Palliation Modalities for Elderly Patients with Terminal Illnesses establishes the foundational philosophy of the book, arguing for a care model that addresses the physical, psychological, social, and spiritual domains of suffering simultaneously.

Chapter 2: The Quality of Life in Terminal Care: A Multidimensional Approach for Elderly Patients defines and operationalizes the concept of quality of life, providing a framework for assessing and improving patient well-being beyond traditional clinical metrics.

Chapter 3: Symptom Burden in Elder Palliative Care for Non-palliative Specialists serves as a vital practical guide for front-line clinicians, demystifying the assessment and management of common, distressing symptoms in the elderly palliative population.

Chapter 4: Non-Hypoxic Dyspnea in Terminal Care tackles a particularly distressing and complex symptom, offering specialized strategies for palliative management to alleviate suffering and improve daily living.

Chapter 5: Physical Therapy in Palliative and End-of-Life Care for the Elderly redefines the role of rehabilitation in terminal care, demonstrating how physical therapy can maintain function, manage pain, and promote dignity even in the latest stages of disease.

Chapter 6: Physical Therapy Modalities in Management of Bedsores in Elderly focuses on a common and preventable complication, detailing evidence-based preventive and therapeutic strategies to preserve skin integrity and patient comfort.

Chapter 7: Integrating AI-Powered Wearables into Palliative Care Management looks toward the future, exploring how continuous remote monitoring and data analytics can proactively manage symptoms and personalize care plans for elderly patients.

Chapter 8: Home Health Care for Patients: Major Challenges and Strategic Solutions examines the practicalities and barriers of providing high-quality terminal care in the patient's home, offering actionable solutions for one of the most preferred care settings.

Chapter 9: Mindfulness-Based Interventions for Caregivers of Terminally Elderly Patients: Reducing Burden, Enhancing Resilience, and Supporting Compassionate Care outlines the theoretical foundations and empirical evidence of MBIs in geriatric palliative care, presenting a practical "Mindfulness Care Pathway" featuring formal and brief practices adaptable for busy caregivers.

Chapter 10: Cultural and Religious Dimensions of Dying underscores the essential role of cultural humility, providing crucial guidance for honoring diverse beliefs, rituals, and practices surrounding death and dying, thereby ensuring care is both clinically and culturally competent.

CONCLUSION

In conclusion, this book impacts the field by synthesizing specialized clinical knowledge with holistic and systemic perspectives. It contributes to the subject matter by moving the discourse on terminal care from a generalized concept to a set of concrete, actionable strategies tailored to the unique physiology and needs of the elderly patient. By bridging the gap between physical therapy and palliation, between technology and compassion, and between clinical care and cultural respect, this volume provides a roadmap for a more dignified, comfortable, and person-centric end-of-life journey. It is our firm belief that the insights contained within these chapters will empower professionals to transform the experience of terminal care for the growing population of elderly patients and their families.

Marwa Mohammed Eleawa

Department of Physical Therapy, Applied Science Private University, Amman, Jordan

Chapter 1
Holistic Palliation Modalities for Elderly Patients With Terminal Illnesses

Irumba Pauline
https://orcid.org/0009-0001-0235-4131
Mountains of the Moon University, Uganda

Rugumayo Charles
Mountains of the Moon University, Uganda

Tugume Daniel
Mountains of the Moon University, Uganda

ABSTRACT

Current trends in geriatric palliative care require expert team engagement with acknowledgement of challenges and opportunities for improvement. The unique requirements of elderly patients across different societal settings need practical consideration. As such, models for delivery of geriatric palliative care services should be feasible, with consideration of the population demographics. Healthcare disparities still affect geriatric palliative care. Training and the need for global standardization of geriatric palliative care is also discussed.

DOI: 10.4018/979-8-3373-4099-9.ch001

1.0 INTRODUCTION

Nearly fifty million people are expected to die globally over decades due to life threatening terminal illnesses, of which over eighty percent of the deaths are likely to occur among elderly patients from countries with low developmental index (Murray & Lopez, 1997; Sleeman et al., 2019). Consequently, WHO (2020) estimated nearly sixty million people with a significant elderly population in need of terminal care. Specialized care for elderly terminally ill patients requires dedicated teams of both trained health professionals, and supporting individuals like carers (Loosen et al., 2023; Peralta et al., 2022). Palliative care (PC) definition explains the what, who, when, how, and why (Mercadante et al., 2018)? Through several modifications since 1982, PC focuses on improving the quality of life (QOL) of adults, children, and families in the face of a life threatening and debilitating illness (WHO, 2020). Loosen et al. (2023) emphasizes improvement in all forms of suffering from the point when an illness becomes incurable.

Globally, studies and guidelines are mostly concentrated with cancer related palliative care with most evidence existing in the developed countries and Abu-Odah et al. (2022) reports gaps in developing parts of the world. Chronic diseases affecting elderly populations that require palliative care include; diabetes mellitus, AIDS, chronic obstructive pulmonary disease, and congestive cardiac failure, end stage renal disease, cancer, parkinsonism, multiple sclerosis, dementia and rheumatoid arthritis (Hudson et al., 2021; WHO, 2020). Several countries in Africa have reported complex circumstances faced while offering any of the palliative care services especially among the elderly populations (Adonteng-Kissi, 2021; Biney et al., 2024). Limitations similar to those in Africa also prevail elsewhere in countries with low developmental index in parts of Asia and Latin America (Cheong et al., 2019; Wang et al., 2024; Zertuche-Maldonado et al., 2020) which could compromise care.

Individualised patient centred care (Hui & Bruera, 2020; Hui et al., 2018) through models such as specialist palliative care could improve care. However their application could be affected by health system structure, and resource limitation (Anderson & Grant, 2017). An up-to-date detailed account on appropriate care models in certain settings based on the resources will be discussed in this chapter. There will be emphasis to identify gaps for improvement and further research to improve therapeutic interventions in geriatric palliative care.

All definitions should emphasize better quality of life rather than the quantity of life while acknowledging that dying is a normal process in spite of fears surrounding the concept of death (Alcalde & Zimmermann, 2022; Borasio, 2011; Radbruch et al., 2020; WHO, 2002). Although the WHO definition clearly answers What "an approach", when "faced with a challenging life-threatening illness (Sepúlveda et al., 2002)", how "through prevention and relief of suffering by means of early identification, assessment, and treatment (Sepúlveda et al., 2002)", why "to improve the quality of life of patients and families (Sepúlveda et al., 2002)" depending on several applications, differences in its practicality exist between the developed and developing world. Recent evidence suggest limitations in the application of this definition especially in resource limited settings especially developing countries(Krakauer, 2025; Phillips & Currow, 2019). The need to address several domains of care across diverse demographics categories of elderly patients under palliation remain a necessity. Significant suffering in most adults over 60 years is due to debilitating symptoms, and high costs of treatment (Knaul et al., 2025; Sleeman et al., 2019). Thence, availability, and accessibility to appropriate standard terminal care services requires both human and non-human resources. For optimal care of elders under palliation, feasible action-oriented models of care should be universal in the health sector (Centeno & Arias-Casais, 2019).

2.0 INSIGHTS INTO GLOBAL PERSPECTIVES ABOUT GERIATRIC PALLIATIVE CARE

Although PC is an important aspect of healthcare, it remains out of reach in nearly half of the countries globally (Brant & Silbermann, 2021), and geriatric palliative care remain a growing global concern (Pauline et al., 2024; Voumard et al., 2018). Even when available, specific needs of old frail individuals are not observed which affects their quality of life while under care (de Nooijer et al., 2020; Lei et al., 2022; Stow et al., 2019). The aging population continues to rise in North America with concerns on what should be delivered when nearing death, and countries like Canada, USA have initiated strategies to continuously identify areas of improvement in elderly PC (Antonacci et al., 2020; Robinson et al., 2017). Deficits for improvement have included but not limited to more consultations towards the end of life during hospital admission, healthcare disparities especially for marginalized populations, and inaccessibility (Jones et al., 2021; Roeland et al., 2016; Wachterman & Sommers, 2021). Healthcare disparities affecting elders with life limiting chronic illness also extend to Latin American countries with key challenges quite similar including limited accessibility to palliative care, policies and funds, insufficient solid evidence among others (Paiva et al., 2023; Pergolizzi Jr et al., 2024; Robledo et al., 2022).

Residential aged facilities have been a mainstay in many European countries for offering palliative care (PC) to aged people (Mitchell et al., 2024). Several improvement have been noted in geriatric PC; however shortfalls such as discrepancy in the access, and utilization of PC services among elderly people, of which almost all countries used PC in towards death (Axelsson, 2022; Cerullo et al., 2024). Furthermore, equal access and utilization of palliation services by people in people in

European countries remain a significant challenge just like in American countries. Gaps in training of nurses and doctors for providing PC services in Europe, together with appropriate policies to improve delivery have been recommended in studies in the continent(Hagelin et al., 2022; Hökkä et al., 2021; Martins Pereira et al., 2021; Paal et al., 2019). Marginalization also plummets older persons efforts to get PC services, for example non-Western Migrant workers in Europe were impended by the system to access PC (Shabnam et al., 2022).

Although there is progress in PC among several Asian Countries, there exists vivid evidence about insufficiency in hospice and PC services with low awareness still among the contributing factors(Lee et al., 2019; Lee et al., 2024; Wang et al., 2024). Cultural differences pose a need for a different approach for PC which calls for harmonization, and sensitization. Access and utilization of geriatric PC services often vary in Asian countries based on the developmental index. For example nations like China, Japan, and South Korea have increased efforts to improve PC services with achievements over decades although scarcity of appropriate PC services still prevail in parts of the respective countries (Iida et al., 2022; Lam et al., 2021; Lee et al., 2019; Lu et al., 2018; Sakurai, 2025; Yang et al., 2025; Zhang et al., 2022). The Association of South East Asian Nations (ASEAN) endorsed strategies to enhance care for aged population but financial sustainability hinder the effectiveness of this initiative (Vo & Fong, 2025; Yeung & Thang, 2018).Geriatric palliative care in developing Asian countries such as Cambodia and Vietnam is strained by resource limitations, applicable palliation strategies due to low research in the subject area(Kaiser et al., 2025; Kaiser et al., 2023; Nguyen et al., 2023).

In Africa, high income nations still require further development of policies to optimize PC (Henry et al., 2024). What is more to this, addressing aged persons needs as a distinct discipline (geriatric nursing and medicine) still remain a relatively new entity in Africa compared countries in the Global North (Adamek et al., 2022; Nukunu et al., 2024). Developing countries including those in Sub Saharan Africa require great advocacy and investment to improve palliation services (Brant & Silbermann, 2021). Few African countries have integrated palliation services in their healthcare system (Nkhoma et al., 2025).Multimorbidity among African geriatric patients can pose catastrophe. This becomes eminent especially due to tribal system that is different in the African cultures. Even the basic of palliative care concept like communication could be complicated by limited capacity for translation(Nkhoma et al., 2025). Overall, Africa needs a strategic, feasible work plan that enhances research, and practice oriented to specific geriatric palliative care needs(Afolabi et al., 2021).

3.0 CORE COMPONENTS OF PALLIATIVE CARE

Palliation services may reduce healthcare inequalities through addressing distinct healthcare needs. It focuses on an integral diverse multilevel form of care for an individual's visible and invisible concerns affecting the totality of health. Assessment, and management should address problems affecting the person physically, psychosocially and spiritually(WHPCA, 2020). Specific consideration is given to promote a balance between the physical and non-physical aspects (Figure 1) that constitute being healthy which is not mere absence of disease as defined by World Health Organization (Larsen, 2022). The external environment in which old persons live could influence their health outcomes either positively or negatively. Frailty due to chronic disease, and old age make them more vulnerable to effects of drastic changes in the environment(Davies & Bhutta, 2022; Katz et al., 2025)

Figure 1. Understanding the interactive impact of milieu to a patient

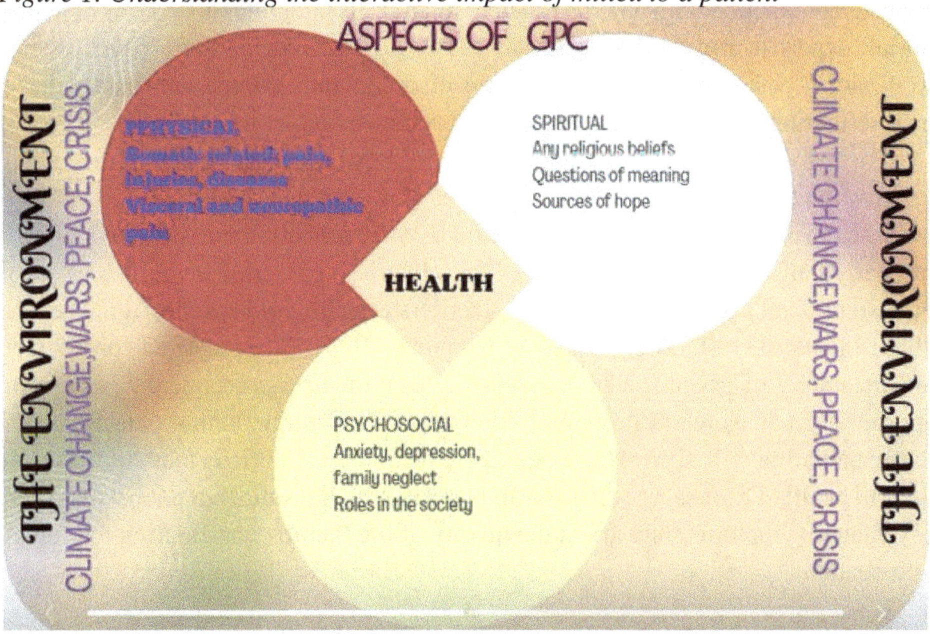

3.1 Physical Considerations for Geriatric Patients

Normally, physical complaints among geriatric patients are often distinct from those of other age groups mainly due to multimorbidity throughout the diagnostic process (Gülalp et al., 2009; Takechi et al., 2022). Age related body changes, together with medications tend to affect the overall functioning of the body which complicates functionality drastically when affected by a chronic life limiting disease. Debilitating common symptoms (Chai et al., 2014) include breathlessness, constipation, diarrhoea, headache, pain, urinary and feacal incontinence. These and others will be discussed further in the next section below. Complexity in diagnosis and treatment could arise due to somatization, where psychosocial disorders manifest physically. Symptoms which cannot be explained by a clear clinical presentation could be classified under somatoform disorders(Van Driel et al., 2018). Consequently, clinicians' diagnostic approaches to these complex conditions are heavily dependent on their training in PC.

3.2 Psychosocial Considerations in Geriatric Palliative Care

Psychosocial well-being of an individual occurs at different levels beginning with intrapersonal level, interpersonal level and the skills perspective. Intrapersonal domain includes positivity in emotions, and feeling, interpersonal domain involves balanced interaction with others in society; then skills integrates all aspects of learning and expertise in executing duties(UNICEF, 2019).Deviation from "psychosocial well-being" casts uncertainty for mental disorder. Internalized and externalized manifestations include depression, anxiety and misconduct respectively.

Existing evidence suggests that old people above 65 years have unnoticed personality defects that tend to affect their overall mental health(Holzer et al., 2022). Most health professionals including general medical practitioners tend to be unaware of nearly half of psychological illness (psychiatric disorders) leaving uncertainty on a significant proportion of mental disorders affecting old people(Aguiar et al., 2022; Ighodaro et al., 2015; Yaghi & Chahine, 2023). There is need for a wider understanding of psychosocial aspects of elders; thence appreciate deviations for appropriate management(Steffens & Zdanys, 2022). Contrary to this, elderly people under palliation will always have pending psychological deficits that culminate to their ill health. Distressing somatoform features which result from poorly managed psychiatric symptoms shall affect the quality of life thereby contributing to premature death.

3.3 Spiritual Considerations in Geriatric Palliative Care

Spirituality has been a subtle concept for decades especially due to its relationship with religion which is indeed a distinct entity. However, the relationship between these two is quite adherent in that they aid their existence in a significant proportion of people influencing, most people globally. Is there a consensus on the definition of spirituality? Actually, (Lepherd, 2015) wrote that "spirituality is owned by everyone but what is it? It means that with or without religion, an individual has spirituality which suggests that religion can be a gateway to achieve spirituality. Harris et al. (2018) and Dik et al. (2024) proposed that spirituality refers to "relationship with the sacred" while religion "entails ritualistic, institutionalized, and coded spirituality that is accepted in a given society". In addition, (Dik et al., 2024) explains sacred as broad term that refers to the drive to search for meaning in life as appreciated by the individual. Spirituality can be expressed in ways such as engagement in religious practices, belief in God, gods, family, humanism, appreciation of nature and arts among others.

Spiritual care if incorporated in geriatric PC could yield better outcomes (Ukpo et al., 2024). However, integration of spiritual care should not be from a biased approach; for example, imposition of certain religious beliefs to an elderly patient either without a religious denomination or belonging to a different religion. This requires thorough spiritual assessment which could be done in phases. Firstly, the basic assessment that helps identify patient's needs; then a more focused assessment which could require expertise from a specially trained spiritual leader if needed (Elizabeth, 2015; Ferrell & Paice, 2019). Different models if properly used have been of immense value in spiritual assessment and subsequent management. Such models include PC-7 model (Fitchett et al., 2020; Galchutt, 2024), SPIRIT model (Maugans, 1996), HOPE model (Anandarajah & Hight, 2001), FICA model(Borneman et al., 2010), FACT model(LaRocca-Pitts, 2015) and MVAST model(Skalla, 2006). Healthcare professionals caring for geriatric patients under palliation must have great insight on how to assess for spiritual needs and provide appropriate interventions (Nissen et al., 2021).

4.0 COMMUNICATION WITH ELDERLY PATIENTS UNDER PALLIATION

Communication is very crucial for effective palliative care. Communication is the fundamental element to all aspects of palliative nursing for example; healthcare professional (nurse, doctor, social worker)-patient-family relationship, interprofessional relationship, assessment of the patient (physically, psychologically), implementation and evaluation of care plans. Precisely, communication is a mediating variable for effective palliative care. The mediation of communication extends to include other stake holders for optimal PC.

Subject to geriatric PC, therapeutic and effective forms of communication should take precedence. This creates a baseline; thence a pillar for appropriate management in PC (Engel et al., 2023; Ifrim et al., 2022). There is an overarching need to clearly apply both verbal and non-verbal communication styles in different cultures of patients. With culture at hand, cultural consciousness adds a stride during interaction with geriatric patients and families from a different cultural background. Culturally competent communication means communicating while aware and knowledgeable of the sociodemographic factors that may determine individual beliefs (Feinberg et al., 2021; Teal & Street, 2009). Linked to this is the ability to solve related challenges amicably for the good of the patient (Aririguzoh, 2022). Communicating effectively is easier said than done as several studies have identified a poor prognosis of patients with chronic illness due poor communication practices (Frydenberg & Brekke, 2012; Guppy et al., 2024; Taran, 2011; Yao et al., 2021). When communication is effective, it aids the therapeutic effects.

Elderly patients tend to have challenges with communication often related to age related changes(Gravell, 2024), and having a chronic illness that adds complexity to communication. Formal training in communications skills for geriatric PC is still lacking globally (Hirano & Kang, 2023; Kelley et al., 2012). Henceforth, developing feasible therapeutic communication models specific for the elderly people under PC should be considered. TAGEET, a therapeutic communication model which was proposed (McCarthy et al., 2021) to help achieve therapeutic communication during nurse- patient interaction in the wave of COVID-19 could be applied to geriatric PC with or without modification. COMFORT model when studied in diverse settings globally, resulted in findings that suggest significant improvement in communication of health professionals with their patients (Goldsmith & Wittenberg, 2024; Mahdiabadi et al., 2023; Wittenberg et al., 2019; Wittenberg et al., 2018). Tailored communication techniques that incorporate the carer(s), and family members' perspectives have been reported to promote effective communication (Wittenberg et al., 2016; Wittenberg et al., 2017). The tool "Family Care giver Communication tool (FCCT)" by Wittenberg et al. (2016) enables tailored approaches in communication that are caregiver/family member oriented. The FCCT tool has two major components: conformity and conversation. The former entails frequency and common topics conversed while the later involves several family beliefs, attitudes, roles, values. Collectively, four different types of communication: carrier caregiver, lone, partner and manager arise from the high and low components of conformity and conversation(Wittenberg et al., 2016).

Figure 2. Tabulated mnemonics to guide good communication

Author(s)	Mnemonic	Interpretation
(McCarthy et al., 2021)	**T** (Tune in)	Awareness of self and environment
	A (Approach and Introduce)	Introduction and creation of rapport
	G (Ground self)	Relax and gain confidence
	E (Engage and respond)	Interact with the patient consideration of verbal and non-verbal communication clues
	E (End encounter)	Paraphrase and clarify
	T (Tune out)	Pause and reflect
(Wittenberg et al., 2019)	**C** (Connect)	Gain mutual understanding in communication
	O (Options)	Possible choices for care
	M (Making meaning)	Being compassionate and totally present for the patient, caregiver and family
	F (Family, caregivers)	Acknowledge the role of the family, and enhance their support
	O (Openings)	Honesty, non-judgmental while acknowledging their concerns and maintaining confidentiality
	R (Relating)	Embrace conflicting goals of the patient, caregivers and health professional while adjusting to the new state of health.
	T (Team)	Multidisciplinary teamwork to optimize outcomes of PC

In breaking bad news which can begin at the point of diagnosis, the SPIKES mnemonic explained below, is a very crucial approach (Meitar & Karnieli-Miller, 2022; Naderi et al., 2022);

S- Setting (private room, space, silent, with adequate lighting)

P-Perception (Assess perception of the current situation using open ended questions)

I-Invitation (Get invitation and ascertain the extent o information required)

K-Knowledge (Give clear information, precise and allow comprehension)

E-Empathy (Address emotions empathetically)

S-Strategy and Summary (Provide the next course of action/steps/treatment)

Another mnemonic "NURSE" by Pollak et al. (2007) emphasizes empathy during breaking bad news due to a chronic, life changing illness. It a great tool for optimizing communication during a trying moment.

N-Name (Mention the patient's emotion)

U-Understand (Show empathy due to the emotion)

R-Respect (Acknowledge and appreciate the patient's strength)

S-Support (Be there for the patient)

E-Explore (Request the patient to explain the emotion)

With different models above, making an informed choice is key for effective communication. Certain situations may require combination of more than one models to communicate effectively while instances like delivery of undesirable information to the patient concerning diagnosis can effectively be done with SPIKES approach.

Despite the limited formal training in communication applicable to geriatric PC, customization of the already existing communication model can yield good results among practitioners. Kelley et al. (2012) findings suggested improved communications skills after attending customized training on communication techniques. Cultural difference in communication styles should be acknowledged. Health professionals should be devoid of judgmental and ethnocentric tendencies for open and transparent communication. To further improve communication across cultures, the health professional should develop cultural relativism, cultural competence, and cultural humility (Atomei et al., 2024; Brown et al., 2021).

Preparation for inevitable barriers despite training is a good practice. Findings from (Sungur et al., 2022) suggested barriers due to inadequate translation by family members blocked access to accurate information which increased uncertainty regarding needs, and cultural differences about the interpretation of health and disease from the perspective of the patient. Overall, hindrances to therapeutic communication can be originate from the patient, caregiver, healthcare professionals, and healthcare systems (Jack et al., 2024; Kuipers et al., 2021). Fears of own mortality, personal attachment with the patient, unrealistic hope for treatment success, and stress from the healthcare professional are common obstacles to therapeutic communication. Health systems could also create hurdles that disrupt the communication. They include but not limited to; limited privacy for patients and family, limited trained health professionals for geriatric PC.

5.0 APPROACH TO SYMPTOMATOLOGY IN GERIATRIC PALLIATIVE CARE

The elderly people under palliation mostly present with a complex and multimorbid clinical picture with evidence of detoriation (Mo et al., 2021; Regnard & Dean, 2022). This mainly due to frailty that comes with old age compounded with conditions that require palliation. For every patient, an open minded approach should be considered to comprehensively assess the patient (Dharmarajan, 2021). Several studies (Chen et al., 2021; Garcia et al., 2021; Veronese et al., 2022) have proposed comprehensive geriatric assessment to help identify symptoms including those rarely reported to facilitate targeted interventions which improve outcomes for PC patients. Screening tools have been tested and reported to be effective in comprehensive geriatric assessment (Garcia et al., 2021). Although this form of assessment has higher efficacy in a hospital setting modified versions could help for geriatric patients outside a hospital setting. Focused geriatric assessment enables identification of clues that would have been otherwise missed during a routine visit (Loh et al., 2018).

6.0 MODELS OF GERIATRIC PALLIATIVE CARE

Timely initiation of "specialist palliative care (SPC)" improves patient outcomes including less pain and suffering compared to general medical care without palliative care (Hui & Bruera, 2020; Hui et al., 2018). The current general palliative care models need testing, and evaluation to understand if they can be incorporated in geriatric palliative care (Chapman et al., 2021). Delivery of optimal geriatric palliative care requires organized, feasible, systematic and flexible approaches that integrates the unique differences among patients, their carers ad families. Variations could be physical, psychological, internalized, or externalized. These include the clinical presentation at the point of care, location and resources to aid the process of "care"(Hui et al., 2018), thence different feasible PC models should be adopted and utilized(Higginson, 2015). Several models of timely PC are summarized with specifications in **Table 2** below. Considering national and international dynamics in healthcare, either a feasible or customized model that optimizes health benefits of geriatric patients under palliation should advocated for. Studies about such models could aid modification to fit societal differences.

Figure 3. Tabulated major models of geriatric palliative care: mnemonic "SGg"

Author(s)	Model of delivery	Insight on its approach
(Eve & Higginson, 2000)	Specialist Palliative Care	Involves treatment and care offered by health professionals specially trained in PC
(Eve & Higginson, 2000; Shipman et al., 2008)	Generalist Palliative Care	Entails treatment and care offered by health professionals without specialized training in PC.
(Sanon et al., 2019)	Geriatric Emergency Departments	Modified from the traditional emergency departments to incorporate unique needs of frail geriatric patients.
(Evans et al., 2019) reported a similarity in the approaches for service delivery. Although all models were focused on the individual receiving care to improve the quality of life, crucial differences were observed. These models service delivery models were; Integrated Geriatric Care and Integrated Palliative Care. Integrated Geriatric Care mainly assessed earlier trajectory of functional decline, with interest in promoting functionality while Integrated Palliative Care assessed functional decline in later stages while ameliorating presenting symptoms.		

Both Specialist and Geriatric PC can be sub divided into more specific model units(Hui & Bruera, 2020; Luckett et al., 2014; Wiencek & Coyne, 2014). These include Outpatient clinics, ambulatory clinics, Inpatient clinics, acute care palliative units, hospice centers, care from personal homes and community palliative care services. Certain models (Hui & Bruera, 2020; Wiencek & Coyne, 2014) existing worldwide have been modified to suite the local needs (Kalantari et al., 2021). This facilitates access and utilization of palliation services according the needs and expectations of both service providers, their clients (patient, carers, and family) and relevant stake holders. Examples of such models have existed in countries like United States of America (SAFECare model, (Ansryan et al., 2018), MediCaring models(Montgomery & Lynn, 2014), France (COPA model, (Vedel et al., 2009)), Spain/Austria (IHMIS model, (Gandarillas & Goswami, 2018), and in Hong Kong (Hong Kong Model, (Leung et al., 2004). Almost all models were studied and implemented in the developed parts of the world. This leaves uncertainty in poor and developing countries globally. Models that consider resource limitations, societal and cultures need to be developed and studied in the different setup to ascertain their scope and feasibility. Other models proposed have focused on elderly patients at their homes; HOMEMEDS(Meredith et al., 2002), Hospital at Home in Leff et al. (2005) and Transitional Care Model as reported by Naylor et al. (2004) are examples of models targeting patients while at home.

7.0 INSIGHT ON ADVANCES IN GERIATRIC PALLIATIVE CARE; CHALLENGES AND FUTURE PROSPECTS

Geriatric palliative care (GPC) is an important discipline for improving outcomes for health the elderly despite lack of global recognition (Antonacci et al., 2020; Brant & Silbermann, 2021; Saracino et al., 2018). Most nations in the Global South with limited resources still have little to no geriatric palliative care services (Brant & Silbermann, 2021). Even when there are PC models that have been implemented in resource rich Global North, it may not be practical to directly apply them in resource limited Global South. Hurdles that may affect direct transfer and application could arise from limited resources and distinct cultural perspectives. While aging together with its vulnerability, and growing need for palliation services are a global concept, their interpretation, appreciation could be largely influenced by societal demands (Nkhoma et al., 2025). Advocacy and coordinated awareness campaigns through key stake holders through health sector, and governmental political leaders enabled incorporation of PC several African countries health sector (Grant et al., 2017). A combination of both geriatric care (GC) and PC in nations of the Global South gained attention in recent years with no formal practice in most countries

(Omoyeni & Gwyther, 2018; Sadiq et al., 2025; Samba et al., 2023). Despite this integral approach, palliative care if available, is mainly in major hospitals in urban centres, thence a challenge for the rural and hard to reach areas. However, there is inaccessibility to PC by inhabitants living in rural areas of nations in both Global North and South (Cai & Lalani, 2022; Fasolino et al., 2024; Grant et al., 2017). Tailored models should be funded with continuous implementation studies to better adopt to the demands and needs of elderly patients under palliation irrespective of their location in each nation.

Education and training in geriatrics and palliative care should be further developed, standardized and implemented as a discipline to enhance its practice (Fields et al., 2022; Grant et al., 2017; Gurwitz, 2023). The training in both geriatrics and palliative is unique, targeting the special needs, physical and psychological deviations of elderly. The uniqueness of training applies to both health professionals, doctors, nurses and social workers(Michel & Cha, 2015; Pelleg et al., 2021; Thiel et al., 2021). Africa which needs the highest demand of this training has PC integrated as part of undergraduate health training programs in just 29 of the 54 nations and policies on PC in only 26 countries (Agom et al., 2021; Bastos et al., 2024; Rawlinson et al., 2014). Although evidence of educational training on PC exists in some countries in Asia-Pacific region (Liu et al., 2021; Mills et al., 2021), gaps in training affect delivery of optimal care to elders under palliation (Bhattacharyya et al., 2024; Chu et al., 2024). Similar gaps in training have affected delivery of GPC services in South American nations (Pergolizzi Jr et al., 2024; Vargas-Escobar et al., 2022). Conversely, better educational strategies in PC have been noted in most countries of Europe, and North America despite less uniformity; for example GPC is not yet recognised as an independent discipline in all nations Europe and North America (Abu-Odah et al., 2022; Suija et al., 2024; Wolf & Wedding, 2025). If geriatric palliative care is to gain full recognition, and acceptance, intense awareness, research and training as a distinct program should be started in all countries. Training materials should be developed with consideration of the population demographics including the cultural and economic differences. Aging is a global growing phenomenon that we need to face with an open mind, with interest on how we can improve health outcomes amidst frailty.

Multidisciplinary approach in GPC is used in most countries especially those with a wide range of specialization. Specialists in varying areas of geriatrics, medicine, and palliative care play crucial while using models of PC including general and specialist (Alanazi et al.; Castagna et al., 2024; Irumba et al., 2024; Krishnaswami et al., 2022). Overall patients who receive collaborative care from health professionals with different scope of practice achieve higher patient satisfaction, less psychological disorders with better outcomes as opposed to single approach. Everyone involved in the caring process needs thorough explanation not only about the condition but also identification and roles of each healthcare professional (Borgstrom et al., 2024).

Subject to the above, we infer that GPC is a growing discipline in infancy that has not gained adequate global attention despite existence of independent disciplines of palliative care, geriatric and gerontological care. In addition, both geriatric care and palliative care are still almost non-existent in some parts of the world. There is limited data, training together with limited expertise in GPC which are among the key challenges restricting access and utilization of GPC. The suggested models could enhance access, utilization of GPC if their feasibility is considered together with the sociodemographic characteristics of the population being served.

REFERENCES

Abu-Odah, H., Molassiotis, A., & Liu, J. Y. W. (2022). Global palliative care research (2002-2020): Bibliometric review and mapping analysis. *BMJ Supportive & Palliative Care*, *12*(4), 376–387. PMID: 34373283

Adamek, M. E., Gebremariam Kotecho, M., Chane, S., & Gebeyaw, G. (2022). Challenges and assets of older adults in Sub-Saharan Africa: Perspectives of gerontology scholars. *Journal of Aging & Social Policy*, *34*(1), 108–126. PMID: 34160333

Adonteng-Kissi, B. (2021). Chronic life-limiting illness and informal care in Ghana: experiences of older people and their family carers.

Afolabi, O. A., Nkhoma, K., Maddocks, M., & Harding, R. (2021). What constitutes a palliative care need in people with serious illnesses across Africa? A mixed-methods systematic review of the concept and evidence. *Palliative Medicine*, *35*(6), 1052–1070. PMID: 33860715

Agom, D. A., Onyeka, T. C., Iheanacho, P. N., & Ominyi, J. (2021). Barriers to the Provision and Utilization of Palliative Care in Africa: A Rapid Scoping Review. *Indian Journal of Palliative Care*, *27*(1), 3–17. DOI: 10.4103/ijpc.Ijpc_355_20 PMID: 34035611

Aguiar, J. P., Gama Marques, J., Leufkens, H. G., & Alves da Costa, F. (2022). Healthcare professionals' Views on the management of medication complexities in the elderly with mental health disorders: A cross-sectional study. *Frontiers in Psychiatry*, *13*, 885216. PMID: 35677869

Alanazi, H. H. F., Alqarni, A. M. S., Alamri, A. A. H., Al-Faridi, S. G., Altawyan, Y. S. S., Al-Harbi, Z. B. B. H., Al Nemer, A. A. R., & Alqahtani, S. F. M. (•••). Palliative Care of Geriatrics-nursing Care Plans: An Updated Review. *International Journal of Health Sciences*, *2*(S1), 444–456.

Alcalde, J., & Zimmermann, C. (2022). Stigma about palliative care: origins and solutions. *ecancermedicalscience, 16*, 1377.

Anandarajah, G., & Hight, E. (2001). Spirituality and medical practice: Using the HOPE questions as a practical tool for spiritual assessment. *American Family Physician*, *63*(1), 81–89. PMID: 11195773

Anderson, R. E., & Grant, L. (2017). What is the value of palliative care provision in low-resource settings? *BMJ Global Health*, *2*(1), e000139. PMID: 28588999

Ansryan, L. Z., Aronow, H. U., Borenstein, J. E., Mena, V., Haus, F., Palmer, K., Chan, E., Swanson, J. W., Mass, S., & Rosen, B. (2018). Systems addressing frail elder care: Description of a successful model. *The Journal of Nursing Administration, 48*(1), 11–17. PMID: 29219905

Antonacci, R., Barrie, C., Baxter, S., Chaffey, S., Chary, S., Grassau, P., Hammond, C., Mirhosseini, M., Mirza, R. M., & Murzin, K. (2020). Gaps in hospice and palliative care research: A scoping review of the North American literature. *Journal of Aging Research, 2020*(1), 3921245. PMID: 33204532

Aririguzoh, S. (2022). Communication competencies, culture and SDGs: Effective processes to cross-cultural communication. *Humanities & Social Sciences Communications, 9*(1), 1–11.

Atomei, O.-L., Sânpălean, M., & Tarcea, M. (2024). Cultural Competence in Dietetic Practice. *Dietetics, 3*(4), 555–567.

Axelsson, B. (2022). The challenge: Equal availability to palliative care according to individual need regardless of age, diagnosis, geographical location, and care level. *International Journal of Environmental Research and Public Health, 19*(7), 4229. PMID: 35409908

Bastos, F., Garralda, E., Montero, A., Rhee, J. Y., Arias-Casais, N., Luyirika, E., Namisango, E., Pereira, J., Centeno, C., & Tripodoro, V. A. (2024). Comprehensive scoping review of palliative care development in Africa: Recent advances and persistent gaps. *Frontiers in Health Services, 4*, 1425353. PMID: 39717493

Bhattacharyya, D. S., Hossain, M. H., Dutta, G. K., Snigdha, M. F., Nowrin, I., & Saif-Ur-Rahman, K. (2024). Service coverage and health workforce allocation strategies for geriatric and palliative care in low and middle-income countries: A systematic review. *Health Sciences Review (Oxford, England)*, •••, 100166.

Biney, A., Sarfo, J. O., Poku, C. A., Deegbe, D. A., & Atibila, F., Ti-enkawol Nachinab, G., Anaba, E., Dzansi, G., & Attafuah, P. Y. A. (2024). Challenges and coping strategies when caring for terminally ill persons with cancer: Perspectives of family caregivers. *BMC Palliative Care, 23*(1), 175. PMID: 39020352

Borasio, G. D. (2011). Translating the World Health Organization definition of palliative care into scientific practice. *Palliative & Supportive Care, 9*(1), 1–2. PMID: 21352612

Borgstrom, E., Schiff, R., Khan, S. A., Hindley, E., Thayabaran, D., Savage, E., Gough, N., & Holti, R. (2024). Practices, issues and possibilities at the interface between geriatrics and palliative care (InGaP): An exploratory study and knotworking. *Health Open Research*, *6*(12), 12.

Borneman, T., Ferrell, B., & Puchalski, C. M. (2010). Evaluation of the FICA tool for spiritual assessment. *Journal of Pain and Symptom Management*, *40*(2), 163–173. PMID: 20619602

Brant, J. M., & Silbermann, M. (2021). Global perspectives on palliative care for cancer patients: Not all countries are the same. *Current Oncology Reports*, *23*, 1–10. PMID: 33829323

Brown, J. V., Spicer, K. J., & French, E. (2021). Exploring the inclusion of cultural competence, cultural humility, and diversity concepts as learning objectives or outcomes in healthcare curricula. *Journal of Best Practices in Health Professions Diversity : Research, Education and Policy*, *14*(1), 63–81.

Cai, Y., & Lalani, N. (2022). Examining Barriers and Facilitators to Palliative Care Access in Rural Areas: A Scoping Review. *The American Journal of Hospice & Palliative Care*, *39*(1), 123–130. DOI: 10.1177/10499091211011145 PMID: 33906486

Castagna, A., Militano, V., Ruberto, C., Manzo, C., & Ruotolo, G. (2024). Comprehensive geriatric assessment and palliative care. *Aging Medicine (Milton, N.S.W.)*, *7*(5), 645–648. PMID: 39507225

Centeno, C., & Arias-Casais, N. (2019). Global palliative care: From need to action. *The Lancet. Global Health*, *7*(7), e815–e816. PMID: 31129121

Cerullo, G., Figueiredo, T., Coelho, C., Campos, C. S., Videira-Silva, A., Carrilho, J., Midão, L., & Costa, E. (2024). Palliative care in the ageing European population: A cross-country comparison. *International Journal of Environmental Research and Public Health*, *21*(1), 113. PMID: 38276807

Chai, E., Meier, D., & Morris, J. (2014). *Geriatric palliative care*. OUP Us.

Chapman, A. E., Elias, R., Plotkin, E., Lowenstein, L. M., & Swartz, K. (2021). Models of care in geriatric oncology. *Journal of Clinical Oncology*, *39*(19), 2195. PMID: 34043453

Chen, Z., Ding, Z., Chen, C., Sun, Y., Jiang, Y., Liu, F., & Wang, S. (2021). Effectiveness of comprehensive geriatric assessment intervention on quality of life, caregiver burden and length of hospital stay: A systematic review and meta-analysis of randomised controlled trials. *BMC Geriatrics*, *21*, 1–14. PMID: 34154560

Cheong, W. L., Mohan, D., Warren, N., & Reidpath, D. D. (2019). Palliative care research in the Asia Pacific region: A systematic review and bibliometric analysis of peer-reviewed publications. *Journal of Palliative Medicine*, *22*(5), 545–552. PMID: 30570416

Chu, W.-M., Tsai, H.-B., Chen, Y.-C., Hung, K.-Y., Cheng, S.-Y., & Lin, C.-P. (2024). Palliative care for adult patients undergoing hemodialysis in Asia: Challenges and opportunities. *Journal of Hospice and Palliative Care*, *27*(1), 1. PMID: 38449832

Davies, B., & Bhutta, M. F. (2022). Geriatric medicine in the era of climate change. *Age and Ageing*, *51*(1), afab199. PMID: 34651175

de Nooijer, K., Penders, Y. W., Pivodic, L., Van Den Noortgate, N. J., Pype, P., & Van den Block, L. (2020). Specialist palliative care services for older people in primary care: A systematic review using narrative synthesis. *Palliative Medicine*, *34*(1), 32–48. PMID: 31564214

Dharmarajan, T. (2021). Comprehensive geriatric assessment. In *Geriatric gastroenterology* (pp. 201–246). Springer.

Dik, B. J., Daniels, D., & Alayan, A. J. (2024). Religion, spirituality, and the workplace: A review and critique. *Annual Review of Organizational Psychology and Organizational Behavior*, *11*(1), 279–305.

Elizabeth, J. T. (2015). *Oxford Textbook of Palliative Nursing* (R. F. Betty., Nessa, C., & Judith, A. P, Ed. 4th Edition ed.). Oxford University Press.

Engel, M., Kars, M. C., Teunissen, S. C., & van der Heide, A. (2023). Effective communication in palliative care from the perspectives of patients and relatives: A systematic review. *Palliative & Supportive Care*, *21*(5), 890–913. PMID: 37646464

Fasolino, T., Mayfield, M. E., Valentine, K., Rosa, W. E., & Koci, A. (2024). Palliative Care in Rural Communities. *AJN The American Journal of Nursing*, *124*(8), 50–55. DOI: 10.1097/01.Naj.0001027716.70431.35 PMID: 39051815

Feinberg, I. Z., Owen-Smith, A., O'Connor, M. H., Ogrodnick, M. M., Rothenberg, R., & Eriksen, M. P. (2021). Strengthening culturally competent health communication. *Health Security*, *19*(S1), S–41–S–49. PMID: 33961489

Ferrell, B. R., & Paice, J. A. (2019). *Oxford textbook of palliative nursing*. Oxford University Press.

Fields, L., Shalev, D., Nathanson, M., & Shapiro, P. A. (2022). Palliative care training for geriatric psychiatry fellows: A national survey project. *The American Journal of Geriatric Psychiatry*, *30*(4), 504–510. PMID: 34535362

Fitchett, G., Hisey Pierson, A. L., Hoffmeyer, C., Labuschagne, D., Lee, A., Levine, S., O'Mahony, S., Pugliese, K., & Waite, N. (2020). Development of the PC-7, a quantifiable assessment of spiritual concerns of patients receiving palliative care near the end of life. *Journal of Palliative Medicine*, *23*(2), 248–253. PMID: 31483184

Frydenberg, K., & Brekke, M. (2012). Poor communication on patients' medication across health care levels leads to potentially harmful medication errors. *Scandinavian Journal of Primary Health Care*, *30*(4), 234–240. PMID: 23050954

Galchutt, P. K. (2024). Spiritual assessment models for palliative care chaplains: A narrative review. *Journal of Health Care Chaplaincy*, *30*(4), 329–345. PMID: 38900925

Gandarillas, M. Á., & Goswami, N. (2018). Merging current health care trends: Innovative perspective in aging care. *Clinical Interventions in Aging*, •••, 2083–2095. PMID: 30425463

Garcia, M. V., Agar, M. R., Soo, W.-K., To, T., & Phillips, J. L. (2021). Screening tools for identifying older adults with cancer who may benefit from a geriatric assessment: A systematic review. *JAMA Oncology*, *7*(4), 616–627. PMID: 33443547

Goldsmith, J. V., & Wittenberg, E. (2024). The COMFORT model: Moving the initiative outside of the academy. *Health Communication*, *39*(14), 3514–3519. PMID: 38450611

Grant, L., Downing, J., Luyirika, E., Murphy, M., Namukwaya, L., Kiyange, F., Atieno, M., Kemigisha-Ssali, E., Hunt, J., Snell, K., Murray, S. A., & Leng, M. (2017). Integrating palliative care into national health systems in Africa: A multi-country intervention study. *Journal of Global Health*, *7*(1), 010419. DOI: 10.7189/jogh.07.010419 PMID: 28685037

Gravell, R. (2024). *Communication problems in elderly people: Practical approaches to management*. Taylor & Francis.

Gülalp, B., Aldinç, H., Karagün, Ö., Çetinel, Y., & Benli, S. (2009). The complaint and outcome of geriatric patient in emergency department. *Turkish Journal of Emergency Medicine, 9*(2), 073–077.

Guppy, J. H., Widlund, H., Munro, R., & Price, J. (2024). Incivility in healthcare: The impact of poor communication. *BMJ Leader*, *8*(1). PMID: 37419661

Gurwitz, J. H. (2023). The Paradoxical Decline of Geriatric Medicine as a Profession. *Journal of the American Medical Association*, *330*(8), 693–694. DOI: 10.1001/jama.2023.11110 PMID: 37540519

Hagelin, C. L., Melin-Johansson, C., Ek, K., Henoch, I., Österlind, J., & Browall, M. (2022). Teaching about death and dying—A national mixed-methods survey of palliative care education provision in Swedish undergraduate nursing programmes. *Scandinavian Journal of Caring Sciences*, *36*(2), 545–557. PMID: 34962307

Harris, K. A., Howell, D. S., & Spurgeon, D. W. (2018). Faith concepts in psychology: Three 30-year definitional content analyses. *Psychology of Religion and Spirituality*, *10*(1), 1.

Henry, M., Asuzu, C., Savard, S., Devault-Tousignant, C., Timmermans, S., Khosravi, K., Amin, A., Albert, J., Krochmalnek, T., & Odiyo, P. (2024). Psychosocial and palliative care in African national cancer control plans: A qualitative study. *Psycho-Oncology*, *33*(5), e6346. PMID: 38743345

Higginson, I. J. (2015). Palliative care delivery models. In N. Cherny, M. Fallon, S. Kaasa, R. K. Portenoy, & D. C. Currow (Eds.), *Oxford Textbook of Palliative Medicine* (pp. 0). Oxford University Press. https://doi.org/DOI: 10.1093/med/9780199656097.003.0012

Hirano, L. A., & Kang, G. (2023). Primary Palliative Care Education for Geriatricians: Lessons Learned. *Current Geriatrics Reports*, *12*(3), 85–92.

Hökkä, M., Melender, H.-L., Lehto, J. T., & Kaakinen, P. (2021). Palliative nursing competencies required for different levels of palliative care provision: A qualitative analysis of health care professionals' perspectives. *Journal of Palliative Medicine*, *24*(10), 1516–1524. PMID: 33720785

Holzer, K. J., Vaughn, M. G., Loux, T. M., Mancini, M. A., Fearn, N. E., & Wallace, C. L. (2022). Prevalence and correlates of antisocial personality disorder in older adults. *Aging & Mental Health*, *26*(1), 169–178. PMID: 33107330

Hudson, P., Collins, A., Boughey, M., & Philip, J. (2021). Reframing palliative care to improve the quality of life of people diagnosed with a serious illness. *The Medical Journal of Australia*, *215*(10), 443. PMID: 34676567

Hui, D., & Bruera, E. (2020). Models of palliative care delivery for patients with cancer. *Journal of Clinical Oncology*, *38*(9), 852–865. PMID: 32023157

Hui, D., Hannon, B. L., Zimmermann, C., & Bruera, E. (2018). Improving patient and caregiver outcomes in oncology: Team-based, timely, and targeted palliative care. *CA: a Cancer Journal for Clinicians*, *68*(5), 356–376. PMID: 30277572

Ifrim, R. A., Klugarová, J., Măguri ă, D., Zazu, M., Mazilu, D. C., & Klugar, M. (2022). Communication, an important link between healthcare providers: A best practice implementation project. *JBI Evidence Implementation, 20*(S1), S41–S48. PMID: 36372792

Ighodaro, A., Stefanovics, E., Makanjuola, V., & Rosenheck, R. (2015). An assessment of attitudes towards people with mental illness among medical students and physicians in Ibadan, Nigeria. *Academic Psychiatry, 39*, 280–285. PMID: 24903130

Iida, K., Ryan, A., Payne, S., Hasson, F., & McIlfatrick, S. (2022). Palliative care in Japanese long-term care facilities. *International Journal of Palliative Nursing, 28*(1), 28–37. PMID: 35094533

Irumba, P., Tugume, D., & Apuulison, D. (2024). Advances in Multidisciplinary Approach for Liver Cancer. *Liver Cancer-Multidisciplinary Approach: Multidisciplinary Approach*, 3.

Jack, K., Ridley, C., & Turner, S. (2024). Effective communication with older people. *Nursing Older People, 36*(3). PMID: 31468756

Jones, T., Luth, E. A., Lin, S.-Y., & Brody, A. A. (2021). Advance care planning, palliative care, and end-of-life care interventions for racial and ethnic underrepresented groups: A systematic review. *Journal of Pain and Symptom Management, 62*(3), e248–e260. PMID: 33984460

Kaiser, A. H., Mao, S., Sundewall, J., Ross, M., Koy, S., Vorn, S., Koeut, P., & Ekman, B. (2025). Assessing the determinants of out-of-pocket health expenditures among Cambodian households in informal employment using survey data. *International Journal for Equity in Health, 24*(1), 33. DOI: 10.1186/s12939-025-02394-6 PMID: 39891289

Kaiser, A. H., Rotigliano, N., Flessa, S., Ekman, B., & Sundewall, J. (2023). Extending universal health coverage to informal workers: A systematic review of health financing schemes in low- and middle-income countries in Southeast Asia. *PLoS One, 18*(7), e0288269. DOI: 10.1371/journal.pone.0288269 PMID: 37432943

Kalantari, A. R., Mehrolhassani, M. H., Shati, M., & Dehnavieh, R. (2021). Health service delivery models for elderly people: A systematic review. *Medical Journal of the Islamic Republic of Iran, 35*, 21. PMID: 34169033

Katz, G. M., Arigoni, D., Rice, M. B., & Stall, N. M. (2025). Addressing the Health Impacts of Climate Change in Older Adults. *JAMA Internal Medicine, 185*(4), 362–363. PMID: 39899284

Kelley, A. S., Back, A. L., Arnold, R. M., Goldberg, G. R., Lim, B. B., Litrivis, E., Smith, C. B., & O'Neill, L. B. (2012). Geritalk: Communication skills training for geriatric and palliative medicine fellows. *Journal of the American Geriatrics Society*, *60*(2), 332–337. PMID: 22211768

Knaul, F. M., Arreola-Ornelas, H., Kwete, X. J., Bhadelia, A., Rosa, W. E., Touchton, M., Méndez-Carniado, O., Enciso, V. V., Pastrana, T., & Friedman, J. R. (2025). The evolution of serious health-related suffering from 1990 to 2021: An update to The Lancet Commission on global access to palliative care and pain relief. *The Lancet. Global Health*, *13*(3), e422–e436. PMID: 40021301

Krakauer, E. L. (2025). Palliative Care: Toward a More Responsive Definition. In *Textbook of palliative care* (pp. 115–119). Springer.

Krishnaswami, A., Bernacki, G. M., & Bhatt, D. L. (2022). Geriatric and palliative care specialists as valued members of the multidisciplinary heart team. *The American Journal of Medicine*, *135*(7), 810–812. PMID: 35134366

Kuipers, S. J., Nieboer, A. P., & Cramm, J. M. (2021). Easier said than done: Healthcare professionals' barriers to the provision of patient-centered primary care to patients with multimorbidity. *International Journal of Environmental Research and Public Health*, *18*(11), 6057. PMID: 34199866

Lam, T.-C., Chan, S.-K., Choi, C.-W., Tsang, K.-C., Yuen, K.-K., Soong, I., Wong, K.-H., Lui, L., Lo, S.-H., & Tong, M. (2021). Integrative palliative care service model improved end-of-life care and overall survival of advanced cancer patients in Hong Kong: A review of ten-year territory-wide cohort. *Journal of Palliative Medicine*, *24*(9), 1314–1320. PMID: 33507834

LaRocca-Pitts, M. (2015). Four FACTs spiritual assessment tool. *Journal of Health Care Chaplaincy*, *21*(2), 51–59. PMID: 25793421

Larsen, L. T. (2022). Not merely the absence of disease: A genealogy of the WHO's positive health definition. *History of the Human Sciences*, *35*(1), 111–131.

Lee, V., Lam, T., Jing, H., Liu, F., Zhang, Y., Huang, J., & Lee, A. (2019). Integrative palliative cancer care in Hong Kong: An overview and an example from the East. *Clinical Oncology*, *31*(8), 589–594. PMID: 31230834

Lee, Y. J., Kim, S.-H., Yoo, S. H., Kim, A.-S., Lin, C.-P., Martina, D., Mori, M., & Suh, S.-Y. (2024). Advance Care Planning in Palliative Care in Asia: Barriers and Implications. *Journal of Hospice and Palliative Care*, *27*(4), 107. PMID: 39691175

Leff, B., Burton, L., Mader, S. L., Naughton, B., Burl, J., Inouye, S. K., Greenough, W. B.III, Guido, S., Langston, C., & Frick, K. D. (2005). Hospital at home: Feasibility and outcomes of a program to provide hospital-level care at home for acutely ill older patients. *Annals of Internal Medicine, 143*(11), 798–808. PMID: 16330791

Lei, L., Lu, Y., Gan, Q., Hu, Z., & Luo, Y. (2022). Awareness and perceptions of palliative care among the elderly: A qualitative study. *Journal of Palliative Care, 37*(2), 204–212. PMID: 35195464

Lepherd, L. (2015). Spirituality: Everyone has it, but what is it? *International Journal of Nursing Practice, 21*(5), 566–574. PMID: 24666816

Leung, A. C.-t., Liu, C.-p., Chow, N. W.-s., & Chi, I. (2004). Cost-benefit analysis of a case management project for the community-dwelling frail elderly in Hong Kong. *Journal of Applied Gerontology, 23*(1), 70–85.

Liu, M. F., Ho, M.-H., Montayre, J., Wang, Y.-W., & Lin, C.-C. (2021). Palliative care development in the Asia pacific region: A review of assessment indicators. *Journal of Pain and Symptom Management, 62*(5), 1008–1014. PMID: 33933621

Loh, K. P., Soto-Perez-de-Celis, E., Hsu, T., de Glas, N. A., Battisti, N. M. L., Baldini, C., Rodrigues, M., Lichtman, S. M., & Wildiers, H. (2018). What every oncologist should know about geriatric assessment for older patients with cancer: Young international society of geriatric oncology position paper. *Journal of Oncology Practice / American Society of Clinical Oncology, 14*(2), 85–94. PMID: 29436306

Loosen, S. H., Schwartz, J., Grewe, S., Krieg, S., Krieg, A., Luedde, T., Batzler, Y.-N., Kostev, K., Neukirchen, M., & Roderburg, C. (2023). Drug landscape in patients receiving general outpatient palliative care in Germany: Results from a retrospective analysis of 10,464 patients. *BMC Palliative Care, 22*(1), 118. PMID: 37596590

Lu, Y., Gu, Y., & Yu, W. (2018). Hospice and palliative care in China: Development and challenges. *Asia-Pacific Journal of Oncology Nursing, 5*(1), 26–32. PMID: 29379830

Luckett, T., Phillips, J., Agar, M., Virdun, C., Green, A., & Davidson, P. M. (2014). Elements of effective palliative care models: A rapid review. *BMC Health Services Research, 14*, 1–22. PMID: 24670065

Mahdiabadi, F. R., Mirzaei, S., Entezari, A., & Nasiriani, K. (2023). The effect of implementing the COMFORT communication model on communication skills of nursing students. *International Journal of Palliative Nursing, 29*(9), 412–420. PMID: 37757811

Martins Pereira, S., Hernández-Marrero, P., Pasman, H. R., Capelas, M. L., Larkin, P., & Francke, A. L. (2021). Nursing education on palliative care across Europe: Results and recommendations from the EAPC Taskforce on preparation for practice in palliative care nursing across the EU based on an online-survey and country reports. *Palliative Medicine*, *35*(1), 130–141. PMID: 32912033

Maugans, T. A. (1996). The spiritual history. *Archives of Family Medicine*, *5*(1), 11–16. PMID: 8542049

McCarthy, B., O'Donovan, M., & Trace, A. (2021). A new therapeutic communication model "TAGEET" to help nurses engage therapeutically with patients suspected of or confirmed with COVID-19. *Journal of Clinical Nursing*, *30*(7-8), 1184–1191. PMID: 33350012

Meitar, D., & Karnieli-Miller, O. (2022). Twelve tips to manage a breaking bad news process: Using SPw-ICE-S–A revised version of the SPIKES protocol. *Medical Teacher*, *44*(10), 1087–1091. PMID: 34057007

Mercadante, S., Gregoretti, C., & Cortegiani, A. (2018). Palliative care in intensive care units: Why, where, what, who, when, how. *BMC Anesthesiology*, *18*, 1–6. PMID: 30111299

Meredith, S., Feldman, P., Frey, D., Giammarco, L., Hall, K., Arnold, K., Brown, N. J., & Ray, W. A. (2002). Improving medication use in newly admitted home healthcare patients: A randomized controlled trial. *Journal of the American Geriatrics Society*, *50*(9), 1484–1491. PMID: 12383144

Michel, J.-P., & Cha, H. B. (2015). Filling the geriatric education gap around the world. *Journal of the American Medical Directors Association*, *16*(12), 1010–1013. PMID: 26410106

Mills, J., Kim, S.-H., Chan, H. Y., Ho, M.-H., Montayre, J., Liu, M. F., & Lin, C.-C. (2021). Palliative care education in the Asia Pacific: Challenges and progress towards palliative care development. *Progress in Palliative Care*, *29*(5), 251–254.

Mitchell, R. J., Wijekulasuriya, S., du Preez, J., Lystad, R., Chauhan, A., Harrison, R., Curtis, K., & Braithwaite, J. (2024). Population-level quality indicators of end-of-life-care in an aged care setting: Rapid systematic review. *Archives of Gerontology and Geriatrics*, *116*, 105130. PMID: 37535984

Mo, L., Geng, Y., Chang, Y. K., Philip, J., Collins, A., & Hui, D. (2021). Referral criteria to specialist palliative care for patients with dementia: A systematic review. *Journal of the American Geriatrics Society*, *69*(6), 1659–1669. PMID: 33655535

Montgomery, A., & Lynn, J. (2014). The MediCaring™ Model: Best plan for frail elders in the longevity era. *The Public Policy and Aging Report, 24*(3), 112–117.

Murray, C. J., & Lopez, A. D. (1997). Alternative projections of mortality and disability by cause 1990–2020: Global Burden of Disease Study. *Lancet, 349*(9064), 1498–1504. PMID: 9167458

Naderi, N. B., Rafiei, S. Z., Pourramzani, A., Mirpour, S. H., Biazar, G., Atrkar-roushan, Z., Mortazavi, M., & Ahmadi, M. (2022). *Physicians.* Skills in Breaking Bad News to Patients With Cancer Using SPIKES Protocol.

Naylor, M. D., Brooten, D. A., Campbell, R. L., Maislin, G., McCauley, K. M., & Schwartz, J. S. (2004). Transitional care of older adults hospitalized with heart failure: A randomized, controlled trial. *Journal of the American Geriatrics Society, 52*(5), 675–684. PMID: 15086645

Nguyen, V., Khanh, Q. T., Hocaoglu, M., Huyen, H. T. M., Thinh, D. H. Q., & Krakauer, E. L. (2023). Integrated hospital-and home-based palliative care for cancer patients in Vietnam: People-centered outcomes. *Journal of pain and symptom management, 66*(3), 175–182. e173.

Nissen, R. D., Viftrup, D. T., & Hvidt, N. C. (2021). The process of spiritual care. *Frontiers in Psychology, 12*, 674453. PMID: 34557128

Nkhoma, K. B., Bates, M. J., van Breevoort, D., Chifamba, D. D., Evans, C. J., Kwaitana, D., Mensah, A. B. B., Mnenula, M. C., Mupaza, L., & Opare-Lokko, E. B. A. (2025). Integrating palliative care into primary care for older people with multimorbid serious illness: A multinational qualitative cross-sectional study in Sub-Saharan Africa. *BMJ Public Health, 3*(1). PMID: 40134537

Nukunu, F., Ahwireng, S. O., Gandaa, M., Donkor, W., & Odoi, P. (2024). Legal and Ethical Issues in Geriatric Care in Ghana. *JL Pol'y & Globalization, 140*, 20.

Omoyeni, E., & Gwyther, L. (2018). Assessing the palliative care needs of elderly patients seen at The University College Hospital, Ibadan, Nigeria (TH321A). *Journal of Pain and Symptom Management, 55*(2), 571–572.

Paal, P., Brandstötter, C., Lorenzl, S., Larkin, P., & Elsner, F. (2019). Postgraduate palliative care education for all healthcare providers in Europe: Results from an EAPC survey. *Palliative & Supportive Care, 17*(5), 495–506. PMID: 30683163

Paiva, C. E., Bonilla-Sierra, P., Tripodoro, V. A., Rodríguez-Nunez, A., De Simone, G., Rodriguez, L. H., de Oliveira Vidal, E. I., Ríos, M. R., Crispim, D. H., & Pérez-Cruz, P. (2023). How to advance palliative care research in South America? Findings from a delphi study. *Journal of Pain and Symptom Management, 65*(3), 193–202. PMID: 36455800

Pauline, I., David, A., & Daniel, T. (2024). Challenges in Geriatrics Palliative Care: A Global Concern. In *Difficulties and Challenges in Geriatric Health Management* (pp. 83–97). IGI Global.

Pelleg, A. R., Schiller, G., Goldhirsch, S. L., Fernandez, H. M., & Lindenberger, E. C. (2021). Geriatrics and palliative medicine leadership is needed now more than ever: What are the training gaps? *Journal of the American Geriatrics Society, 69*(4), 1063–1070. PMID: 33580716

Peralta, T., Castel-Branco, M. M., Reis-Pina, P., Figueiredo, I. V., & Dourado, M. (2022). Prescription trends at the end of life in a palliative care unit: Observational study. *BMC Palliative Care, 21*(1), 65. PMID: 35505394

Pergolizzi, J.Jr, LeQuang, J. A. K., Wagner, M., & Varrassi, G. (2024). Challenges in Palliative Care in Latin America: A Narrative Review. *Cureus, 16*(5). PMID: 38899235

Phillips, J. L., & Currow, D. (2019). Challenges and future directions of palliative care. *Textbook of palliative care*, 111–130.

Pollak, K. I., Arnold, R. M., Jeffreys, A. S., Alexander, S. C., Olsen, M. K., Abernethy, A. P., Sugg Skinner, C., Rodriguez, K. L., & Tulsky, J. A. (2007). Oncologist communication about emotion during visits with patients with advanced cancer. *Journal of Clinical Oncology, 25*(36), 5748–5752. PMID: 18089870

Radbruch, L., De Lima, L., Knaul, F., Wenk, R., Ali, Z., Bhatnaghar, S., Blanchard, C., Bruera, E., Buitrago, R., & Burla, C. (2020). Redefining palliative care—A new consensus-based definition. *Journal of Pain and Symptom Management, 60*(4), 754–764. PMID: 32387576

Rawlinson, F., Gwyther, L., Kiyange, F., Luyirika, E., Meiring, M., & Downing, J. (2014). The current situation in education and training of health-care professionals across Africa to optimise the delivery of palliative care for cancer patients. *ecancermedicalscience, 8*, 492.

Regnard, C., & Dean, M. (2022). *A guide to symptom relief in palliative care*. CRC Press.

Robinson, M. R., Al-Kindi, S. G., & Oliveira, G. H. (2017). Trends in palliative care use in elderly men and women with severe heart failure in the United States. *JAMA Cardiology*, *2*(3), 344–344. PMID: 27926774

Robledo, L. M. G., Cano-GutiéRrez, C., & Garcia, E. V. (2022). Healthcare for older people in Central and South America. *Age and Ageing*, *51*(5), afac017. PMID: 35604089

Roeland, E. J., Triplett, D. P., Matsuno, R. K., Boero, I. J., Hwang, L., Yeung, H. N., Mell, L., & Murphy, J. D. (2016). Patterns of palliative care consultation among elderly patients with cancer. *Journal of the National Comprehensive Cancer Network : JNCCN*, *14*(4), 439–445. PMID: 27059192

Sadiq, F. U., Yu-Lyu, Y., Hung-En, L., Eka, P. M. A., Sneha, P., & Shih, Y.-H. (2025). The benefits, barriers, and specific needs of palliative care for adults with cancer in sub-Saharan Africa: A systematic review. *Global Health Action*, *18*(1), 2485742. DOI: 10.1080/16549716.2025.2485742 PMID: 40208058

Sakurai, Y. (2025). A Comparative Analysis of End-of-Life Care for Older Adults in East Asia, the US and Europe: With a Particular Focus on Family Involvement, Advance Directives and ACP. *Yokohama International Society and Social Science Research*, *29*(3), 107–124.

Samba, E. I., Mensah, G. B., Frimpong, P. O., Addy, A., & Otoo, J. (2023). The State of Gerontological and Geriatric Studies in Sub-Saharan Africa and Ghanaian Studies: Literature Review. *International Journal for Multidisciplinary Research*

Saracino, R. M., Bai, M., Blatt, L., Solomon, L., & McCorkle, R. (2018). Geriatric palliative care: Meeting the needs of a growing population. *Geriatric Nursing*, *39*(2), 225–229. PMID: 29042070

Sepúlveda, C., Marlin, A., Yoshida, T., & Ullrich, A. (2002). Palliative care: The World Health Organization's global perspective. *Journal of Pain and Symptom Management*, *24*(2), 91–96. PMID: 12231124

Shabnam, J., Timm, H. U., Nielsen, D. S., & Raunkiaer, M. (2022). Palliative care utilization among non-western migrants in Europe: A systematic review. *Journal of Immigrant and Minority Health*, *•••*, 1–19. PMID: 34709528

Skalla, K. A. (2006). Spiritual assessment of patients with cancer: the moral authority, vocational, aesthetic, social, and transcendent model. *Number 4/July 2006*, *33*(4), 745–751.

Sleeman, K. E., De Brito, M., Etkind, S., Nkhoma, K., Guo, P., Higginson, I. J., Gomes, B., & Harding, R. (2019). The escalating global burden of serious health-related suffering: Projections to 2060 by world regions, age groups, and health conditions. *The Lancet. Global Health*, *7*(7), e883–e892. PMID: 31129125

Steffens, D. C., & Zdanys, K. F. (2022). *The American Psychiatric Association Publishing Textbook of Geriatric Psychiatry*. American Psychiatric Pub.

Stow, D., Spiers, G., Matthews, F. E., & Hanratty, B. (2019). What is the evidence that people with frailty have needs for palliative care at the end of life? A systematic review and narrative synthesis. *Palliative Medicine*, *33*(4), 399–414. PMID: 30775957

Suija, K., Mason, S. R., Elsner, F., & Paal, P. (2024). Palliative care training in medical undergraduate education: A survey among the faculty. *BMC Palliative Care*, *23*(1), 19. PMID: 38233862

Sungur, H., van den Muijsenbergh, M. E., van Weert, J. C., & Schouten, B. C. (2022). Caring for older culturally and linguistically diverse patients with Cancer: Healthcare Providers' perceived barriers to communication. *Journal of Geriatric Oncology*, *13*(6), 862–870. PMID: 35589543

Takechi, H., Tsuzuki, A., Matsumoto, K., Fukui, A., Kawakita, H., Yoshino, H., & Kanada, Y. (2022). Differences in the frequency of subjective geriatric complaints along with aging and their associations with physical function, multimorbidity, and mood: A cross-sectional study. *PLoS One*, *17*(2), e0263889. PMID: 35148335

Taran, S. (2011). An examination of the factors contributing to poor communication outside the physician-patient sphere. *McGill Journal of Medicine : MJM : an International Forum for the Advancement of Medical Sciences by Students*, *13*(1), 86. PMID: 22363186

Teal, C. R., & Street, R. L. (2009). Critical elements of culturally competent communication in the medical encounter: A review and model. *Social Science & Medicine*, *68*(3), 533–543. PMID: 19019520

Thiel, M., Mattison, D., Goudie, E., Licata, S., Brewster, J., & Montagnini, M. (2021). Social work training in palliative care: Addressing the gap. *The American Journal of Hospice & Palliative Care*, *38*(8), 893–898. PMID: 32969240

Ukpo, S. D., Imohiosen, C. E., Owot, J. A., & Ajuluchukwu, P. (2024). The impact of religious and spiritual counseling on mental health outcomes in geriatric care. *International Journal of Multidisciplinary Research and Growth Evaluation*, *5*(6), 1538–1547.

UNICEF. (2019). *Mental Health and Psychosocial Technical Note*

Van Driel, T., Hilderink, P., Hanssen, D., De Boer, P., Rosmalen, J., & Oude Voshaar, R. (2018). Assessment of somatization and medically unexplained symptoms in later life. *Assessment*, *25*(3), 374–393. PMID: 28745072

Vargas-Escobar, L. M., Sánchez-Cárdenas, M. A., Guerrero-Benítez, A. C., Suarez-Prieto, V. K., Moreno-García, J. R., Cañón Piñeros, Á. M., Rodríguez-Campos, L. F., & León-Delgado, M. X. (2022). Barriers to access to palliative care in Colombia: A social mapping approach involving stakeholder participation. *INQUIRY: The Journal of Health Care Organization, Provision, and Financing*, *59*, 00469580221133217. PMID: 36317765

Vedel, I., De Stampa, M., Bergman, H., Ankri, J., Cassou, B., Mauriat, C., Blanchard, F., Bagaragaza, E., & Lapointe, L. (2009). A novel model of integrated care for the elderly: COPA, Coordination of Professional Care for the Elderly. *Aging Clinical and Experimental Research*, *21*, 414–423. PMID: 20154510

Veronese, N., Custodero, C., Demurtas, J., Smith, L., Barbagallo, M., Maggi, S., Cella, A., Vanacore, N., Aprile, P. L., & Ferrucci, L. (2022). Comprehensive geriatric assessment in older people: An umbrella review of health outcomes. *Age and Ageing*, *51*(5), afac104. PMID: 35524746

Vo, M. T. H., & Fong, B. Y. F. (2025). Long-Term Care Initiatives in Southeast Asian Countries with Emerging Ageing Population and the Sustainability of Health and Social Care Systems. In *The Handbook of Public Health in the Asia-Pacific* (pp. 1–32). Springer.

Voumard, R., Rubli Truchard, E., Benaroyo, L., Borasio, G., Büla, C., & Jox, R. (2018). Geriatric palliative care: A view of its concept, challenges and strategies. *BMC Geriatrics*, *18*, 1–6. PMID: 30236063

Wachterman, M. W., & Sommers, B. D. (2021). Dying poor in the US—Disparities in end-of-life care. *Journal of the American Medical Association*, *325*(5), 423–424. PMID: 33528526

Wang, Y., Zhang, X., Huang, Y., & Ma, X. (2024). Palliative care for cancer patients in asia: Challenges and countermeasures. *Oncology Reviews*, *17*, 11866. PMID: 38293617

WHO. (2002). *National cancer control programmes: policies and managerial guidelines*. World Health Organization.

WHO. W. H. O. (2020). *Palliative Care*. WHO. Retrieved 23/04/2025 from https://www.who.int/news-room/fact-sheets/detail/palliative-care

WHPCA. W. P. C. A. (2020). *Global Atlas of Palliative Care* (2nd Edition ed.).

Wiencek, C., & Coyne, P. (2014). Palliative care delivery models. Seminars in oncology nursing, Wittenberg, E., Ferrell, B., Goldsmith, J., & Ruel, N. H. (2016). Family Caregiver Communication Tool: A New Measure for Tailoring Communication with Cancer Caregivers: For submission to Psycho Oncology. *Psycho-Oncology, 26*(8), 1222.

Wittenberg, E., Goldsmith, J. V., Ragan, S. L., & Parnell, T. A. (2019). *Communication in Palliative Nursing: The COMFORT Model.* Oxford University Press., DOI: 10.1093/med/9780190061326.001.0001

Wittenberg, E., Kravits, K., Goldsmith, J., Ferrell, B., & Fujinami, R. (2017). Validation of a model of family caregiver communication types and related caregiver outcomes. *Palliative & Supportive Care, 15*(1), 3–11. PMID: 27032294

Wittenberg, E., Reb, A., & Kanter, E. (2018). Communicating with patients and families around difficult topics in cancer care using the COMFORT communication curriculum. Seminars in oncology nursing, Wolf, C., & Wedding, U. (2025). Geriatric Oncology Highlights from the European Society for Medical Oncology Annual Meeting 2024. *Oncology Research and Treatment.*

Yaghi, G., & Chahine, B. (2023). Potentially inappropriate medications use in a psychiatric elderly care hospital: A cross-sectional study using Beers criteria. *Health Science Reports, 6*(5), e1247. PMID: 37234198

Yang, Y., Liang, X., Liu, Q., & Liu, J. (2025). Navigating limited resources: Experiences of caregivers for elderly terminal cancer patients in a region with limited palliative care services. *Supportive Care in Cancer, 33*(3), 207. PMID: 39971822

Yao, M., Zhou, X.-y., Xu, Z.-j., Lehman, R., Haroon, S., Jackson, D., & Cheng, K. K. (2021). The impact of training healthcare professionals' communication skills on the clinical care of diabetes and hypertension: A systematic review and meta-analysis. *BMC Family Practice, 22*, 1–23. PMID: 34261454

Yeung, W.-J. J., & Thang, L. L. (2018). Long-Term care for older adults in ASEAN plus three: The roles of family, community, and the state in addressing unmet eldercare needs. *Journal of Aging and Health, 30*(10), 1499–1515. PMID: 30239253

Zertuche-Maldonado, T., Figueroa, S. A. V., Cantisani, A. F., Lim, F., & Silva, M. F. (2020). Management of palliative care in Latin America. *Journal of Alternative Medical Research, 12*(1), 63–75.

Zhang, X., Zhang, X., Li, Y., Chen, T., Wang, Y., Siow, L., Wang, Y., Ming, W.-K., Sun, X., & Wu, Y. (2022). Factors affecting acceptance of palliative care in mainland China: A national cross-sectional study. *The Lancet. Oncology, 23*, S3.

Chapter 2

The Quality of Life in Terminal Care: A Multidimensional Approach for Elderly Patients

Mohammed El Rhanbouri
https://orcid.org/0009-0006-9643-5181
Morpho-Science Research Laboratory, Faculty of Medicine and Pharmacy, Cadi Ayyad University, Marrake, Morocco

Mounia Amane
https://orcid.org/0000-0002-9273-4284
Higher Institute of Nursing Professions and Technical Health of Marrakech, Morocco

Hanane Aimad
Higher Institute of Nursing Professions and Technical Health of Marrakech, Morocco

Fatima Ezzahra Madihi
Higher Institute of Nursing Professions and Technical Health of Marrakech, Morocco

Amina El Fahli
Higher Institute of Nursing Professions and Technical Health of Marrakech, Morocco

Mohamed Khalyfa
https://orcid.org/0009-0009-0902-0132
Laboratoire Sciences de Santé et Technologies, ISSS-UH1 Settat, Morocco

Samia Boussaa
https://orcid.org/0000-0002-5599-1097
Higher Institute of Nursing Professions and Technical Health of Rabat, Morocco

ABSTRACT

Quality of life (QoL) in terminal care for elderly patients is a multifaceted concept that includes not only physical symptoms but also psychological, social, and spiritual aspects of well-being. With the global aging population and rising rates of

DOI: 10.4018/979-8-3373-4099-9.ch002

chronic, incurable diseases, understanding and addressing QoL is critical in the final stages of life. Factors influencing QoL in terminal care include effective symptom management, emotional support, and the importance of social connections. The ethical challenges of respecting patient autonomy and making end-of-life decisions are also discussed. An integrated approach combining medical care, psychological support, and social interaction is essential for improving the quality of life, preserving dignity, and providing comfort to elderly patients. The chapter emphasizes a holistic approach to terminal care that acknowledges the complexity of the patient experience and adapts to their evolving needs.

INTRODUCTION

The aging of the global population, coupled with the rise of chronic and incurable diseases, highlights the need to rethink care strategies for older adults nearing the end of life. With the rapid increase in life expectancy, it has become essential to focus on the quality of life (QOL) of elderly patients in their final years. QOL, a complex and multidimensional concept introduced in 1964 (Mercier & Filion, 2006), is not limited to managing physical symptoms but also encompasses psychological, social, and spiritual dimensions that directly influence the well-being of patients in palliative care (Sepúlveda et al., 2002; WHO, 1993).

The concept of end-of-life care refers to care provided to patients with serious or terminal illnesses for whom recovery is no longer possible. The objective becomes managing symptoms and improving QOL. In this context, QOL is defined as an individual's overall experience in various aspects of life, influenced by their health condition, social interactions, emotional well-being, and satisfaction in meaningful areas of existence (Gijsberts et al., 2019). According to the World Health Organization (WHO), QOL "is the perception an individual has of their position in life, in the context of the culture and value systems in which they live" (WHO, 1997).

Research conducted over the last few decades shows that, although pain and symptom management are crucial, QOL in end-of-life care cannot be reduced to these aspects alone. It is now widely recognized that improving patients' QOL requires a holistic approach that considers not only physical symptoms but also the emotional, social, and spiritual needs of patients. The integration of palliative care into the care trajectory of elderly patients at the end of life is therefore essential to provide care that is adapted and respectful of the patient's preferences (Breitbart et al., 2004; Fowlie & Berkeley, 1987).

Demographic aging, which is expected to see the number of people over 65 years of age reach 1.5 billion by 2050 (United Nations, 2019), implies an increased demand for palliative and end-of-life care tailored to the needs of the elderly. These projections highlight the urgent need for an approach that is both accessible and personalized to support elderly individuals in this phase of life.

This review aims to examine the challenges and opportunities related to managing QOL in end-of-life care for older adults, based on a thorough analysis of recent research in the field of palliative care. The primary objective is to provide a comprehensive overview of the different dimensions of QOL in end-of-life care and offer recommendations for improving current practices. This chapter addresses key concepts of QOL, assessment tools used, factors influencing this quality, and the ethical challenges associated with the care of elderly individuals at the end of life.

QOL, in the context of end-of-life care, refers to the overall physical, psychological, social, and spiritual dimensions that contribute to the patient's well-being as life comes to an end. This concept is inherently subjective because it depends on the patient's perception of their health, expectations, and life priorities. The World Health Organization (WHO) defines QOL as "the perception an individual has of their position in life in the context of the culture and value systems in which they live" (WHO, 1997). This definition highlights the importance of personal and cultural context in how individuals assess their QOL, especially at the end of life.

DIMENSIONS OF QOL IN END-OF-LIFE CARE

QOL in end-of-life care is based on a multidimensional approach that integrates the physical, psychological, social, and spiritual aspects of patients' well-being (OECD, 2023). Each dimension plays a significant role in the care of older adults at the end of life, influencing their comfort, dignity, and overall satisfaction.

Physical Dimension

Managing physical symptoms is a central element of QOL in end-of-life care. Pain, fatigue, insomnia, dyspnea, and nausea are among the most common symptoms experienced by patients at the end of life. Palliative care aims to alleviate these symptoms and improve the patient's physical comfort. Several studies show that effective pain management is crucial for improving QOL in this context. Pharmacological interventions such as opioids, combined with non-pharmacological strategies like relaxation and physiotherapy, enable more comprehensive symptom control. However, managing pain and other physical symptoms alone is not sufficient to ensure satisfactory QOL. It is also necessary to consider environmental adjustments, such as room temperature, bed or chair ergonomics, and lighting, all of which can impact the patient's overall comfort. Green et al (2020) highlights that simple yet effective physical environment modifications, such as optimizing lighting and adjusting room temperature, can enhance patient well-being and contribute to better symptom management (Green et al., 2020).

Cognitive disorders, particularly dementia such as Alzheimer's disease, significantly complicate the physical dimension of QOL in end-of-life care for elderly patients. Dementia, a leading cause of death in older adults, often coexists with geriatric syndromes like frailty, sarcopenia (muscle loss), and falls, exacerbating vulnerability and reducing functional independence. Systematic reviews indicate that patients with advanced dementia receive suboptimal end-of-life care, including inadequate pain control and limited palliative interventions, due to challenges in symptom communication and assessment (Miranda et al., 2019; Sampson et al., 2018). Frailty amplifies these issues by increasing susceptibility to falls and immobility, which in turn heighten risks of pressure ulcers, infections, and delirium, further diminishing QoL. Integrating geriatric-specific strategies, such as frailty screening (e.g., via the Clinical Frailty Scale) and fall prevention protocols, into palliative care can mitigate these effects, but evidence highlights underutilization in dementia populations, calling for tailored multidisciplinary approaches (Clegg et al., 2013; Turner & Clegg, 2014).

Psychological Dimension

Emotional suffering, such as anxiety, depression, and fear of death, are significant factors influencing the QOL of patients in end-of-life care. Numerous studies have shown that patients near the end of life, particularly those with cancer, are exposed to high levels of psychological stress (Green et al., 2020).. Additionally, experiences of anxiety and depression can be exacerbated by factors such as social isolation, uncertainties related to the disease progression, and changes in family roles (Zhao et al., 2022). Psychological support is therefore crucial in this context. Cognitive-behavioral therapies, for example, have been shown to be effective in reducing symptoms of anxiety and depression in palliative care patients (Anderson et al., 2008; Green et al., 2020). Furthermore, giving patients the opportunity to explore their emotions, express their fears and concerns about death, and participate in support groups can provide them with emotional relief. Caregivers' work in this area also involves identifying signs of psychological distress and responding appropriately (Umar et al., 2023).

Social Dimension

Social relationships play a vital role in the overall well-being of end-of-life patients. Social isolation, which can result from illness or aging, is a major negative factor for the QOL of elderly individuals in end-of-life care. Many studies have shown that regular social interactions improve patients' emotional states and can reduce feelings of loneliness (Bradley et al., 2022). Family visits and interactions with loved one's help maintain social connections, which can strengthen patients' emotional resilience. Support from loved ones is also important for patients in palliative care. Additionally, participating in community activities, such as charitable visits or virtual contacts through online platforms, can be an effective way to combat social isolation and improve QOL. The biopsychosocial model, as described by Engel (1977), emphasizes the importance of integrating social dimensions into the follow-up of palliative care patients (Engel, 1977).

Family caregivers play a pivotal role in the social dimension of QOL for elderly patients in end-of-life care, often acting as primary sources of emotional and practical support, yet their own burden can inadvertently diminish patient well-being. Systematic reviews highlight that caregivers experience high levels of stress, fatigue, and depression, which correlate with poorer patient outcomes, including increased isolation and reduced QoL (Adelman et al., 2014; Schulz et al., 2016). In dementia contexts, caregivers manage complex behaviors and decision-making, amplifying distress; interventions like respite care and training programs have been shown to improve both caregiver resilience and patient satisfaction (Schulz & Czaja, 2018).

Cultural beliefs, values, and practices profoundly permeate every aspect of end-of-life care, shaping perceptions of QOL and influencing decisions on treatment, family involvement, and rituals. Systematic reviews reveal that in collectivist cultures (e.g., Asian or Latin American), family-centered decision-making prioritizes harmony and filial piety, potentially delaying palliative referrals to avoid perceived abandonment, while individualistic Western cultures emphasize patient autonomy and advance directives (Fang et al., 2016; Kwak & Salmon, 2007). These differences impact QoL by affecting pain expression, spiritual comfort, and end-of-life preferences—e.g., some Indigenous groups view death as a communal transition requiring specific ceremonies (Hampton et al., 2011). Culturally competent care, incorporating tools like cultural assessments, enhances QoL by reducing disparities and respecting diverse values, yet barriers in multicultural settings underscore the need for training in cultural humility (Cain et al., 2018; Crawley et al., 2002)

Spiritual Dimension

The spiritual dimension is often overlooked in traditional care, but it is of paramount importance for many patients at the end of life. The search for meaning, reconciliation with oneself and the beyond, as well as maintaining a spiritual connection, are key elements for many individuals when facing death (Amoah, 2011; Kang et al., 2023). Spirituality in palliative care is not limited to a religious framework but also encompasses personal and philosophical aspects, which allow patients to find comfort and accept the end of their life more peacefully. Spiritual practices, such as prayer, religious rituals, or philosophical discussions on the meaning of life and death, can be integrated into palliative care to meet the spiritual needs of patients (Gijsberts et al., 2019). Including caregivers in this process, in collaboration with spiritual counselors or chaplains, is essential to providing comprehensive support for end-of-life patients (Koper et al., 2019).

THEORETICAL MODELS OF QOL

QOL in end-of-life care is a complex and multidimensional concept that encompasses various aspects of the human experience. To better understand and assess this notion, several models have been proposed. Among the most influential is the conceptual model of QOL developed by Wilson and Cleary in 1995, which offers a systematic approach to linking objective clinical variables to subjective health perceptions. This model divides health outcomes into five hierarchical levels, each representing a specific dimension of health, ranging from measurable biological and physiological parameters to subjective assessments of well-being. These levels include biological and physiological factors, symptoms, functioning, general health perceptions, and, finally, global QOL (Wilson & Cleary, 1995).

As we move from left to right in the model, we observe that each level becomes progressively more integrated and harder to define and measure. The causal relationships between these levels suggest that traditional clinical variables, such as physiological and symptomatic measurements, influence QOL related health measures (QoLS). This model highlights the increasing complexity of the health experience, where biological aspects evolve into subjective health perceptions as patients interact with their environment. This model has proven effective in evaluating QoLS, particularly in populations with chronic illnesses, and remains a valuable tool for understanding the determinants of patients' QoL.

Another influential model in this field is the one developed by Carol Estwing Ferrans. This model is based on an individualistic approach, recognizing that QoL depends on each individual's unique experience. Thus, each person is seen as the only appropriate judge of their own QoL, with their values and priorities directly influencing their evaluation of well-being. From this perspective, QoL is defined in terms of satisfaction with aspects of life that the individual deems important. This model grouped related elements into four main domains: health and functioning, psychological/spiritual, social and economic, and family. These four dimensions cover various facets of human experience and allow for a more comprehensive assessment of an individual's well-being (Ferrans, 1996).

To measure QoL in these different domains, Ferrans and Marjorie Powers developed the Quality-of-Life Index (QLI) in 1985, a tool designed to assess satisfaction in each of these domains. The QLI stands out for its individualized approach, measuring not only satisfaction in each domain but also the importance the individual places on these dimensions. Thus, the scores reflect not only the patient's satisfaction but also their priorities, offering a personalized assessment of their well-being (Ferrans, 1990; Ferrans & Powers, 1985)

These models emphasize the importance of personalized and multidimensional evaluation of QoL in end-of-life care. In this context, current approaches stress the need to adapt assessment tools to the specific needs and preferences of patients. It is crucial that these evaluations account for the patient's evolving health status and changing priorities as the end-of-life approaches. This approach allows for more comprehensive and humane care, responding precisely to the expectations of each patient, particularly in palliative care.

Despite their strengths, theoretical models like Wilson and Cleary's (1995) and Ferrans' (1996) have limitations when applied to elderly patients in end-of-life care, particularly those with geriatric complexities such as multimorbidity and cognitive decline. Wilson and Cleary's hierarchical framework, while integrating biological to subjective elements, often underemphasizes social and spiritual domains in frail populations, where environmental interactions are limited by mobility issues or dementia, leading to incomplete QoL assessments (Bakitas et al., 2020). Similarly, Ferrans' individualistic model relies on self-reported priorities, which becomes problematic in advanced dementia where patients cannot articulate values, potentially biasing evaluations toward proxy reports and reducing accuracy. Critiques from recent reviews suggest adapting these models for geriatrics by incorporating frailty indices and cultural modifiers, as their general palliative focus overlooks age-specific vulnerabilities like sarcopenia's impact on functioning (Clegg et al., 2013). Enhancing these with practical geriatric adaptations could provide a more robust, synthetic framework for end-of-life care.

ASSESSMENT TOOLS FOR QOL IN END-OF-LIFE CARE

Assessing the QoL in patients in end-of-life care is a major challenge due to the complexity and subjectivity of the various factors that contribute to it. While quantitative approaches have been developed to measure QoL, it is essential to recognize that QoL at the end of life is a deeply personal experience influenced by physical, psychological, social, and spiritual factors. Many instruments have been designed to quantify these aspects and assist healthcare professionals in tailoring care to the individual needs of patients.

Multidimensional Tools

Multidimensional tools are designed to assess QoL across all its dimensions: physical, emotional, social, and spiritual. These instruments are particularly useful in palliative care, as they allow for a comprehensive assessment of the patient's well-being. Among the most widely used tools are:

EORTC QLQ-C30

The EORTC QLQ-C30 is one of the most commonly used questionnaires for assessing the QoL of cancer patients, but it is also widely applied in other palliative care contexts. It was developed by the European Organization for Research and Treatment of Cancer (EORTC) and is designed to measure the QoL of patients undergoing treatment or in palliative care. It includes functional scales (e.g., physical activity, role), symptom scales (e.g., pain, fatigue, nausea), and a global QoL scale (Aaronson et al., 1993).

This questionnaire is often supplemented with disease-specific scales (e.g., QLQ-LC13 for lung cancer) to tailor the assessment to the patient's particular condition. The strength of the QLQ-C30 lies in its ability to provide information on the overall impact of the disease and treatment on the patient's life while being relatively simple to administer. However, some studies suggest that this tool lacks consideration of the spiritual and social dimensions of quality of life, making it incomplete for holistic evaluation (Fayers & Bottomley, 2002).

McGill Quality of Life Questionnaire (MQOL)

The McGill Quality of Life Questionnaire (MQOL) is another widely used tool in palliative care, especially for patients in end-of-life care. This questionnaire stands out for its holistic approach to QoL, including physical, psychological, social, and spiritual dimensions. It measures factors such as pain, symptoms, social interaction, and the sense of life, with a particular focus on the spiritual dimension (Cohen et al., 1995).

The MQOL has been validated in several studies and is often preferred for patients at the end of life because it allows for a more complete assessment of overall well-being, particularly in terms of existential concerns. However, it can be more complex to administer than other tools, and some criticisms highlight that the patients' responses may be influenced by their emotional state at the time of the evaluation.

The WHOQOL

The WHOQOL (World Health Organization Quality of Life) is another relevant instrument, although less specific to palliative care. It assesses QoL across six dimensions: physical, psychological, level of living, social relationships, environment, and independence. While WHOQOL is widely used in international research on QoL, it has been adapted for palliative care contexts, particularly concerning social interactions and spiritual support (WHO, 1997).

One of the advantages of this tool is its ability to be used in diverse cultural contexts, as it has been validated in numerous languages and is applicable to a wide range of populations. However, its application in palliative care has been criticized for not adequately capturing the emotional and spiritual suffering specific to the end of life (Caliskan et al., 2019).

Comparing multidimensional tools like the EORTC QLQ-C30, MQOL, and WHOQOL reveals strengths and limitations in their suitability for elderly palliative populations, necessitating critical adaptation for geriatric complexities. The EORTC QLQ-C30 excels in oncology-specific symptom assessment (e.g., pain, fatigue) with high reliability (Cronbach's $\alpha > 0.70$), but its self-report format limits use in cognitively impaired elderly, where proxy versions introduce bias, and it underemphasizes spiritual domains (Aaronson et al., 1993; Fayers & Bottomley, 2002). . In contrast, the MQOL integrates existential well-being effectively for end-of-life, showing strong validity in advanced disease (r=0.60-0.80), yet its brevity may overlook geriatric syndromes like frailty, reducing applicability in multimorbid older adults (Cohen et al., 1995). The WHOQOL offers broad cultural sensitivity across domains but requires lengthy administration, challenging for frail elderly with fatigue or dementia, and lacks end of life-specific items (Skevington et al., 2004; WHO, 1997). Critically, studies like Green et al. (2020) demonstrate efficacy in younger, cognitively intact groups, but for elderly, tools must be adapted (e.g., simplified versions or integrated with dementia proxies) to avoid underestimating QoL, emphasizing practical geriatric tailoring for accurate, non-reductive assessments (Burks et al., 2021).

Qualitative Tools: Interviews and Discussions

In addition to quantitative instruments, qualitative tools play a crucial role in assessing the QoL of patients in end-of-life care. Semi-structured interviews and focus group discussions are commonly used methods to gain deeper insights into the subjective perceptions of patients. These methods help address dimensions such as personal preferences, existential concerns, and overall patient satisfaction with their care.

Research shows that qualitative data collected through interviews can provide rich information on how patients experience their end of life and their expectations regarding care. Such information is essential for caregivers to adapt treatments and care plans to better meet patients' needs (McCABE et al., 2007).

Advantages and Limitations of Quality-of-Life Assessment Tools

QoL assessment tools in end-of-life care offer several advantages, primarily by providing systematic and standardized evaluations of patients' well-being. These tools offer valuable data that can guide clinical decision-making and help adjust treatments based on patients' needs. Furthermore, they allow for tracking the progression of QoL over time and comparing the effects of different interventions.

However, these tools are not without limitations. One major challenge lies in the subjective nature of QoL, which can be influenced by the patient's emotional state at the time of evaluation, their health status, and their personal values (Van Hecke et al., 2018). Additionally, most existing tools still underestimate the spiritual and social dimensions of QoL, which are essential in palliative care contexts (Gijsberts et al., 2019).

FACTORS INFLUENCING QOL IN END-OF-LIFE CARE

Numerous interconnected factors influence QoL in end-of-life care. These factors include physical, emotional, social, and spiritual aspects, which determine the well-being of patients approaching the end of life. Since each patient is unique, these dimensions may evolve as the disease progresses. Therefore, it is crucial to consider each factor in an integrated manner to provide tailored and personalized care. The main factors identified in the scientific literature are as follows:

Pain and Symptom Management

Pain management is a central aspect of end-of-life care. Pain is one of the most common and debilitating symptoms for patients nearing the end of life, especially those suffering from cancer or other severe diseases. According to Hedman et al. (2024), up to 81% of palliative care patients experience pain in the final stages of life

(Hedman et al., 2024). Pain can be acute or chronic, and controlling it is essential to ensure an acceptable QoL.

Palliative care aims to provide maximum pain relief through a combination of pharmacological treatments (opioids, analgesics) and non-pharmacological methods (relaxation, physiotherapy, acupuncture). Studies by Candy et al. (2015) and Corli et al. (2019) show that opioids are effective for pain control but can cause undesirable side effects such as drowsiness and constipation (Candy et al., 2015; Corli et al., 2019). Therefore, care teams must adjust treatments based on individual patient needs, considering their tolerance to medications and any side effects.

In addition to pain, other physical symptoms such as dyspnea (difficulty breathing), insomnia, nausea, and fatigue can also affect patients' QoL in end-of-life care (Cella, 1994). An integrated approach, combining different treatments and strategies to relieve these symptoms, is essential for ensuring patient comfort. Environmental modifications, such as temperature and lighting adjustments in the room, have also been shown to improve overall patient comfort (Bae & Kim, 2024)

Psychological Support and Emotional Well-Being

Emotional disorders such as anxiety, depression, and fear of death are common in patients nearing the end of life. Green et al. (2020) highlight that anxiety and depression are the main causes of psychological distress in palliative care patients, impacting their overall well-being and perception of QoL. Fear of suffering, the fear of the unknown, and a sense of losing control are factors that exacerbate these emotional symptoms (Green et al., 2020).

Psychological support is therefore crucial. According to Anderson et al. (2008) et Green et al. (2020), interventions such as cognitive-behavioral therapy (CBT), psychotherapy, and the integration of support groups can reduce symptoms of depression and anxiety, thereby improving patients' QoL (Anderson et al., 2008; Green et al., 2020). Person-centered care approaches, which allow patients to express their emotions and discuss concerns (Khaldouni et al., 2025), have also been shown to reduce anxiety and enhance emotional well-being.

Furthermore, the perception of control is essential for emotional management. Montori et al. (2023) suggest that allowing patients to actively participate in their care decisions, particularly in terms of treatment and symptom management, improves their sense of autonomy and emotional well-being (Montori et al., 2023).

Social Relationships and Social Isolation

Social isolation is a major negative factor for QoL in end-of-life care, particularly for elderly patients. Hanna et al. (2022) show that loneliness and isolation can intensify emotional suffering, increase stress levels, and reduce overall satisfaction with care (Hanna et al., 2022). Social interactions with family, friends, and the community are essential for maintaining patients' morale and providing the necessary emotional support.

Integrating loved ones into the care process, as well as facilitating regular visits and virtual contact, helps combat social isolation. Support groups, where patients can share their experiences with others facing similar situations, are also beneficial for maintaining social connections and providing mutual emotional support (Kim & Kim, 2024). These interactions reduce anxiety and promote a sense of security and belonging.

Spiritual and Cultural Dimensions

Spirituality plays a vital role in the QoL of patients in end-of-life care, especially when it comes to understanding and managing existential aspects of dying. Gijsberts et al. (2019) indicate that spirituality, whether religious or not, helps patients find meaning in their suffering and accept death. Spiritual care, including practices such as prayer, rituals, and philosophical discussions on life and death, helps patients maintain inner peace (Gijsberts et al., 2019).

Furthermore, taking into account cultural and spiritual differences is crucial in providing quality palliative care. Each culture has its own beliefs and practices regarding the end of life, and it is essential to respect these beliefs when making palliative care decisions. Amoah (2011) and Koper et al. (2019) emphasize that integrating spiritual and cultural needs into end-of-life care promotes greater respect for the patient and more comprehensive care (Amoah, 2011; Koper et al., 2019).

Autonomy and Shared Decision-Making

Autonomy is a fundamental factor in the QoL of patients in end-of-life care. Allowing patients to actively participate in decisions regarding their care and treatments directly impacts their satisfaction and emotional well-being. Sepúlveda et al. (2002) assert that autonomy, and the ability to choose between different care options, significantly improves the QoL of palliative care patients (Sepúlveda et al., 2002).

The shared decision-making process, where caregivers collaborate with patients and their families to develop a care plan, is essential for ensuring that care respects the patient's wishes and minimizes unnecessary suffering (Svendsen et al., 2024). This approach also ensures that treatments are neither overly invasive nor unnecessary, thus maintaining the patient's dignity until the end of life.

ETHICAL CHALLENGES IN END-OF-LIFE CARE

End-of-life care for the elderly raises numerous ethical questions. These dilemmas are not limited to medical decisions regarding treatments and interventions but also encompass issues related to patient autonomy, pain management, and how to respect patients' end-of-life choices. The complexity of these situations, particularly the need to balance respecting the patient's wishes with minimizing suffering, requires deep ethical reflection and informed decision-making.

Patient Autonomy and Advance Directives

Autonomy is one of the most fundamental ethical principles in healthcare. It involves allowing individuals to make informed decisions regarding their own treatment and care. In end-of-life care, autonomy becomes particularly important, as patients must be able to clearly express their preferences regarding the end of life, including decisions about resuscitation, artificial feeding, or discontinuing treatments.

Advance directives play a critical role in preserving patient autonomy at the end of life. These documents, which outline a patient's wishes for end-of-life care, ensure that their desires will be respected even when they are no longer able to communicate (House et al., 2025). However, in cases of dementia or cognitive disorders, determining the patient's true will can be challenging, particularly when advance directives are absent or unclear (Perreault, 2018).

This raises the question of how healthcare professionals can intervene to "protect" a patient from suffering they may no longer understand, while still respecting their autonomy. Von Roenn (2013) addresses this issue within the context of deciding whether to continue or stop treatments, highlighting the tension between autonomy and beneficence (Von Roenn, 2013). Care teams must navigate this area carefully, listening to the patient's wishes while balancing medical and ethical imperatives.

Shared Decision-Making

Shared decision-making is another key concept in end-of-life care. This process involves active collaboration between the patient, their family, and the medical team to make decisions regarding treatment options. The goal is to ensure that the patient remains at the center of their care journey, even in the face of serious illness.

However, in complex contexts like those found in end-of-life care, shared decision-making can face several obstacles. For example, families may have expectations that differ from the patient's wishes, or doctors may find themselves in a position where they must guide discussions without imposing their own values (Azoulay et al., 2014). Diverging opinions between family members and healthcare professionals can lead to conflicts, particularly when dealing with sensitive decisions regarding the cessation of treatments.

A study by Feinberg (2014) shows that when decisions are shared and family members are involved in the process, there is greater satisfaction with care, even as end-of-life approaches (Feinberg, 2014). However, this requires open communication, active listening to the patient's and family's values and preferences, and careful management of potential disagreements.

Euthanasia and Assisted Suicide

One of the most controversial ethical debates in end-of-life care concerns euthanasia and assisted suicide. While euthanasia involves deliberately ending a patient's life to relieve suffering, assisted suicide allows the patient to make the decision to end their life with the help of a physician (Emanuel, 2000). These practices raise profound questions about respect for human dignity, the role of physicians, and the boundaries of medical intervention.

Laws regarding euthanasia and assisted suicide vary significantly from country to country. In some nations, these practices are legal, provided they meet strict criteria (e.g., Belgium, the Netherlands, and Canada). However, in many other countries, they remain illegal, often due to ethical and religious considerations. Rossi et al. (2010) explains that euthanasia raises questions about the role of caregivers in a patient's death, particularly the fear of "crossing a moral line" that could render the practice acceptable (Rossi, 2010). The ethical dilemmas surrounding these practices are even more complex when patients are unable to clearly communicate their wishes due to cognitive impairments or dementia.

Advocates of euthanasia and assisted suicide argue that these practices respect patient autonomy by providing an informed choice in the face of unbearable suffering. However, opponents contend that end-of-life care should prioritize respect for human dignity and that medicine should focus on alleviating suffering rather than determining the outcome of life itself (Quah et al., 2023). This debate continues to divide medical and ethical communities, and there is no clear consensus on how to address these issues in the context of palliative care.

Respecting Dignity and End-of-Life Choices

Respecting the dignity of patients at the end of life is at the heart of palliative care ethics. Dignity is a broad concept that encompasses respecting the patient's wishes, maintaining their autonomy to the extent possible, and ensuring they are treated with care and humanity throughout their care journey (Grignoli et al., 2018). According to Rossi et al. (2010), dignity in palliative care is not merely about avoiding pain but about providing emotional, psychological, and spiritual support while respecting the patient's values and beliefs (Rossi, 2010).

An essential aspect of respecting dignity is managing symptoms and adapting care to the patient's condition. This includes not only addressing pain but also considering the patient's wishes regarding the cessation or continuation of treatments, the decision to admit the patient to a hospital or continue home care, and the type of support the family wishes to receive.

INTERVENTIONS TO IMPROVE QOL IN END-OF-LIFE CARE

Improving QoL in end-of-life care relies on interventions that address symptom management, emotional and psychological support, and spiritual and social care. Palliative care must respond to varied needs by considering the physical, emotional, social, and spiritual dimensions of the patient. Interventions should be tailored to individual preferences, necessitating continuous evaluation of the patient's condition. Interdisciplinary care, combining medicine, psychology, nursing, and spirituality, plays a central role in enhancing the QoL.

Pharmacological Interventions: Symptom Management

Pharmacological interventions form the cornerstone of pain and symptom management in end-of-life care. Pain, in particular, is one of the most frequent and debilitating symptoms for patients nearing the end of life. Medications are often necessary to alleviate this suffering.

Pain Management: Opioids and Other Medications

Opioids, such as morphine and hydromorphone, are the most commonly used medications for pain management in palliative care. According to Leppert & Nosek (2019), these medications are effective for controlling moderate to severe pain but can cause side effects such as constipation, drowsiness, and respiratory depression, requiring careful dosage management (Leppert & Nosek, 2019).

Other medications, such as non-steroidal anti-inflammatory drugs (NSAIDs) and antidepressants or anticonvulsants, may also be used to treat neuropathic pain or as adjuncts in pain management. A study by Al-Ansari et al. (2021) shows that combining opioids with adjunct medications helps better control opioid-resistant pain (Al-Ansari et al., 2021).

Treatment of Non-Physical Symptoms

Beyond pain, many other symptoms can affect the QoL of patients in end-of-life care, such as dyspnea (difficulty breathing), nausea, fatigue, and sleep disturbances. Specific medications, such as bronchodilators for dyspnea and antiemetics for nausea, are used depending on the patient's symptoms (Cella, 1994). Managing fatigue and sleep disturbances in end-of-life care involves a mix of pharmacological and non-pharmacological treatments. Henderson et al. (2006) recommend using medications like benzodiazepines to improve sleep, while being mindful of potential side effects such as confusion and hypotension (Henderson et al., 2006).

Non-Pharmacological Interventions

Non-pharmacological interventions also play a vital role in enhancing patient comfort and QoL. These interventions aim to alleviate physical and emotional symptoms while reducing dependence on medications.

Nursing Care and Physical Activity

Nursing care is crucial in managing physical and emotional symptoms in palliative care. Comfort measures, such as patient positioning, skin care, and wound management, help reduce pain and improve overall comfort (Cowdell et al., 2014).

Light physical activities, tailored to the patient's disease stage, can also help reduce fatigue and improve mood. Research by Oldervoll et al. (2006) has shown that adapted physical exercises can improve QoL by reducing anxiety, depression, and fatigue in palliative care patients (Oldervoll et al., 2006).

Complementary Therapies: Relaxation and Acupuncture

Complementary therapies are often used alongside pharmacological treatments to enhance QoL in palliative care. Studies have shown that approaches such as meditation, relaxation, and acupuncture can help reduce pain, anxiety, and symptoms of post-traumatic stress disorder in terminally ill patients (Dingley et al., 2021). These non-invasive methods can provide additional relief to patients, particularly those who have contraindications to pharmacological treatments or prefer a more natural approach.

Spiritual and Psychosocial Care

Spiritual and psychosocial support is essential in providing a holistic approach to palliative care. As Amoah (2011) and Kang et al. (2023) highlight, the spiritual dimension is often overlooked in clinical practice, yet it plays a significant role in the experience of patients nearing the end of life (Amoah, 2011; Kang et al., 2023).

Spiritual Support

Spiritual care in palliative care aims to help patients find meaning and cope with existential issues related to the end of life. According to Koper et al. (2019), it is essential to consider the patient's religious or philosophical beliefs to offer respectful support (Koper et al., 2019). This includes practices such as prayer, religious rituals, or discussions about the meaning of life and death.

Spiritual care is generally provided by spiritual counselors or chaplains, but doctors, nurses, and other caregivers can also play a role in addressing the spiritual concerns of patients. Fawole et al. (2013) show that integrating spiritual care into clinical practice improves QoL at the end of life by providing patients with valuable moral and emotional support (Fawole et al., 2013).

Psychosocial Support: Psychotherapeutic Interventions

Psychological support is also critical in maintaining the emotional well-being of patients in end-of-life care. Psychotherapeutic interventions, such as CBT, are effective for treating anxiety, depression, and other emotional disorders associated with the end of life (Anderson et al., 2008). Additionally, support groups can provide patients with a space to share their experiences and support one another, helping to reduce feelings of isolation and enhance emotional well-being (McCABE et al., 2007).

Interdisciplinary Care and Care Coordination

One of the key characteristics of effective palliative care is the interdisciplinary approach. Palliative care teams consist of doctors, nurses, psychologists, social workers, spiritual counselors, and other healthcare professionals who work together to provide care tailored to the patient's needs. This approach allows for comprehensive and personalized care that addresses the physical, emotional, social, and spiritual dimensions of QoL (Bökberg et al., 2019)

Coordinating care between different professionals is essential to ensure continuity of care and consistent support throughout the palliative care journey. According to Fawole et al. (2013), effective communication among team members helps better understand the patient's needs, adjust interventions, and improve the end-of-life experience (Fawole et al., 2013).

The interventions aimed at improving QoL in end-of-life care are numerous and varied. A holistic and integrated approach, combining pharmacological and non-pharmacological treatments, as well as spiritual and psychosocial care, is essential to meet the complex needs of patients nearing the end of life. Addressing physical symptoms, emotional and spiritual support, and coordinating care through interdisciplinary teams are key to ensuring optimal comfort and dignity for elderly patients in end-of-life care.

FUTURE PERSPECTIVES AND RECOMMENDATIONS FOR IMPROVING QOL IN END-OF-LIFE CARE

The evolution of end-of-life and palliative care worldwide involves ongoing re-evaluation of existing practices to address the growing needs of aging populations and those suffering from chronic diseases. The field of palliative care continues to develop with the emergence of new technologies, therapeutic approaches, and a better understanding of the emotional, spiritual, and social needs of patients. Future perspectives and recommendations for improving QoL in end-of-life care should focus on integrating these innovations while improving access to care and training for healthcare professionals.

Innovations in QOL Assessment

One of the primary challenges in end-of-life care remains the precise and comprehensive assessment of QoL. While current assessment tools focus mainly on physical and emotional dimensions, there is a need to develop new instruments that include spiritual, social, and environmental aspects. Digital technologies and mobile applications offer exciting possibilities for real-time assessment of patients' QoL.

Digital Measurement Tools and Real-Time Self-Assessment

Recent innovations in mobile applications and wearable devices enable continuous monitoring of patients' QoL. These tools can be used to collect data on pain, mood, mobility, and other symptoms directly from the patients themselves. A study by Chan et al. (2025) demonstrated that the use of mobile applications in palliative care allows patients to provide valuable information about their condition, facilitating real-time decision-making by caregivers (Chan et al., 2025).

Remote monitoring systems, such as telemedicine platforms or wearable sensors, can also allow continuous observation of patients' vital signs and overall health, ensuring a prompt response to concerning symptoms. These innovations have the potential to enhance the responsiveness of care teams and ensure that patients receive appropriate care at every stage of their journey (van den Brink et al., 2007)

Psychosocial and Spiritual Measurements

It is also necessary to integrate assessment tools that measure the psychological and spiritual dimensions of QoL. The use of tailored questionnaires, such as the McGill QoL Questionnaire, which assesses psychological suffering, existential concerns, and social support, should be encouraged in clinical practices to ensure a comprehensive evaluation of the patient's condition in end-of-life care (Cohen et al., 1995).

Training Healthcare Professionals

Training healthcare professionals is another crucial area for improving QoL in end-of-life care. Many studies have found that healthcare providers' competency in palliative care and symptom management is often insufficient, which can negatively affect the quality of care (Bökberg et al., 2019; Tark et al., 2020). It is imperative that medical schools, nursing schools, and other training institutions include specific courses on palliative care, pain management, and emotional support.

Interdisciplinary Training and Collaborative Practice

The interdisciplinary model in palliative care, involving doctors, nurses, psychologists, social workers, and spiritual counselors, must be promoted. Collaboration between these professionals is essential to ensure comprehensive patient care. A study by Wang & Ding (2025) shows that interdisciplinary teams enhance the effectiveness of palliative care and promote better QoL for patients (Wang & Ding, 2025).

Continuing education programs for healthcare providers should include modules on the use of digital technologies, spiritual and psychological support approaches, and new practices in palliative care. These programs will help professionals adapt to patients' evolving needs and respond more effectively to the challenges of end-of-life care.

Accessibility and Coverage of Palliative Care

Access to palliative care remains a significant challenge. In many regions, particularly in developing countries or rural areas, access to palliative care remains limited. Salikhanov et al. (2023) highlighted that the lack of infrastructure and qualified personnel in these areas contributes to inadequate end-of-life care (Salikhanov et al., 2023).

Increasing Access to Home-Based Palliative Care

Home-based palliative care represents an effective alternative to hospital care for elderly patients who wish to remain at home at the end of life. A study by Gomes et al. (2016) demonstrated that home-based palliative care provides a more comfortable and personalized environment while reducing the costs associated with hospital care (Gomes et al., 2016). Public policies are needed to support the integration of these services into the community, providing sufficient resources to train home-care staff and ensuring access to necessary medications.

Public Health Policies and Universal Coverage

Public health policies must focus on expanding access to palliative care worldwide. The WHO (2014) recommends integrating palliative care into primary healthcare systems and implementing educational programs for patients and families on symptom management and end-of-life support. Moreover, policies that ensure equitable access to medications, such as opioids, must be established to guarantee that all patients, regardless of location, can receive adequate pain relief (WHO, 2014).

Technological Innovation and Care Improvement

Technological innovations are playing an increasingly important role in improving palliative care. The use of telemedicine for remote consultations, home monitoring of vital symptoms through wearable devices (Gordon et al., 2022), and the application of artificial intelligence (AI) to predict patients at high risk of short-term mortality and plan end-of-life care (Xie & Butcher, 2023) offer promising prospects for enhancing care quality.

Technologies can also be used to improve communication between patients, their families, and caregivers. Online support platforms and mobile applications can help patients and their loved ones better understand care options and actively participate in decisions. Additionally, virtual reality (VR) has recently shown its potential in treating pain and anxiety by offering patients means of escapism and relaxation, thus helping to reduce emotional stress (Gaina et al., 2024).

End-of-life care for elderly individuals is at the heart of an evolving field. Technological innovations, improving healthcare professionals' training, and expanding access to palliative care are major pathways to ensuring better QoL for patients at the end of life. It is essential to continue adapting practices to meet the diverse needs of patients and their families while accounting for demographic changes and scientific advances. However, ethical challenges like data privacy and algorithmic bias in diverse elderly populations must be addressed to ensure equitable access, positioning AI as a tool for proactive, personalized end-of-life planning (Obermeyer et al., 2019; Topol, 2019).

CONCLUSION

QoL in end-of-life care is a complex and multidimensional concept that encompasses physical, emotional, social, and spiritual aspects of patients' end-of-life experiences. As the global population ages, the demand for quality palliative and terminal care continues to rise. In light of these challenges, it is necessary to understand the different factors that influence patients' QoL in end-of-life care and adopt practices based on a holistic approach to care.

Integrating palliative care into healthcare systems, providing continuing education for healthcare professionals, and expanding access to palliative care are essential priorities for ensuring quality care. Technological innovations, such as telemedicine, mobile applications for self-assessment of symptoms, and the use of virtual reality, offer new avenues for improving end-of-life care quality. These innovations, combined with interdisciplinary practices and better care coordination, can transform the end-of-life experience by enabling more individualized and responsive care.

Recommendations for improving QoL in end-of-life care include the implementation of public health policies that support universal access to palliative care, the training of interdisciplinary teams, and the integration of spiritual and psychological care into care pathways. Furthermore, promoting a patient-centered approach, where patients' values and preferences are respected throughout their care journey, is essential.

Finally, it is imperative to continue researching QoL in end-of-life care to better understand the needs of patients and families and to refine assessment tools that more comprehensively and accurately measure the impact of palliative care. By evolving care practices and addressing the ethical and practical challenges that arise, we can significantly improve the QoL for patients at the end of their lives and offer them a dignified end, respecting their desires and needs.

REFERENCES

Aaronson, N. K., Ahmedzai, S., Bergman, B., Bullinger, M., Cull, A., Duez, N. J., Filiberti, A., Flechtner, H., Fleishman, S. B., Haes, J. C. J. M. D., Kaasa, S., Klee, M., Osoba, D., Razavi, D., Rofe, P. B., Schraub, S., Sneeuw, K., Sullivan, M., & Takeda, F. (1993). The European Organization for Research and Treatment of Cancer QLQ-C30 : A Quality-of-Life Instrument for Use in International Clinical Trials in Oncology. *Journal of the National Cancer Institute*, *85*(5), 365–376. DOI: 10.1093/jnci/85.5.365 PMID: 8433390

Adelman, R. D., Tmanova, L. L., Delgado, D., Dion, S., & Lachs, M. S. (2014). Caregiver Burden : A Clinical Review. *Journal of the American Medical Association*, *311*(10), 1052. DOI: 10.1001/jama.2014.304 PMID: 24618967

Al-Ansari, A. M., Abd-El-Gawad, W. M., AboSerea, S. M., ElShereafy, E. E. S., Ali, F. A. S., & ElSayed, M. A. E. (2021). The pattern of change in opioid and adjuvant prescriptions for cancer pain before and after referral to a comprehensive program in the Palliative Care Center in Kuwait. *BMC Palliative Care*, *20*(1), 25. DOI: 10.1186/s12904-021-00717-2 PMID: 33536013

Amoah, C. F. (2011). The central importance of spirituality in palliative care. *International Journal of Palliative Nursing*, *17*(7), 353–358. DOI: 10.12968/ijpn.2011.17.7.353 PMID: 21841704

Anderson, T., Watson, M., & Davidson, R. (2008). The use of cognitive behavioural therapy techniques for anxiety and depression in hospice patients : A feasibility study. *Palliative Medicine*, *22*(7), 814–821. DOI: 10.1177/0269216308095157 PMID: 18755828

Azoulay, E., Chaize, M., & Kentish-Barnes, N. (2014). Involvement of ICU families in decisions : Fine-tuning the partnership. *Annals of Intensive Care*, *4*(1), 37. DOI: 10.1186/s13613-014-0037-5 PMID: 25593753

Bae, S., & Kim, D. (2024). Improving home-like environments in long-term care units : An exploratory mixed-method study. *Scientific Reports*, *14*(1), 13243. DOI: 10.1038/s41598-024-62328-0 PMID: 38853152

Bakitas, M. A., Dionne-Odom, J. N., Ejem, D. B., Wells, R., Azuero, A., Stockdill, M. L., Keebler, K., Sockwell, E., Tims, S., Engler, S., Steinhauser, K., Kvale, E., Durant, R. W., Tucker, R. O., Burgio, K. L., Tallaj, J., Swetz, K. M., & Pamboukian, S. V. (2020). Effect of an Early Palliative Care Telehealth Intervention vs Usual Care on Patients With Heart Failure : The ENABLE CHF-PC Randomized Clinical Trial. *JAMA Internal Medicine, 180*(9), 1203–1213. DOI: 10.1001/jamainternmed.2020.2861 PMID: 32730613

Bökberg, C., Behm, L., & Ahlström, G. (2019). Quality of life of older persons in nursing homes after the implementation of a knowledge-based palliative care intervention. *International Journal of Older People Nursing, 14*(4), e12258. DOI: 10.1111/opn.12258 PMID: 31298499

Bradley, N., Dowrick, C., & Lloyd-Williams, M. (2022). Feasibility of Patient Reported Outcome Measures in Psychosocial Palliative Care : Observational Cohort Study of Hospice Day Care and Social Support Groups. *International Journal of Environmental Research and Public Health, 19*(20), 13258. DOI: 10.3390/ijerph192013258 PMID: 36293835

Breitbart, W., Gibson, C., Poppito, S. R., & Berg, A. (2004). Psychotherapeutic Interventions at the End of Life : A Focus on Meaning and Spirituality. *Canadian Journal of Psychiatry, 49*(6), 366–372. DOI: 10.1177/070674370404900605 PMID: 15283531

Burks, H. B., Des Bordes, J. K. A., Chadha, R., Holmes, H. M., & Rianon, N. J. (2021). Quality of Life Assessment in Older Adults with Dementia : A Systematic Review. *Dementia and Geriatric Cognitive Disorders, 50*(2), 103–110. DOI: 10.1159/000515317 PMID: 34167127

Cain, C. L., Surbone, A., Elk, R., & Kagawa-Singer, M. (2018). Culture and Palliative Care : Preferences, Communication, Meaning, and Mutual Decision Making. *Journal of Pain and Symptom Management, 55*(5), 1408–1419. DOI: 10.1016/j.jpainsymman.2018.01.007 PMID: 29366913

Caliskan, H., Sengul Aycicek, G., Ozsurekci, C., Dogrul, R. T., Balci, C., Sumer, F., Ozcan, M., Karabulut, E., Halil, M., Cankurtaran, M., & Yavuz, B. B. (2019). Turkish validation of a new scale from older people's perspectives : Older people's quality of life-brief (OPQOL-brief). *Archives of Gerontology and Geriatrics, 83*, 91–95. DOI: 10.1016/j.archger.2019.04.002 PMID: 30991155

Candy, B., Jones, L., Larkin, P. J., Vickerstaff, V., Tookman, A., & Stone, P. (2015). Laxatives for the management of constipation in people receiving palliative care. *Cochrane Database of Systematic Reviews, 2020*(1). Advance online publication. DOI: 10.1002/14651858.CD003448.pub4 PMID: 25967924

Cella, D. F. (1994). Quality of life : Concepts and definition. *Journal of Pain and Symptom Management, 9*(3), 186–192. DOI: 10.1016/0885-3924(94)90129-5 PMID: 8014530

Chan, W.-L., Tai, Y.-L., Siu, W.-K. S., Hou, H. L.-Y., Yuen, K.-K., & Lee, V. H.-F. (2025). Use of mobile app "SUPPORT+" to enhance community palliative care in patients with advanced cancer : A prospective study. *Palliative Care and Social Practice, 19*, 26323524251351036. DOI: 10.1177/26323524251351036 PMID: 40606554

Clegg, A., Young, J., Iliffe, S., Rikkert, M. O., & Rockwood, K. (2013). Frailty in elderly people. *Lancet, 381*(9868), 752–762. DOI: 10.1016/S0140-6736(12)62167-9 PMID: 23395245

Cohen, S. R., Mount, B. M., Strobel, M. G., & Bui, F. (1995). The McGill Quality of Life Questionnaire : A measure of quality of life appropriate for people with advanced disease. A preliminary study of validity and acceptability. *Palliative Medicine, 9*(3), 207–219. DOI: 10.1177/026921639500900306 PMID: 7582177

Corli, O., Santucci, C., Corsi, N., Radrezza, S., Galli, F., & Bosetti, C. (2019). The Burden of Opioid Adverse Events and the Influence on Cancer Patients' Symptomatology. *Journal of Pain and Symptom Management, 57*(5), 899–908.e6. DOI: 10.1016/j.jpainsymman.2019.02.009 PMID: 30776537

Cowdell, F., Jadotte, Y. T., Ersser, S. J., Danby, S., Walton, S., Lawton, S., Roberts, A., Gardiner, E., Ware, F., & Cork, M. (2014). Hygiene and emollient interventions for maintaining skin integrity in older people in hospital and residential care settings. *Cochrane Database of Systematic Reviews*. Advance online publication. DOI: 10.1002/14651858.CD011377 PMID: 32006460

Crawley, L. M., Marshall, P. A., Lo, B., & Koenig, B. A., & for the End-of-Life Care Consensus Panel. (2002). Strategies for Culturally Effective End-of-Life Care. *Annals of Internal Medicine, 136*(9), 673–679. DOI: 10.7326/0003-4819-136-9-200205070-00010 PMID: 11992303

Dingley, C., Ruckdeschel, A., Kotula, K., & Lekhak, N. (2021). Implementation and outcomes of complementary therapies in hospice care : An integrative review. *Palliative Care and Social Practice, 15*, 26323524211051753. DOI: 10.1177/26323524211051753 PMID: 34723183

Emanuel, E. J. (2000). Attitudes and Desires Related to Euthanasia and Physician-Assisted Suicide Among Terminally Ill Patients and Their Caregivers. *Journal of the American Medical Association, 284*(19), 2460. DOI: 10.1001/jama.284.19.2460 PMID: 11074775

Engel, G. L. (1977). The Need for a New Medical Model : A Challenge for Biomedicine. *Science, 196*(4286), 129–136. DOI: 10.1126/science.847460 PMID: 847460

Fang, M. L., Sixsmith, J., Sinclair, S., & Horst, G. (2016). A knowledge synthesis of culturally- and spiritually-sensitive end-of-life care : Findings from a scoping review. *BMC Geriatrics, 16*, 107. DOI: 10.1186/s12877-016-0282-6 PMID: 27193395

Fawole, O. A., Dy, S. M., Wilson, R. F., Lau, B. D., Martinez, K. A., Apostol, C. C., Vollenweider, D., Bass, E. B., & Aslakson, R. A. (2013). A Systematic Review of Communication Quality Improvement Interventions for Patients with Advanced and Serious Illness. *Journal of General Internal Medicine, 28*(4), 570–577. DOI: 10.1007/s11606-012-2204-4 PMID: 23099799

Fayers, P., & Bottomley, A. (2002). Quality of life research within the EORTC—The EORTC QLQ-C30. *European Journal of Cancer, 38*, 125–133. DOI: 10.1016/S0959-8049(01)00448-8 PMID: 11858978

Feinberg, L. F. (2014). Moving Toward Person- and Family-Centered Care. *The Public Policy and Aging Report, 24*(3), 97–101. DOI: 10.1093/ppar/pru027

Ferrans, C. E. (1990). Development of a quality of life index for patients with cancer. *Oncology Nursing Forum, 17*(3, Suppl), 15–19. PMID: 2342979

Ferrans, C. E. (1996). Development of a conceptual model of quality of life. *Scholarly Inquiry for Nursing Practice, 10*(3), 293–304. PMID: 9009823

Ferrans, C. E., & Powers, M. J. (1985). Quality of life index : Development and psychometric properties. *Advances in Nursing Science, 8*(1), 15–24. DOI: 10.1097/00012272-198510000-00005 PMID: 3933411

Fowlie, M., & Berkeley, J. (1987). Quality of Life—A Review of the Literature. *Family Practice, 4*(3), 226–234. DOI: 10.1093/fampra/4.3.226 PMID: 3311862

Gaina, A.-M., Stefanescu, C., Szalontay, A.-S., Gaina, M.-A., Poroch, V., Mosoiu, D. V., Stefanescu, B.-V., Axinte, M., Tofan, C.-M., & Magurianu, L. A. (2024). A Systematic Review of Virtual Reality's Impact on Anxiety During Palliative Care. *Healthcare (Basel, Switzerland), 12*(24), 2517. DOI: 10.3390/healthcare12242517 PMID: 39765944

Gijsberts, M.-J. H. E., Liefbroer, A. I., Otten, R., & Olsman, E. (2019). Spiritual Care in Palliative Care : A Systematic Review of the Recent European Literature. *Medical Sciences (Basel, Switzerland)*, *7*(2), 25. DOI: 10.3390/medsci7020025 PMID: 30736416

Gomes, B., Calanzani, N., Curiale, V., McCrone, P. P., Higginson, I. J., & Brito, M. D. (2016). Effectiveness and cost-effectiveness of home palliative care services for adults with advanced illness and their caregivers. *São Paulo Medical Journal = Revista Paulista de Medicina*, *134*(1), 93–94. DOI: 10.1590/1516-3180.20161341T2 PMID: 26786605

Gordon, B., Mason, B., & Smith, S. L. H. (2022). Leveraging Telehealth for Delivery of Palliative Care to Remote Communities : A Rapid Review. *Journal of Palliative Care*, *37*(2), 213–225. DOI: 10.1177/08258597211001184 PMID: 33730904

Green, E. P., Lai, Y., Pearson, N., Rajasekharan, S., Rauws, M., Joerin, A., Kwobah, E., Musyimi, C., Jones, R. M., Bhat, C., Mulinge, A., & Puffer, E. S. (2020). Expanding Access to Perinatal Depression Treatment in Kenya Through Automated Psychological Support : Development and Usability Study. *JMIR Formative Research*, *4*(10), e17895. DOI: 10.2196/17895 PMID: 33016883

Grignoli, N., Di Bernardo, V., & Malacrida, R. (2018). New perspectives on substituted relational autonomy for shared decision-making in critical care. *Critical Care*, *22*(1), 260. DOI: 10.1186/s13054-018-2187-6 PMID: 30309384

Hampton, M., Baydala, A., Bourassa, C., McKenna, B., & Saul, G., MckKay-McNabb, K., Goodwill, K., Clark, V., & Christiansen, J. (2011). Seven Years of Completing the Circle. *End-of-Life Care With Aboriginal Families.*, *43*(3), 119–125.

Hanna, J. R., McConnell, T., Harrison, C., Patynowska, K. A., Finucane, A. M., Hudson, B., Paradine, S., McCullagh, A., & Reid, J. (2022). 'There's something about admitting that you are lonely' – prevalence, impact and solutions to loneliness in terminal illness : An explanatory sequential multi-methods study. *Palliative Medicine*, *36*(10), 1483–1492. DOI: 10.1177/02692163221122269 PMID: 36081273

Hedman, C., Fürst, P., Strang, P., Schelin, M. E. C., Lundström, S., & Martinsson, L. (2024). Pain prevalence and pain relief in end-of-life care – a national registry study. *BMC Palliative Care*, *23*(1), 171. DOI: 10.1186/s12904-024-01497-1 PMID: 39004730

Henderson, M., MacGregor, E., Sykes, N., & Hotopf, M. (2006). The use of benzodiazepines in palliative care. *Palliative Medicine*, *20*(4), 407–412. DOI: 10.1191/0269216306pm1151oa PMID: 16875110

House, S. A., Schoo, C., & Ogilvie, W. A. (2025). Advance Directives. In *StatPearls* [Internet]. StatPearls Publishing., https://www.ncbi.nlm.nih.gov/books/NBK459133/

Kang, K.-A., Kim, D.-B., Koh, S.-J., Park, M.-H., Park, H. Y., Yoon, D. H., Yoon, S.-J., Lee, S.-J., Choi, J.-E., Han, H.-S., & Chun, J. (2023). Spiritual Care Guide in Hospice Palliative Care. *Journal of Hospice and Palliative Care*, *26*(4), 149–159. DOI: 10.14475/jhpc.2023.26.4.149 PMID: 38075589

Khaldouni, S., Amane, M., Lamtali, S., Boussaa, S., El Rhanbouri, M., Oussous, A., & Laghouasli, F. (2025). Implementation of Advanced Nursing Practices Through the Adoption of a Patient-Centered Approach. In Amane, M., & Boussaa, S. (Eds.), *Advanced Nursing Practices for Clinical Excellence* (pp. 305–348). IGI Global., DOI: 10.4018/979-8-3693-6730-8.ch014

Kim, Y., & Kim, D.-H. (2024). Interventions for family involvement enhance end-of-life care for hospitalized patients : An integrative review. *BMC Nursing*, *23*(1), 917. DOI: 10.1186/s12912-024-02538-z PMID: 39695593

Koper, I., Pasman, H. R. W., Schweitzer, B. P. M., Kuin, A., & Onwuteaka-Philipsen, B. D. (2019). Spiritual care at the end of life in the primary care setting : Experiences from spiritual caregivers - a mixed methods study. *BMC Palliative Care*, *18*(1), 98. DOI: 10.1186/s12904-019-0484-8 PMID: 31706355

Kwak, J., & Salmon, J. (2007). Attitudes and preferences of Korean-American older adults and caregivers on end-of-life care. *Journal of the American Geriatrics Society*, *55*(11). Advance online publication. DOI: 10.1111/j.1532-5415.2007.01394.x PMID: 17727642

Leppert, W., & Nosek, K. (2019). Comparison of the Quality of Life of Cancer Patients with Pain Treated with Oral Controlled-Release Morphine and Oxycodone and Transdermal Buprenorphine and Fentanyl. *Current Pharmaceutical Design*, *25*(30), 3216–3224. DOI: 10.2174/1381612825666190717091230 PMID: 31333114

McCABE, C., Begley, C., Collier, S., & McCANN, S. (2007). Methodological issues related to assessing and measuring quality of life in patients with cancer : Implications for patient care. *European Journal of Cancer Care*, *0*(0), 070611034311001-??? DOI: 10.1111/j.1365-2354.2007.00809.x

Mercier, C., & Filion, J. (2006). La qualité de la vie : Perspectives théoriques et empiriques. *Sante Mentale au Quebec*, *12*(1), 135–143. DOI: 10.7202/030380ar PMID: 16946975

Miranda, R., Bunn, F., Lynch, J., Van Den Block, L., & Goodman, C. (2019). Palliative care for people with dementia living at home : A systematic review of interventions. *Palliative Medicine, 33*(7), 726–742. DOI: 10.1177/0269216319847092 PMID: 31057088

Montori, V. M., Ruissen, M. M., Hargraves, I. G., Brito, J. P., & Kunneman, M. (2023). Shared decision-making as a method of care. *BMJ Evidence-Based Medicine, 28*(4), 213–217. DOI: 10.1136/bmjebm-2022-112068 PMID: 36460328

Obermeyer, Z., Powers, B., Vogeli, C., & Mullainathan, S. (2019). Dissecting racial bias in an algorithm used to manage the health of populations. *Science, 366*(6464), 447–453. DOI: 10.1126/science.aax2342 PMID: 31649194

OECD. (2023). *Time for Better Care at the End of Life*. OECD., DOI: 10.1787/722b927a-

Oldervoll, L. M., Loge, J. H., Paltiel, H., Asp, M. B., Vidvei, U., Wiken, A. N., Hjermstad, M. J., & Kaasa, S. (2006). The Effect of a Physical Exercise Program in Palliative Care : A Phase II Study. *Journal of Pain and Symptom Management, 31*(5), 421–430. DOI: 10.1016/j.jpainsymman.2005.10.004 PMID: 16716872

Perreault, L. (2018). Les directives anticipées des personnes atteintes d'une démence de type Alzheimer : Comment faire pour bien faire? *BioéthiqueOnline, 5*. Advance online publication. DOI: 10.7202/1044261ar

Quah, E. L. Y., Chua, K. Z. Y., Lua, J. K., Wan, D. W. J., Chong, C. S., Lim, Y. X., & Krishna, L. (2023). A Systematic Review of Stakeholder Perspectives of Dignity and Assisted Dying. *Journal of Pain and Symptom Management, 65*(2), e123–e136. DOI: 10.1016/j.jpainsymman.2022.10.004 PMID: 36244639

Rossi, I. (2010). Culture palliative : Pour anticiper et accueillir la mort. *Revue internationale de soins palliatifs, 25*(1), 37-43. DOI: 10.3917/inka.101.0037

Salikhanov, I., Katapodi, M. C., Kunirova, G., & Crape, B. L. (2023). Improving palliative care outcomes in remote and rural areas of LMICs through family caregivers : Lessons from Kazakhstan. *Frontiers in Public Health, 11*, 1186107. DOI: 10.3389/fpubh.2023.1186107 PMID: 37601198

Sampson, E. L., Candy, B., Davis, S., Gola, A. B., Harrington, J., King, M., Kupeli, N., Leavey, G., Moore, K., Nazareth, I., Omar, R. Z., Vickerstaff, V., & Jones, L. (2018). Living and dying with advanced dementia : A prospective cohort study of symptoms, service use and care at the end of life. *Palliative Medicine, 32*(3), 668–681. DOI: 10.1177/0269216317726443 PMID: 28922625

Schulz, R., & Czaja, S. J. (2018). Family Caregiving : A Vision for the Future. *The American Journal of Geriatric Psychiatry: Official Journal of the American Association for Geriatric Psychiatry, 26*(3), 358–363. DOI: 10.1016/j.jagp.2017.06.023 PMID: 28774786

Schulz, R., Eden, J., & Adults, C. on F. C. for O., Services, B. on H. C., Division, H. and M., & National Academies of Sciences, E. (2016). Family Caregiving Roles and Impacts. In *Families Caring for an Aging America*. National Academies Press (US). https://www.ncbi.nlm.nih.gov/books/NBK396398/

Sepúlveda, C., Marlin, A., Yoshida, T., & Ullrich, A. (2002). Palliative Care. *Journal of Pain and Symptom Management, 24*(2), 91–96. DOI: 10.1016/S0885-3924(02)00440-2 PMID: 12231124

Skevington, S. M., Lotfy, M., & O'Connell, K. A.WHOQOL Group. (2004). The World Health Organization's WHOQOL-BREF quality of life assessment : Psychometric properties and results of the international field trial. A report from the WHOQOL group. *Quality of Life Research: An International Journal of Quality of Life Aspects of Treatment, Care and Rehabilitation, 13*(2), 299–310. DOI: 10.1023/B:QURE.0000018486.91360.00 PMID: 15085902

Svendsen, S. J., Grov, E. K., & Staats, K. (2024). Patients' experiences with shared decision-making in home-based palliative care – navigation through major life decisions. *BMC Palliative Care, 23*(1), 101. DOI: 10.1186/s12904-024-01434-2 PMID: 38627710

Tark, A., Estrada, L. V., Tresgallo, M. E., Quigley, D. D., Stone, P. W., & Agarwal, M. (2020). Palliative care and infection management at end of life in nursing homes : A descriptive survey. *Palliative Medicine, 34*(5), 580–588. DOI: 10.1177/0269216320902672 PMID: 32153248

Topol, E. J. (2019). High-performance medicine : The convergence of human and artificial intelligence. *Nature Medicine, 25*(1), 44–56. DOI: 10.1038/s41591-018-0300-7 PMID: 30617339

Turner, G., & Clegg, A. (2014). Best practice guidelines for the management of frailty : A British Geriatrics Society, Age UK and Royal College of General Practitioners report. *Age and Ageing, 43*(6), 744–747. DOI: 10.1093/ageing/afu138 PMID: 25336440

Umar, Z., Tahir, Z., & Nizami, A. (2023). Impact of severe mental illnesses on health-related quality of life among patients attending the Institute of Psychiatry, Rawalpindi from 2019 to 2021 : A cross-sectional study. *PLoS One, 18*(8), e0289080. DOI: 10.1371/journal.pone.0289080 PMID: 37535604

United Nations. (2019). *World Population Prospects, The 2019 Revision - Volume I : Comprehensive Tables*. UN. DOI: 10.18356/15994a82-en

van den Brink, J. L., Moorman, P. W., de Boer, M. F., Hop, W. C. J., Pruyn, J. F. A., Verwoerd, C. D. A., & van Bemmel, J. H. (2007). Impact on quality of life of a telemedicine system supporting head and neck cancer patients : A controlled trial during the postoperative period at home. *Journal of the American Medical Informatics Association : JAMIA*, *14*(2), 198–205. DOI: 10.1197/jamia.M2199 PMID: 17213498

Van Hecke, N., Claes, C., Vanderplasschen, W., De Maeyer, J., De Witte, N., & Vandevelde, S. (2018). Conceptualisation and Measurement of Quality of Life Based on Schalock and Verdugo's Model : A Cross-Disciplinary Review of the Literature. *Social Indicators Research*, *137*(1), 335–351. DOI: 10.1007/s11205-017-1596-2

Von Roenn, J. H. (2013). Advance Care Planning : Ensuring That the Patient's Voice Is Heard. *Journal of Clinical Oncology*, *31*(6), 663–664. DOI: 10.1200/JCO.2012.46.8181 PMID: 23284035

Wang, M., & Ding, X. (2025). Integrated palliative care improves the quality of life of advanced cancer patients. *BMC Palliative Care*, *24*(1), 162. DOI: 10.1186/s12904-025-01800-8 PMID: 40483417

WHO. (1993). Study protocol for the World Health Organization project to develop a Quality of Life assessment instrument (WHOQOL). *Quality of Life Research: An International Journal of Quality of Life Aspects of Treatment, Care and Rehabilitation*, *2*(2), 153–159. PMID: 8518769

WHO. (1997). *WHOQOL Measuring Quality of Life*. World Health Organization. https://iris.who.int/handle/10665/63482

WHO. (2014). *Renforcement des soins palliatifs en tant qu'élément du traitement intégré à toutes les étapes de la vie.*

Wilson, I. B., & Cleary, P. D. (1995). Linking clinical variables with health-related quality of life. A conceptual model of patient outcomes. *Journal of the American Medical Association*, *273*(1), 59–65. PMID: 7996652

Xie, W., & Butcher, R. (2023). *Artificial Intelligence Decision Support Tools for End-of-Life Care Planning Conversations : CADTH Horizon Scan*. Canadian Agency for Drugs and Technologies in Health. https://www.ncbi.nlm.nih.gov/books/NBK599854/

Zhao, X., Tong, S., & Yang, Y. (2022). The Correlation Between Quality of Life and Positive Psychological Resources in Cancer Patients : A Meta-Analysis. *Frontiers in Psychology*, *13*, 883157. DOI: 10.3389/fpsyg.2022.883157 PMID: 35783766

Chapter 3
Symptom Burden in Elder Palliative Care for Non-Palliative Specialists

Adil Hamad Alharthi
https://orcid.org/0000-0001-6124-5907
King Fahad Armed Forces Hospital, Saudi Arabia

ABSTRACT

What makes a sensation turn into a symptom? You might guess duration, severity, or temporal relation to the disease, would make the patient decide to share it with his healthcare provider or his family and turn it into a symptom and you're right, but this is only part of the symptom story as symptoms are not only diverse, but multi-dimensional as well. Because each one of us is unique, we experience, understand, express and suffer from symptoms differently. In a sense this is about our uniqueness and how it is significantly reflected on our older age and our terminal illness.

INTRODUCTION

Proper symptom assessment is the hallmark of medicine because it results in the correct diagnosis and proper management (Kalantar-Zadeh et al., 2022). In the same way it is the essence of palliative care because if done appropriately, it will result in the reduction of patient suffering and the successful quality of life (Aghaei et al., 2021).

Due to the growing number of older people in the community, the non-malignant elderly needing palliative care population is outgrowing palliative specialists' availability and palliative centers' accessibility (Llop Medina, 2024). Therefore, the best practical way to ensure the delivery of high-quality care to those patients is by

DOI: 10.4018/979-8-3373-4099-9.ch003

equipping non-palliative specialist healthcare providers in primary and secondary care with palliative care skills, knowledge, and capabilities (Yao et al., 2025).

This chapter will discuss the concept of symptom burden and its specific and interesting relation with Multimorbidity and palliative care in the elderly population, aiming to upgrade the awareness and knowledge of healthcare providers who are managing those terminally ill patients. Then we will discuss some details about pain in palliative Care. Details needed for the non-palliative specialist.

SYMPTOM BURDEN

Symptom burden is the overall impact of physical and emotional symptoms experienced by a patient characterized by the prevalence (how many), frequency (how often) and severity (how bad), which can negatively affect daily life, progress and quality of life (Gapstur, 2007).

At its beginning, palliative care primarily started for cancer patients only, it was Paramount to assess and measure the improvement of patient suffering (Strang, 2022). Specifically, of this vulnerable and delicate group. Quality care is interested in assessing the above improvement using measurable quality standards to properly assess and compare each improvement and to properly investigate such improvements on a global scale using evidence-based medicine.

Patient reported outcomes PROs are used to study Symptom burden. Many tools used to asses PROs, the most common and accurate are the Edmonton symptom assessment system ESAS and the memorial symptom assessment scale MSAS (Donlan, 2024).

In the following chapter, we will review different studies investigating important concepts of symptom burden and pain control in palliative care, later we will discuss the important concepts that we learned in the field of symptom burden and pain control in palliative care, in order to improve our knowledge, understanding and behavior towards appropriately managing palliative care patients.

MULTIMORBIDITY

Multimorbidity is the presence of two or more chronic diseases in the same individual (Skou et al., 2022). In the elderly population this concept became the norm rather than the exception. Multiple retrospective and cross-sectional studies around the world found that the prevalence of multimorbidity in the elder population is high and the older the patients are the higher the multimorbidity figure they suffer from (Zhao et al., 2023).

This concept is very important because healthcare providers primary basic training depends on the single disease theory. On the other hand, the multimorbidity theory is deferent and it depends more on early prognostic risk identification, polypharmacy identification, disease to disease and disease to drug interaction rather than on differential diagnosis capabilities alone (Skou et al., 2022).

Multimorbidity Challenges

The known definition of multimorbidity is heterogeneous. It's not clear whether organ failure or physical limitation should be included in the multimorbidity definition or only chronic diseases (Roubaud-Baudron & Guerville, 2022). This makes the definition heterogeneous, and that is a limitation and challenge to studying it and will cause different populations to end up with different study outcomes.

An interesting umbrella review study went through an electronic search to assess studies about symptom management in multimorbidity and had important findings (Cheng & Christensen, 2024). It found that multimorbidity definition is heterogeneous, and that was the major challenge in collecting symptom management outcomes. It also found that the lack of standardization in measurement and reporting of symptoms related to multimorbidity is another major challenge, but they did conclude that in spite of the multiple barriers and challenges, it's confirmed that quality of life, low physical function and mood are predominant outcomes which are negatively affected by multimorbidity (Cheng & Christensen, 2024).

In conclusion a universal standard definition that is clear, measurable and non-heterogeneous is needed to standardize multimorbidity studies in order to compare different studies and come out with systemic reviews to understand it better on a larger scale.

Multimorbidity and Symptom Burden

Compared to malignancy, non-malignant terminally ill patient symptom burden is understudied, generally due to difficulties to identify time to initiate palliative care need (Booker, 2024). Some studies investigated the relationship between multimorbidity and symptom burden in the elderly and found interesting results. A Danish study tried to answer the question does multimorbidity have an additive effect, meaning do more diseases in Multimorbidity cause more symptoms? By using a questionnaire on more than 47,000 participants they found that multimorbidity has an additive effect. The more diseases in multimorbidity the more symptoms the patient may have (Willadsen et al., 2021).

The National health and aging trend study NHATS was a US prospective cohort study in which more than 7000 participants aged 65 or older living in community or residential care were interviewed. This large study found that the prevalence of 0, 1, 2, 3 and four or more symptoms in the population were 25%, 27%, 21%, 14% and 13.5% respectively, pain and fatigue were the most distressing symptoms. They also found that high symptom counts were associated with reduced physical activity. Patient with 1, 2, 3 and four or more symptoms had a gate speed of 0.04, 0.06, 0.09 and 0.13 m/s slower, respectively (Patel et al., 2018).

The same US study mentioned above examined symptom burden for older people with and without dementia. By interviewing more than 1000 patients above 65 years old in a cross-sectional study, the mean age was 80.6 years. They found out that the most reported symptoms in dementia patients were low energy 68%, pain 59%, limited movement 56%, poor coordination 55%. They also found that dementia and probable dementia were associated with significant greater likelihood of high burden of physical and psychiatric symptoms. They came with a conclusion that greater social engagement is associated with better mental outcome, and also older adults with dementia are at risk of high symptom burden and limited social participation (Amjad et al., 2019).

A Swedish cross-sectional study that interviewed more than 370 community dwelling elders by using the memorial symptom assessment scale MSAS, this scale emphasizes the presence, severity and distress associated with terminally ill patients. They found that in their population, there was a mean of 8 symptoms per person. They also found that seven out of 10 complained of pain, which had the highest severity and was the most associated with distress. They also found that symptom burden and severity were associated with the likelihood of depression and poor vision as well (Eckerblad et al., 2015).

Another Australian study was also studying Symptom burden influencers in multimorbidity, but this time in a rural low-income population. They found that functional impairment and mental health conditions are the greatest influencers of capacity and symptom burden severity. They also found that there is an important interactive role of function and psychological factors in multimorbidity patients (Hardman et al., 2021).

An interesting Swedish descriptive study that was investigating symptom management strategies of older patient with multimorbidity, they found that they could have active strategies which are the ones that they choose to implement to control symptoms and passive strategies which are the ones they are unable to avoid. The active strategies are more effective in symptom management and related to better mental health and well-being than the passive strategies which should be discovered, treated and avoided (Eckerblad et al., 2020).

A retrospective cohort Pakistani study reviewed the health records of 600 elder patients, and found that most patients had moderate to severe multimorbidity. They also had severe levels of polypharmacy (using five or more medications) they also found that most were in moderate nutritional range and a large percentage were at risk of malnutrition. The study concluded that the management of Elders with multimorbidity is complex and screening for nutritional status in Elders with multimorbidity is needed (Qamar et al., 2025).

The above studies clearly show that multimorbidity in elderly is strongly related to a larger symptom burden, not only in the number of symptoms, but in relation to the severity as well

It shows that symptom burden in multimorbidity is strongly related to emotional and psychological stress as influencers. Also understanding the patient's concerns about their symptoms, and their adaptive strategies toward their symptoms is crucial for understanding and implementing treatment plans for their symptom management.

Malignant Versus Non-Malignant Terminally Ill Patients

Palliative care was initially related to malignant diseases. The incorporation of the non-malignant terminally ill concept is relatively recent, and this concept is still struggling for proper implementation, and in need for more studies (Michels et al., 2023). A Danish study involving about 44,000 patients, compared the palliative care needs for cancer versus non-cancer patients and they found that 50% of the cancer patients were referred to palliative care and only 4% of the non-cancer were referred to palliative care. They also found that the cancer patients show better physical function than the non-cancer patient. On the other hand, non-cancer patients were manifesting more physical limitations, and their symptoms were characteristically more severe in nature and in number, and their symptoms are more likely to be associated insomnia and fatigue (Hansen et al., 2024).

A retrospective study in three public palliative care departments in Northern Italy, studied end-stage non-cancer diseases and found that there is a clear under representation of non-cancer patients in palliative care in spite of the availability of proper assessment tools. They also found a clear discrepancy between non-cancer patients needing palliative care and those actually receiving the care. The study ended with a conclusion that there is a clear delay in the early initiation of palliative care to those non-cancer terminally ill patients (Romanò et al., 2022).

Another multicenter randomized control trial that was performed in four European cities (Amadora of Portugal, Inverness of UK, Thessaloniki of Greece and Valencia of Spain) used the NATPD (The needs assessment tool for progressive disease), 183 patients and their caregiver participated, and later 29 healthcare providers were involved and the aim of the study was to identify reasons of delayed integration of elder non-malignant patients in palliative care. In the end of the study healthcare providers acknowledged that the NATPD tool is user friendly. They were encouraged to initiate healthy discussions with the patient and their caregivers while using it, and in the study the percentage of palliative care referrals of non-malignant terminally ill patients were higher than the community referrals (Doñate-Martínez et al., 2025).

An interesting cross-sectional multicenter German study that was investigating the predictors of short-term survival (26 days) in non-cancer terminally ill patients, reviewed more than 6000 cases and found that performance status was the strongest predictor of short-term survival. It also found that the type of disease was irrelevant to short term survival in their large population of patients (Just et al., 2021).

The above studies clearly show that in relation to non-cancer terminally patients there is a discrepancy between those needing palliative care and those receiving it. They also show that there are proper skills and tools that can be used to assist healthcare providers to initiate early integration of palliative care for non-cancer terminally ill patients. The studies also show that non-cancer terminally ill patient's symptoms and needs are the same or more severe than their cancer counterparts.

Among the reasons for delayed initiation of palliative care in non-cancer terminally ill patients are lack of training of healthcare providers. Major differences in disease trajectories of cancer versus non-cancer diseases leading to difficulties in prognostication. Most studies were done in developed European countries; situation is considered to be far more disastrous in the developing world of Asia and Africa.

Symptom Complexity in Palliative Care

Symptom complexity is one of the characteristics of malignant and non-malignant symptoms. understanding its features, knowing how to assess it and appreciating it, is a cornerstone in the process of implementing a management (Jensen et al., 2022). we will review some of the studies to get an idea and come out with conclusions and recommendations.

An interesting cross-sectional Egyptian study was investigating elder female patients requiring palliative care by using the abbreviated version of the memorial symptom assessment scale MSAS-SF (Elsawy et al., 2024). The study showed that lack of appetite, pain, lack of energy and difficulty in concentration were the most distressing symptoms, the study showed that there was some difference according to the symptom burden in relation to the patient's perspective versus the caregiver and the attending physician perspective. According to the caregiver, the most distressing symptoms were pain and lack of appetite, and according to the attending physician, the most distressing symptoms were pain, dyspnea, and lack of energy. The study also found that caregivers may overestimate the symptom burden and attending physicians may underestimate the symptom burden. The study concluded that elder females receiving palliative care had a high symptom burden, and that symptom burden may vary according to the diagnosis and comorbidity as well (Kamal Elmasry et al., 2024).

Another retrospective Canadian study was investigating the negative outcomes of symptom complexity in terminal care patients by using the Edmonton Symptom assessment system revised ESAS-r. The study found that cancer patients had a high symptom complexity. It found that the more complexity, the more likely the patients would use emergency department services. The study also noted that appropriate screening tools are needed to prevent patient deterioration and emergency department overload (Watson et al., 2023).

A prospective cohort study investigating more than 300 Advanced heart failure patients in a university hospital in Japan, the median age was 79 years. The study found that distressing symptoms in advanced heart failure patients were anxiety 28%, drowsiness 26%, tiredness 25% and depression 22%. Very interestingly it showed that the ESAS sum score didn't show significant association with the severity of heart failure i.e. NYHA class, BNP level, length of hospital stay, weight reduction during hospital among the population group. This study shows the concept of non-disease specific PROs. Which is expected to exist in some or most non-malignant terminally ill patients with the multimorbidity. This concept could be very important to improve patient well-being, and quality of life (Tanaka et al., 2025).

Another study was investigating more than 270 Danish speaking patients referred to a palliative specialty center looking for symptom prioritization and whether it improved their well-being or not. They found that some symptoms like pain will overshadow other symptoms. They found that in half of the patient pain was the priority symptom. They also found that fatigue was underappreciated as a priority symptom because different patients express it by different means. They also found that patients who prioritize a symptom can achieve a better outcome, this was approved with pain, but was found inconclusive with fatigue (Strömgren et al., 2006).

An interesting Danish study interviewed more than 2000 patient with non-cancer terminally ill disease by using the write three symptom/problem WISP to investigate if non-cancer terminally ill patients need open-ended questions, and to understand their symptom burden better. They found that by using the WISP tool most of their patients expressed associated symptoms of edema, dizziness, cough, existential problems and dyspnea. They concluded that malignant thermally ill patients need open- ended question tools to discover and understand the full scope of their associated symptoms and thus to deliver a higher quality management to them (Leslye Rojas-Concha et al., 2024).

The above studies highlight some of the symptom complexity features of terminally patient, examples are symptom prioritization, non-disease specific PRO's, stakeholders' different perspectives of patient symptoms, some of the negative outcomes of the symptom burden like overuse of the emergency department services. The above have preventive and management Importance in order to improve the quality of life and well-being in elderly with terminal illness.

Psychological Distress in Palliative Care

As mentioned before terminally ill patients complain of the total Symptom burden which is the sum of physical symptoms and emotional symptoms. Ignoring the emotional or psychological component of the terminally ill patient's symptoms, will result in partial understanding of their symptom burden that will result in incomplete management and continuation of their suffering (Vaiphei, 2025). Many studies proved the existence of the emotional and psychological factor in malignant and non-malignant terminally ill patients. Some we already discussed above, but we will discuss two more here for confirmation.

A literature searches integrated review, investigated factors influencing symptom complexity in palliative care in 32 peer reviewed articles and found that there are 29 influential factors distributed in different domains. In the physical domain they are mainly pain, reduced physical function, and fatigue. In the psychological domain most, influential factors are anxiety, depression, abnormal mental health i.e. emotional distress, mood disorders, and grief (Ohinata et al., 2022).

Another interesting prospective multicenter Chinese study that investigated the prevalence of somatic systemic disorder SSD in more than 9000 elderly participants living in Shanghai. Somatic systemic disorders defined as distressing or disturbing physical symptoms, accompanied by excessive thoughts, feelings or behaviors related to the symptom or to the health problem. They found that the prevalence of SSD in Shanghai is higher in older people compared to the young 63% to 45% respectively. They also found that elder participant suffered from more severe SSD compared to the young 20% versus 12% respectively. The conclusion was that elder participants in Shanghai were more vulnerable to have SSD. Also, the importance of SSD screening in the elderly population (Wu et al., 2022).

Symptom Burden in End-of-Life Care

End of life care is a special and very important part of palliative care. It's characterized by complex symptoms, exaggerated emotional burden and emotional vulnerability. Controlling patients stress and symptoms carry challenges, overcoming such challenges need multidisciplinary treatment groups and non-pharmacological interventions, both show reduction in patient suffering and improvement in well-being (Kawalpreet et al., 2024). A cross-sectional study used the integrated palliative care outcome scale IPOS on more than 1500 end of life terminally ill patient in Hong Kong. The main age was 77.4 years. They found that the most distressing symptoms were poor mobility, family anxiety, weakness and lack of energy. The main influencing factors were terminal illness and patients age. They concluded that high risk groups for high symptom burden are non-cancer terminally ill elders, and they should be considered for screening (Fordjour et al., 2024).

Another retrospective Canadian cohort study investigated more than 20,000 non-cancer patients using home care services in the last six months in Ontario Canada. The question was whether distressing symptoms differ according to the disease or not. Patients were divided into four groups, cardiovascular, neurological, renal, and respiratory. Cognitive impairment was found in 50% of all group patients, but the highest level of cognitive impairment was found in the neurological group. The study found that pain was moderately to severely distressing in the end of life. The study also found that there are differences in distressing symptoms, according to deferent diseases (Conen et al., 2021).

Another smaller Canadian study investigated advanced metastatic cancer patient by using the ESAS questionnaire median age was 60 years. Symptom burden was linked to prognosis, quality of life and performance status. Patient defined symptom burden as loss of function and psychological suffering. The study concluded that emotional symptoms screening should be done in the terminally ill patient (Gill et al., 2012).

Symptom Burden Management

Due to the complexity of symptom burden in malignant and non-malignant terminally ill patients and it's multidimensional components, managing it is a challenging and difficult task (Jensen et al., 2022). We will present two large studies, investigating challenges and barriers to symptom burden management in terminally ill patients using focused groups of different concerned stakeholders similar to a multidisciplinary team. A large study involved, seven Dutch academic hospitals and the Netherland comprehensive center organization, and the aim was improving Multidimensional symptom management defined as the simultaneous assessment treatment and reassessment of multiple symptoms while considering physical, psychological and spiritual aspects (Delgado-Guay & Harding, 2021). they reviewed files using a focused group of different concerned stakeholders, including patient representatives, general community nurses, general hospital nurses, general hospital physicians, and palliative care physicians. Among their findings is that general clinicians are unaware about assessing non-physical problems and they focus on pharmacological interventions only.

They found that most terminally ill patients find that non-physical problems are more difficult to discuss, and they may use subtle or indirect cues in the history (van der Stap et al., 2022).

Another similar UK study using the ground therapy approach specifically semi-standard focus groups to identify barriers and facilitators to symptom management. The focus groups involved, nurses, doctors, Allied healthcare professionals. They found that many protocols and approaches target physical symptom management alone in related to terminal illness. They also found that only being treated in an in-patient specialty palliative word can itself improve the terminal patient well-being, which is called the simple things i.e. friendly welcome, feeling cared of, being informed about what will happen.

They recommended steps to improve symptom management in palliative care that start with encouraging patient to engage with palliative care service (Chapman et al., 2022).

The above two large studies came up with some recommendations to overcome symptom management challenges. Healthcare providers must have sufficient palliative care skills, which can be achieved by using some tools as the ESAS or the PCOS tool (Vetter, 2022). Improving patient-clinician communication is important by educating patients and properly training clinicians. Early discovery and dissolving of inter-disciplinary communication barriers. Simple none expensive measures could improve symptom management, for example showing empathy and compassion toward the patient and their family. Early identification of psychological disorders by screening is needed, one proper example is using the distress thermometer or the IPOS tool. High quality research for pharmacological and non-pharmacological interventions is needed for the difficult to treat symptoms like for example, fatigability in terminally ill patients. Encouraging the family to engage in the management plan is an important step in symptom management. (van der Stap et al., 2022, Chapman et al., 2022).

Pain in Palliative Care

Pain is a complicated multidimensional symptom that is highly prevalent in palliative care, causing much of suffering and poor quality standards (Gomes-Ferraz et al., 2022). We will review some basic principles related to pain in palliative care to improve the none-palliative specialists' knowledge, attitude, and skills towards it.

Malignant Versus Non-Malignant Pain

Palliative pain is common in both malignant and non-malignant patients. In malignant patients pain is divided into three types, cancer related pain, cancer treatment related pain and chronic non-malignant pain (CNMP) (Kovačević et al., 2022). Chronic non-malignant pain is commonly found in cancer patients. It also often coexists with other types of pain as well, unfortunately chronic non-malignant pain in general is under-appreciated, understudied and under-treated as well, regardless whether it's in cancer patients or non-cancer patients (Hui et al., 2020).

A large Swedish retrospective study from the Swedish registry of palliative care (SRPC) collected data from 2011 - 2022 of more than 300,000 patients in the last week of life. They found that severe pain was 35% prevalent in cancer patients Versus 17 - 21% in non-cancer patients which were (congestive heart failure, COPD and dementia patients), there could of been a limitation that the staff may have asked the cancer patients more intensely than the non-cancer patients, which was a potential bias (Hedman et al., 2024).

Another cross-sectional Korean study investigated more than 110 patients admitted in a tertiary hospital in Seoul, using different tools one of the findings is that the palliative need and satisfaction of non-cancer patients was 3.66 +/- 0.62 and that of terminal cancer patient was 3.58 +/- 0.31. It also showed that non-malignant patients had psychological needs that was higher than cancer patient, it also showed that non-malignant patients anxiety and depression level was higher than cancer patients, and it concluded that non-malignant patients need screening to assess their palliative needs and satisfaction level (Jang et al., 2022).

The above two studies, give us an idea about the importance of pain in both malignant and non-malignant palliative patients, unfortunately pain in non-malignant palliative patients is under-investigated, under-appreciated and under-treated as well. This puts a demand on all healthcare professionals to properly screen for pain in non-malignant palliative patients specifically.

Psychological Aspects of Pain

As we learned before, every symptom in palliative care has a psychological and emotional part that needs to be assessed in order to control it appropriately, due to the importance and high prevalence of pain in palliative care patients we will review some important psychological facts about pain in palliative care.

It's important to appreciate that pain is a complex component of both psychological and physiological parts. The socio-cultural background of the patient is strongly related to the pain severity. Psychological distress is an important part of chronic pain assessment (Vaiphei, 2021).

Assessing the patients coping strategies is an important step in understanding the scope and severity of his distress, active coping strategies, e.g. distraction strategies are adaptive in nature, on the other hand passive coping strategies depend on withdrawal or losing control to external forces, and they result in more pain and depression (Bondarchuk et al., 2023).

One important cognitive error concept is the concept of pain catastrophizing, which is a negative distorted perception of pain as awful and unbearable that results in more pain and depression. Studies involving functional MRI found that pain catastrophizing caused increased activity in pain anticipation areas, and pain attention areas as well.

Another cognitive error concept is Kinesiophobia which is an excessive irrational and debilitating fear of physical movement and activity resulting from a feeling of vulnerability to pain injury or re-injury. One explanation is that hypervigilance of the avoidance behavior became an anticipation rather than a response to pain.

Another important concept in relation to pain is Anxiety, which is a general term that includes uneasiness, apprehension, nervousness and fear. It's highly prevalent with chronic pain. A Brazilian study investigated more than 400 chronic pain patients, it found that 54% have both depression and anxiety. Those with both depression and anxiety experienced higher pain severity. They also found that disability days were more when chronic pain had anxiety, depression, or both respectively (Physiopedia, 2025).

An important concept in relation to the psychological assessment and management is cognitive behavioral therapy (CBT) which is a form of psychotherapy aimed at correcting cognitive distortion and negative behaviors that lead to psychological symptoms and is one of the cornerstone multidisciplinary management aspects of pain in palliative care, (Wilaras, 2024).

Chronic Non-Malignant Pain and Palliative Care

As we said previously, chronic non-malignant pain is a very common and prevalent type of pain in both cancer and non-cancer patients, understanding it is crucial in pain control (Kernick et al., 2023). A systemic review of more than 400 studies investigating chronic non-malignant pain in cancer patients, found that the prevalence in USA is generally 20%, globally the prevalence is 14 - 34% depending on the different participants and their different backgrounds. They found that chronic non-malignant pain is less likely to be treated with opioids compared to cancer pain. They also found that sometimes it's difficult to isolate chronic non-malignant pain from other types of pain in cancer patients (Kernick et al., 2023).

Another cross-sectional study investigating more than 200 patients with cancer, and found that 67 patients had chronic non-malignant pain, of those 31 had isolated chronic non-malignant pain, 20 had concurrent cancer-related pain, 12 had concurrent cancer treatment-related pain and 4 had both. The study concluded that clinicians must be educated about different cancer pains and they must be aware of the strategies of managing chronic non-malignant pain (Hui et al., 2020).

Breakthrough pain

Breakthrough pain is a transitionary exacerbation in an otherwise acceptable analgesic control. its prevalence is around 40 - 80% in cancer patient generally and 58 - 69% in advanced cancer stages. Prevalence was found to be 40% in the outpatient setting and about 80% in hospice. Breakthrough pain has two types, incidental which is predictable for example movement related and spontaneous which is unpredictable (Yeo, 2024).

A Korean survey investigated physicians' perception and management of breakthrough cancer pain using a custom questionnaire developed by the Korean Society for hospice and palliative care. (KSHPC), 100 physicians participated 53% from the oncology department 30% from family medicine and 17% from other departments. They found that there is a gap between the physicians' perception of the difficulty in managing breakthrough cancer pain and the actual perception of the palliative specialist. They concluded that physicians need to be educated about breakthrough pain (Seo et al., 2017).

The WHO Analgesic Ladder

A simple to use tool by all healthcare providers, proposed by the WHO in 1986 (Anekar et al., 2023).

- First step is mild pain, which is treated with non-opioids for example nonsteroidal anti-inflammatory drugs NSAID e.g. paracetamol.
- Second step moderate pain treated with weak opioids for example codeine or tramadol.
- Third step is severe pain, which is treated with strong opioids for example morphine, fentanyl or oxycodone. Adjuvant pain medication can be added to any step to improve pain control, e.g. Antidepressants, Serotonin-epinephrine reuptake inhibitors SNRI, Anti-convulsants and topical therapies

Among the principles of the analgesic ladder is that it should be used by the clock, i.e. regularly or in specific intervals, by the mouth as possible, and by the ladder i.e. to respect the steps.

The analgesic ladder is a monodimensional tool that depends on the physical aspect only so it cannot be the only management of pain in palliative care without the other psychological, social, spiritual aspects, etc. One proposal is the multimodal

Trolly approach to upgrade pain control from monodimensional to multidimensional, but this needs assessment of its practicality and efficiency first.

Some types of pain like neuropathic pain and functional pain disorders have specific mechanisms and different central nervous regions and need specific management strategies other than the analgesic ladder (Anekar et al., 2023).

Adequate Pain Control

We will assess some important concepts to understand adequate pain control in palliative care

In a literature review of chronic non-malignant pain in cancer patients the concept of timely palliative care TPC was found to be paramount in optimizing and personalizing pain management in a timely manner which improved cancer patients' quality of life (Maltoni et al., 2023). In a retrospective German study, more than 4000 cancer patients in palliative care were reviewed between 2015 and 2022 using the symptom and problem checklist (HOPE-SP-CL) they found that moderate to severe pain was 54%, and that 71% of the patient achieved pain relief. They also found that pain prevalence is different between different cancer types, least pain relief was found in patients with bone and cartilage cancer or metastasis (Ramm et al., 2024).

In another retrospective Swedish study using the Swedish registry of palliative care between 2011 and 2015 more than 160,000 patients were reviewed. They found that unrelieved pain was found in about 25%. They found that dying with unrelieved pain is common in both cancer and non-cancer patients. Some risk factors for unrelieved pain in the end of life is absence of end of life conversation, cancer in Bone or lungs and dying in the hospital (Klint et al., 2019). In a retrospective Canadian study, more than 20,000 patients in the last 30 days of life were reviewed and they found that daily severe pain was 17%. They also found that daily pain is common and maybe not proportional to suffering as we expect. They concluded that screening is needed (Hagarty et al., 2020)

Due to the fact that patient discomfort is strongly related to pain perception and experience, an important concept in understanding this is pain modification, which is the body's natural or externally, influenced process of altering or regulating pain signals as they travel along the pain pathway leading to changes in how pain is received (Alorfi, 2023). This can result in either intensification or reduction of pain stimulus. Among the important pain modifiers, family and friends support, religion, personal defense skills, therapeutic strategies. On the social aspect sleep disturbance, appetite, and lower stress tolerance (Sholjakova et al., 2018).

An interesting study in Thailand compared 85 patients with difficult pain management to 85 with active pain management. The median age was 59 and they came up with factors that predicted difficult pain management. The most important were family and anxiety, lack of support, psychological problems, spiritual problems, and unmet needs in descending importance. They concluded that pain is largely multidimensional and must be assessed properly (Sribunlue et al., 2024).

Another large study was investigating the concept of inadequate pain management in palliative patients, after investigating more than 500 patients by using the pain management index PMI, they found that 92% had moderate to severe pain and 77% had inadequate pain management, and they found that inadequate pain management is common in malignant and non-malignant patients. They also found that females are 1.6 time more likely to have inadequate pain management than men. This could be due to different pain sensitivities or different responses to analgesic, etc. They also found that opiophobia and fear of side effects is a potential Cause (Majedi et al., 2019).

Opiophobia is the irrational fear of prescribing opioids for patients with severe pain. In a literature review they found that the important reasons for Opiophobia are concerns about over addiction, concerns about serious side effects, concerns about legal consequences and lack of knowledge about pain management. The above is an old concept documented since the 1970s. The literature review concluded that physician education about pain management and risk of opiophobia is a must (Alattas, 2025).

Another longitudinal observational study in a university hospital in Norway, investigated 130 patients mean age 70, found that palliative cancer patients with high pain spikes at admission experience less improvement in pain intensity during hospitalization compared to patient with low or no pain spikes. It also found that a large variation in pain intensity is considered a poor outcome to pain management (Løhre et al., 2023).

Poor Adherence

Poor adherence is one of the important aspects in palliative pain control (Mercadante et al., 2020), and an important concept to understand in order to achieve high-quality pain control standards. We will review some studies to understand this concept. First a cross-sectional study in a university hospital in north-west Ethiopia reviewed more than 300 palliative patients to investigate factors associated with adherence to cancer management guidelines and found that the prevalence of poor adherence is 21%. Factors related to poor adherence were marital status in which those who are not married had poor adherence, cancer stage and metastasis. They concluded that early screening and early identification of cancer is important for proper pain management (Kibret et al., 2022).

Secondly, a cross-sectional study assessing the adherence to the American Society of clinical oncology ASCO recommendations in palliative care in deferent low- and middle-income countries LMIC recruited 180 healthcare providers 62% females and 51% were less than 45 years, 66% were physicians and 50% Didn't have palliative care education. They found that the barriers to adherence are as follows: 25% insufficient policies, for example limited funding and lack of institutional support. 22% lack of continuous education. 19% shortage of specialized staff and limited home service. 17% stigma and cultural barriers (Bergerot et al., 2025).

Thirdly, a large survey done by the Mary curie Cancer center involved 1000 UK GPs. The GPs found that 61% of the patients had inadequate access to pain control, and that 6 out of 10 patients with pain and terminal illness were not properly managed. Multiple factors were found in relation to this among the patient related barriers were under reporting of pain, under estimation of pain. Non-adherence to analgesics whether intentional or unintentional, false beliefs about pain in palliative care, side effects and over concerns. Among the healthcare practitioner barriers were feeling of lack of skills, failure to prescribe appropriate adjuvant analgesics, neglecting breakthrough pain management, over-concern about opioids, over-prescription, complexity of palliative pain management for example, multimorbidity, polypharmacy, etc (Adam & Murchie, 2014).

CONCLUSION

This short journey through some essential parts of palliative care, by discussing and simplifying complex palliative care concepts, and reviewing its evidence is aiming to send a clear message to all healthcare providers managing terminally ill patients needing palliative care that symptom assessment and management in the terminally ill patients is totally different than that in the non-terminally ill patients.

Upgrading the awareness, the understanding and the knowledge of healthcare providers is paramount for improving their palliative skills and thus delivering high quality care for our terminally ill patients

As we saw above, the terminally ill elder patients, especially the non-malignant ones are characterized by having multimorbidity which is two or more chronic diseases. This is associated with a higher number of symptoms, higher severity of symptoms, higher likelihood of physical limitation and emotional symptoms as well. Upon facing an elder with multimorbidity, which became the norm rather than the exception, the physician should be armed with advanced prognosis skills such as early risk identification, Pollypharmacy risk identification, such as drug to drug, drug to disease or disease to disease interactions, all those skills need proper multidisciplinary teams of physicians, pharmacist and nurses, etc. to improve the quality of care. When this is difficult or unpractical a high-quality physician-pharmacist communication is paramount.

Another concept that we learned was under-appreciation. Non-malignant terminally ill elders suffered clinical and research under-appreciation, which resulted in the delay of palliative care initiation to them, this resulted because of healthcare provider unawareness of palliative care essentials, and due to the difference of disease trajectories in malignancy versus non-malignant diseases. The malignancy disease trajectory is characterized by a sharp decline where's dementia disease trajectory is characterized by a steep and prolonged decline. Lastly, chronic organ failure disease trajectory is characterized by multiple exacerbations and improvements which causes the non-palliative care specialist to get mixed up in judging the proper palliative care initiation for the non-malignant patient with terminal illness.

Another concept that we learned was symptom complexity in palliative care, palliative care patients complain of total symptoms, which is the sum of physical symptoms and emotional symptoms. The psychological and emotional components of the patient's symptomatology is large and strongly related to the physical component, most of the time patients will not feel comfortable discussing non-physical symptoms directly and rather use subtle words or cues. We learned how a proper patient-clinician communication can improve the patient and the clinicians' participation in such history and in the collection of those important non-physical symptoms. We also learned that terminally ill patients' symptom distress may not be related to the disease severity like in the case of the advanced heart failure study what is called the non-specific disease PRO's. We also learned that patients who have multiple symptoms can prioritize one of their symptoms as the most distressing, even if they don't mention it out loud, this prioritization if discovered and managed early can result in a better outcome for some symptoms like pain. We also learned that some tools can be used to improve the healthcare providers' history taking skills, for example, the ESAS tool.

We also learned that palliative care symptom distress has multiple influencers, some are physical like pain. Some are psychological like depression. Some are social like being isolated, or being concerned about younger members of the family, some are spiritual or existential factors which differ upon communities and individuals according to their set of believes, their religion and their practices. We learned that all these must be understood and appreciated by implementing an understanding, empathetic and compassionate conversation with the patient and his family and by involving the family in the management plan and in the multidisciplinary team. We also learned to prepare for the end of life care by a compassionate realistic discussion with the patient and their family to ensure the whole team would expect it and prepare for it, and also to appreciate the emotional liability and exaggerated emotional aspects of the patient in such stage, by approaching complicated and refractory symptoms with empathy and starting an understanding and realistic discussion, and by appreciating and implementing multidisciplinary teams and non-pharmacological interventions. We also learned that due to the complexity of symptom management in the terminal ill patients' multiple challenges and barriers need to be solved, some large studies appreciated such challenges and tried to highlight them by performing multidisciplinary focused groups, they came up with recommendations for proper management and prevention.

We also learned that upgrading healthcare providers with palliative knowledge, and skills using simple measures such as lectures, educational audio-visuals, group or individual case reviews, supervising their palliative clinical skills and capabilities, if that is done properly and sincerely, it can result in improving the suffering of this delicate and vulnerable group of patients, and not only improving their well-being, but improving the overall healthcare centers quality of care as well.

After understanding some concepts of general symptom burden in palliative care we need to test our knowledge by practically choosing one of the important and common symptoms in palliative care and studying it in some details, such practice is important to the non-palliative specialist in order to properly understand the scope of the situation. We will study the symptom of pain in palliative care because pain is the most common symptom and the most symptom causing suffering, and it is one of the most symptoms investigated in palliative care as well. First we learned that pain is common in both cancer and non-cancer palliative care patients, some studies as we saw show that non-malignant palliative care patients suffer more pain and have more psychological needs in relation to pain. We also learned that in cancer patients pain could be in different forms for example there is cancer related pain, cancer treatment related pain, and chronic non-malignant pain.

We also learned that chronic non-malignant pain is common in both cancer and non-cancer patients, and it can manifest with other forms of pain in cancer patients. We also learned some important psychological aspects of pain in palliative care. Of those is understanding the coping strategies of palliative patients suffering pain, for example hunting for passive coping strategies, and treating them to break the vicious cycle of psychological suffering, which is an important task of the multidisciplinary team. We learned that palliative care patients suffering from pain possess cognitive errors that can lead to overestimating the pain severity and can lead to vicious cycles of negative outcome as well, important examples of these cognitive errors are pain catastrophizing, and kinsiophobia. After learning about the important role of cognitive errors in the suffering of palliative patient with pain, we can understand how cognitive behavioral therapy CBT is a rational, effective and safe psychological solution. If performed by a trained healthcare provider, it can alleviate such cognitive errors, that's why it has a pivotal role in palliative pain management.

We also learned about breakthrough pain and we saw how some studies found that healthcare providers underestimate, under-assess and under treat breakthrough pain, which result in poor quality of care standards. After that we learned about the

WHO pain ladder tool, and how it is practical and easy to use for any healthcare provider. Three simple steps, first step in mild pain, non-opioids, second step in moderate pain weak opioids and third step in severe pain, strong opioids. We also learned how to use adjuvant medications to augment each step and improve pain control. In spite of it being simple, easy and practical many healthcare providers globally are not using it due to lack of knowledge or lack of training which is causing more suffering of palliative care patients.

Next, we investigated the important concept of inadequate pain control, and understood that the quality-of-care standards is to provide adequate pain management in palliative care. By studying the reasons and barriers of inadequate pain control we came across some new concepts for example the concept of timely palliative care and how does delaying the appropriate multidimensional management cause more suffering to the patients. We also came across the concept of pain modification and found that many modifiers can either intensify or reduce the pain stimulus. We also came across the concept of Opiophobia and how doctors can augment suffering by improper prescription, that leads to inadequate pain control. And lastly, we examined the concept of poor adherence and we found that this is common in palliative pain management, whether it's patient related or physician related, and we understood that the education of both healthcare providers and patients is a cornerstone in improving adherence and thus achieving better quality standards in treating our elder palliative care patients.

REFERENCES

Adam, R., & Murchie, P. (2014). Why are we not controlling cancer pain adequately in the community? *The British Journal of General Practice*, *64*(626), 438–439. DOI: 10.3399/bjgp14x681229 PMID: 25179046

Aghaei, M. H., Vanaki, Z., & Mohammadi, E. (2021). Inducing a sense of worthiness in patients: The basis of patient-centered palliative care for cancer patients in Iran. *BMC Palliative Care*, *20*(1). Advance online publication. DOI: 10.1186/s12904-021-00732-3 PMID: 33653323

Alattas, I. M. (2025). Opiophobia: A Barrier to Pain Management. *Magalat Game'at al-Malik Abdul Aziz. Al-U'lum al-Tibyat*, *23*(3), 1–7. DOI: 10.4197/med.23-3.1

Alorfi, N. M. (2023). Pharmacological Methods of Pain Management: Narrative Review of Medication Used. *International Journal of General Medicine*, *16*(16), 3247–3256. DOI: 10.2147/IJGM.S419239 PMID: 37546242

Amjad, H., Snyder, S. H., Wolff, J. L., Oh, E., & Samus, Q. M. (2019). Before Hospice: Symptom Burden, Dementia, and Social Participation in the Last Year of Life. *Journal of Palliative Medicine*, *22*(9), 1106–1114. DOI: 10.1089/jpm.2018.0479 PMID: 31058566

Anekar, A. A., Cascella, M., & Hendrix, J. M. (2023). *WHO analgesic ladder*. National Library of Medicine; StatPearls Publishing. https://www.ncbi.nlm.nih.gov/books/NBK554435/

Bergerot, C. D., Soto-Perez-de-Celis, E., Thompson, C., Patel, R., Al-Mondhiry, J., Zhang, T., Dhawan, N., Burbage, D., McCollom, J., Tsang, M., Sedhom, R., & Rosa, W. E. (2025). Navigating Challenges in Palliative Care: A Survey on ASCO Guideline Adherence Among Health Care Providers in Low- and Middle-Income Countries. *JCO Global Oncology*, *11*. Advance online publication. DOI: 10.1200/go-24-00625 PMID: 40403199

Bondarchuk, O., Balakhtar, V., Pinchuk, N., Pustovalov, I., & Pavlenok, K. (2023). Adaptation of Coping Strategies to Reduce the Impact of Stress and Lonelines on the Psychological Well-Being of Adults - Digital Library NAES of Ukraine. *Iitta.gov.ua*. https://lib.iitta.gov.ua/id/eprint/738204/1/1852%2BLaw.pdf

Chapman, E. J., Pini, S., Edwards, Z., Elmokhallalati, Y., Murtagh, F. E. M., & Bennett, M. I. (2022). Conceptualising effective symptom management in palliative care: A novel model derived from qualitative data. *BMC Palliative Care*, *21*(1), 17. DOI: 10.1186/s12904-022-00904-9 PMID: 35115005

Cheng, C., & Christensen, M. (2024). Interventions Addressing Symptoms in Older Adults with Multimorbidity: An Umbrella Review. *Journal of Multidisciplinary Healthcare, 17*, 3181–3192. DOI: 10.2147/jmdh.s452426 PMID: 39006878

Conen, K., Guthrie, D. M., Stevens, T., Winemaker, S., & Seow, H. (2021). Symptom trajectories of non-cancer patients in the last six months of life: Identifying needs in a population-based home care cohort. *PLoS One, 16*(6), e0252814. DOI: 10.1371/journal.pone.0252814 PMID: 34129643

Delgado-Guay, M. O., & Harding, A. (2021). Multidimensional Patient Assessment. *CRC Press EBooks*, 149–166. https://doi.org/DOI: 10.1201/9780429275524-20

Doñate-Martínez, A., Yang, J., Linklater, G., Bradley, C., Reppou, S., Panagiotis, P., Camacho, M., Fernandes, A., Gas, M. E., Giménez-Campos, M. S., Alhambra-Borrás, T., & Garcés-Ferrer, J. (2025). Care professionals' approach to early palliative care for non-malignant diseases shifted from relying on intuition to employing structured needs assessment. *International Journal of Integrated Care, 25*, 99–99. DOI: 10.5334/ijic.icic24047

Eckerblad, J., Theander, K., Ekdahl, A., Unosson, M., Wirehn, A.-B., Milberg, A., Krevers, B., & Jaarsma, T. (2015). Symptom burden in community-dwelling older people with multimorbidity: A cross-sectional study. *BMC Geriatrics, 15*(1). Advance online publication. DOI: 10.1186/1471-2318-15-1 PMID: 25559550

Eckerblad, J., Waldréus, N., Stark, Å. J., & Jacobsson, L. R. (2020). Symptom management strategies used by older community-dwelling people with multimorbidity and a high symptom burden - a qualitative study. *BMC Geriatrics, 20*(1). Advance online publication. DOI: 10.1186/s12877-020-01602-y PMID: 32539798

Elsawy, A., & Elbehery, H., sweed, hala, & Sayed, A. (2024). Symptoms Burden In Elderly Male Patients Receiving Palliative Care .... *Egyptian Journal of Geriatrics and Gerontology, 11*(1), 114–131. DOI: 10.21608/ejgg.2024.350629

Fordjour, G. A., Yin, A., Ka-Ying Hui, V., & Lai, C. (2024). Comparative analysis of symptom burdens and influential factors among diverse terminally-ill patients. *Annals of Palliative Medicine, 13*(3), 513–530. DOI: 10.21037/apm-23-565 PMID: 38769801

Gill, A., Chakraborty, A., & Selby, D. (2012). What is Symptom Burden: A Qualitative exploration of Patient Definitions. *Journal of Palliative Care, 28*(2), 83–89. DOI: 10.1177/082585971202800204 PMID: 22860380

Gomes-Ferraz, C. A., Rezende, G., Fagundes, A. A., & De Carlo, M. M. R. do P. (2022). Assessment of total pain in people in oncologic palliative care: Integrative literature review. *Palliative Care and Social Practice*, *16*, 263235242211252. DOI: 10.1177/26323524221125244 PMID: 36172038

Hagarty, A. M., Bush, S. H., Talarico, R., Lapenskie, J., & Tanuseputro, P. (2020). Severe pain at the end of life: A population-level observational study. *BMC Palliative Care*, *19*(1). Advance online publication. DOI: 10.1186/s12904-020-00569-2 PMID: 32354364

Hansen, M. B., Rojas-Concha, L., Petersen, M. A., Adsersen, M., & Groenvold, M. (2024). Differences in palliative care needs between cancer patients and non-cancer patients at the start of specialized palliative care: A nationwide register-based study. *Palliative Medicine*. Advance online publication. DOI: 10.1177/02692163241269705 PMID: 39194071

Hardman, R., Begg, S., & Spelten, E. (2021). Multimorbidity and its effect on perceived burden, capacity and the ability to self-manage in a low-income rural primary care population: A qualitative study. *PLoS One*, *16*(8), e0255802. DOI: 10.1371/journal.pone.0255802 PMID: 34370758

Hedman, C., Fürst, P., Strang, P., Schelin, M. E. C., Lundström, S., & Martinsson, L. (2024). Pain prevalence and pain relief in end-of-life care – a national registry study. *BMC Palliative Care*, *23*(1). Advance online publication. DOI: 10.1186/s12904-024-01497-1 PMID: 39004730

Hui, D., Abdelghani, E., Chen, J., Dibaj, S., Zhukovsky, D., Dev, R., Tanco, K., Haider, A., Azhar, A., Reddy, A., Epner, D., Arthur, J., Dalal, S., Heung, Y., Reddy, S., De La Cruz, M., Liu, D., & Bruera, E. (2020). Chronic Non-Malignant Pain in Patients with Cancer Seen at a Timely Outpatient Palliative Care Clinic. *Cancers (Basel)*, *12*(1), 214. DOI: 10.3390/cancers12010214 PMID: 31952220

Jang, H., Lee, K., Kim, S., & Kim, S. (2022). Unmet needs in palliative care for patients with common non-cancer diseases: A cross-sectional study. *BMC Palliative Care*, *21*(1). Advance online publication. DOI: 10.1186/s12904-022-01040-0 PMID: 36038840

Jensen, E., Kristensen, J. K., Bjerglund, R. T., Johnsen, S. P., & Thomsen, J. L. (2022). The pathway and characteristics of patients with non-specific symptoms of cancer: A systematic review. *BMC Cancer*, *22*(1). Advance online publication. DOI: 10.1186/s12885-022-09535-y PMID: 35606715

Just, J., Schmitz, M.-T., Grabenhorst, U., Joist, T., Horn, K., Engel, B., & Weckbecker, K. (2021). Factors influencing length of survival in ambulatory palliative care - a cross sectional study based on secondary data. *BMC Palliative Care, 20*(1). Advance online publication. DOI: 10.1186/s12904-021-00762-x PMID: 34001099

Kalantar-Zadeh, K., Lockwood, M. B., Rhee, C. M., Tantisattamo, E., Andreoli, S., Balducci, A., Laffin, P., Harris, T., Knight, R., Kumaraswami, L., Liakopoulos, V., Lui, S.-F., Kumar, S., Ng, M., Saadi, G., Ulasi, I., Tong, A., & Li, P. K.-T. (2022). Patient-centred approaches for the management of unpleasant symptoms in kidney disease. *Nature Reviews. Nephrology, 18*(1). Advance online publication. DOI: 10.1038/s41581-021-00518-z PMID: 34980890

Kamal Elmasry, A., Elawam, A., Sweed, H., & Fahmy Tolba, M. (2024). Symptoms Burden in Elderly Female Patients Receiving Palliative Care. *EJGG.2024 , 11*(1), 86–97. https://ejgg.journals.ekb.eg/article_350627_e60ab735671bde8a1cf6003fa4beb927.pdf

Kawalpreet, K., Rinalben, P., & Ravita, S. (2024). *Managing Anxiety in Palliative Care: Nurses' Non-Pharmacological Intervention.* https://www.theseus.fi/bitstream/handle/10024/886071/Kaur_Parmar_Sharma.pdf?sequence=2

Kernick, L., Glare, P., Hosie, A., Chiu, A., & Kissane, D. W. (2023). Prevalence and management of chronic nonmalignant pain in palliative care populations: A systematic review. *Palliative & Supportive Care, 22*(4), 1–7. DOI: 10.1017/s1478951523000378 PMID: 37039456

Kibret, A. A., Wolde, H. F., Molla, M. D., Aragie, H., Getnet Adugna, D., Tafesse, E., Melese, E. B., Worku, Y. B., & Belay, D. G. (2022). Factors associated with adherence to guidelines in cancer pain management among adult patients evaluated at oncology unit, in the University of Gondar Comprehensive Specialized Hospital, Northwest Ethiopia. *Frontiers in Pain Research (Lausanne, Switzerland), 3.* Advance online publication. DOI: 10.3389/fpain.2022.884253 PMID: 35978991

Klint, Å., Bondesson, E., Rasmussen, B. H., Fürst, C. J., & Schelin, M. E. C. (2019). Dying With Unrelieved Pain—Prescription of Opioids Is Not Enough. *Journal of Pain and Symptom Management, 58*(5), 784–791.e1. DOI: 10.1016/j.jpainsymman.2019.07.006 PMID: 31319106

Kovačević, I., Majerić Kogler, V., Krikšić, V., Ilić, B., Friganović, A., Ozimec Vulinec, Š., Pavić, J., Milošević, M., Kovačević, P., & Petek, D. (2022). Non-Medical Factors Associated with the Outcome of Treatment of Chronic Non-Malignant Pain: A Cross-Sectional Study. *International Journal of Environmental Research and Public Health, 19*(5), 2881. DOI: 10.3390/ijerph19052881 PMID: 35270575

Leslye Rojas-Concha, L., Bang Hansen, M., & Groenvold, M. (2024). Symptoms and problems reported by patients with non-cancer diseases through open-ended questions in specialist palliative care: A national register-based study. *Supportive Care in Cancer*, *32*(2). Advance online publication. DOI: 10.1007/s00520-024-08345-1 PMID: 38305835

Løhre, E. T., Jakobsen, G., Solheim, T. S., Klepstad, P., & Thronæs, M. (2023). Breakthrough and Episodic Cancer Pain from a Palliative Care Perspective. *Current Oncology (Toronto, Ont.)*, *30*(12), 10249–10259. DOI: 10.3390/curroncol30120746 PMID: 38132380

Majedi, H., Dehghani, S. S., Soleyman-Jahi, S., Tafakhori, A., Emami, S. A., Mireskandari, M., & Hosseini, S. M. (2019). (in press). Assessment of Factors Predicting Inadequate Pain Management in Chronic Pain Patients. *Anesthesiology and Pain Medicine, In Press*. Advance online publication. DOI: 10.5812/aapm.97229 PMID: 32280619

Maltoni, M. C., Donati, C. M., Rossi, R., & Morganti, A. G. (2023). Timely Palliative Care Could Be Another Benefit for Cancer Patients with Non-Malignant Pain. *Cancers (Basel)*, *15*(9), 2588. DOI: 10.3390/cancers15092588 PMID: 37174054

Mercadante, S., Adile, C., Tirelli, W., Ferrera, P., Penco, I., & Casuccio, A. (2020). Barriers and Adherence to Pain Management in Advanced Cancer Patients. *Pain Practice*, *21*(4). Advance online publication. DOI: 10.1111/papr.12965 PMID: 33200548

Michels, G., Schallenburger, M., Neukirchen, M., John, S., Janssens, U., Raake, P., Schütt, K., Bauersachs, J., Barchfeld, T., Schucher, B., Delis, S., Karpf-Wissel, R., Kochanek, M., von Bonin, S., Erley, C. M., Kuhlmann, S. D., Müllges, W., Gahn, G., Heppner, H. J., & Wiese, C. H. R. (2023). Recommendations on palliative care aspects in intensive care medicine. *Critical Care*, *27*(1). Advance online publication. DOI: 10.1186/s13054-023-04622-3 PMID: 37723595

Ohinata, H., Aoyama, M., & Miyashita, M. (2022). Complexity in the context of palliative care: A systematic review. *Annals of Palliative Medicine*, *11*(10), 3231–3246. DOI: 10.21037/apm-22-623 PMID: 36226646

Patel, K. V., Guralnik, J. M., Phelan, E. A., Gell, N. M., Wallace, R. B., Sullivan, M. D., & Turk, D. C. (2018). Symptom Burden Among Community-Dwelling Older Adults in the United States. *Journal of the American Geriatrics Society*. Advance online publication. DOI: 10.1111/jgs.15673 PMID: 30548453

Physiopedia. (2025). *Psychological basis of pain*. Physiopedia. https://www.physio-pedia.com/index.php?title=Psychological_basis_of_pain&redirect=no

Qamar, S., Sarfraz, M., Ishtiaq, H., Akbar, A., Khattak, M. I., Raja, S. K., & Khan, M. (2025). The Complexity of Aging: Managing Multimorbidity in Geriatrics. *Cureus*. Advance online publication. DOI: 10.7759/cureus.87615 PMID: 40786252

Ramm, M., Chung, M. L., Schnabel, K., Schnabel, A., Jedamzik, J., Hesse, M., Hach, M., Radbruch, L., Mücke, M., & Conrad, R. (2024). Pain in palliative cancer patients – Analysis of the German National Palliative Care Registry. *Journal of Pain and Symptom Management*. Advance online publication. DOI: 10.1016/j.jpainsymman.2024.10.030 PMID: 39505055

Romanò, M., Oldani, S., Reina, V., Sofia, M., & Castiglioni, C. (2022). Palliative Care for Patients with End-Stage, Non-Oncologic Diseases—A Retrospective Study in Three Public Palliative Care Departments in Northern Italy. *Health Care*, *10*(6), 1031. DOI: 10.3390/healthcare10061031 PMID: 35742082

Roubaud-Baudron, C., & Guerville, F. (2022). Multimorbidity. *Lessons from the ICU*, 111–122. https://doi.org/DOI: 10.1007/978-3-030-94133-8_8

Seo, M. S., Shim, J. Y., Choi, Y. S., Kim, D. Y., Hwang, I. G., Baek, S. K., Shin, J. Y., Lee, J., & Lee, C. G. (2017). Physician's Attitude toward Treating Breakthrough Cancer Pain in Korea. *Han'guk Hosup'isu Wanhwa Uiryo Hakhoe Chi = The Korean Journal of Hospice and Palliative Care*, *20*(1), 18–25. DOI: 10.14475/kjhpc.2017.20.1.18

Sholjakova, M., Durnev, V., Kartalov, A., & Kuzmanovska, B. (2018). Pain relief as an integral part of the palliative care. *Open Access Macedonian Journal of Medical Sciences*, *6*(4), 739–741. DOI: 10.3889/oamjms.2018.163 PMID: 29731950

Skou, S. T., Mair, F. S., Fortin, M., Guthrie, B., Nunes, B. P., Miranda, J. J., Boyd, C. M., Pati, S., Mtenga, S., & Smith, S. M. (2022). Multimorbidity. *Nature Reviews. Disease Primers*, *8*(1), 1–22. DOI: 10.1038/s41572-022-00376-4 PMID: 35835758

Sribunlue, P., Boondet, K., Charoenpol, F., & Pairojkul, S. (2024). Factors Predicting the Difficulty of Pain Management in Patients Receiving First Palliative Care Consultation. *The Journal of Thailand Nursing and Midwifery Council*, *39*(03), 313–327. DOI: 10.60099/jtnmc.v39i03.267495

Strang, P. (2022). Palliative oncology and palliative care. *Molecular Oncology*, *16*(19). Advance online publication. DOI: 10.1002/1878-0261.13278 PMID: 35762045

Strömgren, A. S., Sjogren, P., Goldschmidt, D., Petersen, M. A., Pedersen, L., & Groenvold, M. (2006). Symptom priority and course of symptomatology in specialized palliative care. *Journal of Pain and Symptom Management*, *31*(3), 199–206. DOI: 10.1016/j.jpainsymman.2005.07.007 PMID: 16563314

Tanaka, S., Imaizumi, T., Morohashi, A., Kobayashi, K., Takagi, D., Hattori, K., Yoshito, N., Takeuchi, S., Tsuchikawa, Y., Inoue, T., Nagaya, M., Nishida, Y., Morimoto, R., Kondo, T., Hiraiwa, H., Kazama, S., Okumura, T., & Murohara, T. (2025). Prognostic value of symptom burden as a simple patient-reported outcome measure in older patients with heart failure. *Scientific Reports, 15*(1). Advance online publication. DOI: 10.1038/s41598-025-06615-4 PMID: 40594461

Vaiphei, S. D. (2021). The psychological aspect of pain and symptom management in clinical practices: Scoping review. *Journal of Clinical Medicine of Kazakhstan, 18*(6). https://cyberleninka.ru/article/n/the-psychological-aspect-of-pain-and-symptom-management-in-clinical-practices-scoping-review

Vaiphei, S. D. (2025). *Understanding End-of-Life Care*. Google Books. https://books.google.com/books?hl=en&lr=&id=Q8RIEQAAQBAJ&oi=fnd&pg=PA1&dq=Ignoring+the+emotional+or+psychological+component+of+the+terminally+ill+patient%E2%80%99s+symptoms

van der Stap, L., de Heij, A. H., van der Heide, A., Reyners, A. K. L., & van der Linden, Y. M. (2022). Barriers and facilitators to multidimensional symptom management in palliative care: A focus group study among patient representatives and clinicians. *Palliative & Supportive Care, 21*(4), 1–12. DOI: 10.1017/s147895152200133x PMID: 36177886

Vetter, V. J. (2022). Palliative care screening tools in the gynecologic oncology population: A narrative review. *Annals of Palliative Medicine, 11*(10), 3263–3272. DOI: 10.21037/apm-22-728 PMID: 36226647

Watson, L., Qi, S., Link, C., DeIure, A., Afzal, A., & Barbera, L. (2023). Patient-Reported Symptom Complexity and Acute Care Utilization Among Patients With Cancer: A Population-Based Study Using a Novel Symptom Complexity Algorithm and Observational Data. *Journal of the National Comprehensive Cancer Network : JNCCN, 21*(2), 173–180. DOI: 10.6004/jnccn.2022.7087 PMID: 36791760

Wilaras, A. (2024). Cognitive behavioural interventions for palliative care in adult patients: A scoping review. *Progress in Palliative Care, 32*(6), 1–43. DOI: 10.1080/09699260.2024.2408127

Willadsen, T. G., Siersma, V., Nicolaisdottir, D. R., Jarbol, D., Guassora, A. D., Reventlow, S., & Køster-Rasmussen, R. (2021). Symptom burden in multimorbidity: A population-based combined questionnaire and registry study from Denmark. *BMJ Open, 11*(4), e041877. DOI: 10.1136/bmjopen-2020-041877 PMID: 33849847

Wu, Y., Tao, Z., Qiao, Y., Chai, Y., Liu, Q., Lu, Q., Zhou, H., Li, S., Mao, J., Jiang, M., & Pu, J. (2022). Prevalence and characteristics of somatic symptom disorder in the elderly in a community-based population: A large-scale cross-sectional study in China. *BMC Psychiatry*, *22*(1). Advance online publication. DOI: 10.1186/s12888-022-03907-1 PMID: 35413865

Yao, H., Jingyue, W., Rui, Z., Hou, Y., & Hui, Y. (2025). E-CARE as core competencies for palliative social workers: A systematic review. *BMC Palliative Care*, *24*(1). Advance online publication. DOI: 10.1186/s12904-025-01735-0 PMID: 40490802

Zhao, Y., Wang, J., Zhu, X., Zhang, X., Zhang, Y., Zhang, W., & Dong, Y. (2023). Multimorbidity and polypharmacy in hospitalized older patients: A cross-sectional study. *BMC Geriatrics*, *23*(1), 423. DOI: 10.1186/s12877-023-04109-4 PMID: 37434147

Chapter 4
Non-Hypoxic Dyspnea in Terminal Care:
Palliative Management and Quality of Life in Elderly Patients

Joseph Obiri Asante
https://orcid.org/0000-0002-7042-7371
Jiangsu Food and Pharmaceutical Science College, Huai'an, China & Global Organization of African Academic Doctors (OAAD), Nairobi, Kenya

ABSTRACT

This chapter looks at the many causes of non-hypoxic dyspnea (NHD), outlines structured assessment methods, and presents both pharmacological and non-pharmacological treatment pathways. It does this by using recent research, clinical guidelines, and case studies. A clinical algorithm that combines low-dose morphine, fan therapy, and a systematic 48-hour reassessment is suggested for use in practice, taking into account ethical and communication issues. An interdisciplinary approach that combines targeted symptom control with psychosocial support is necessary for effective NHD management. Studies show that low-dose opioids and other therapies can help with symptoms, while teaching caregivers and giving them advice ahead of time can help with stress and make it easier to cope. To keep elderly patients comfortable and dignified, it is important to address NHD in terminal care. To move forward with best practices, we need standardized clinical pathways, integration into palliative protocols, and more research into neurophysiological mechanisms

DOI: 10.4018/979-8-3373-4099-9.ch004

1. INTRODUCTION

Figure 1. A conceptual schematic abstract

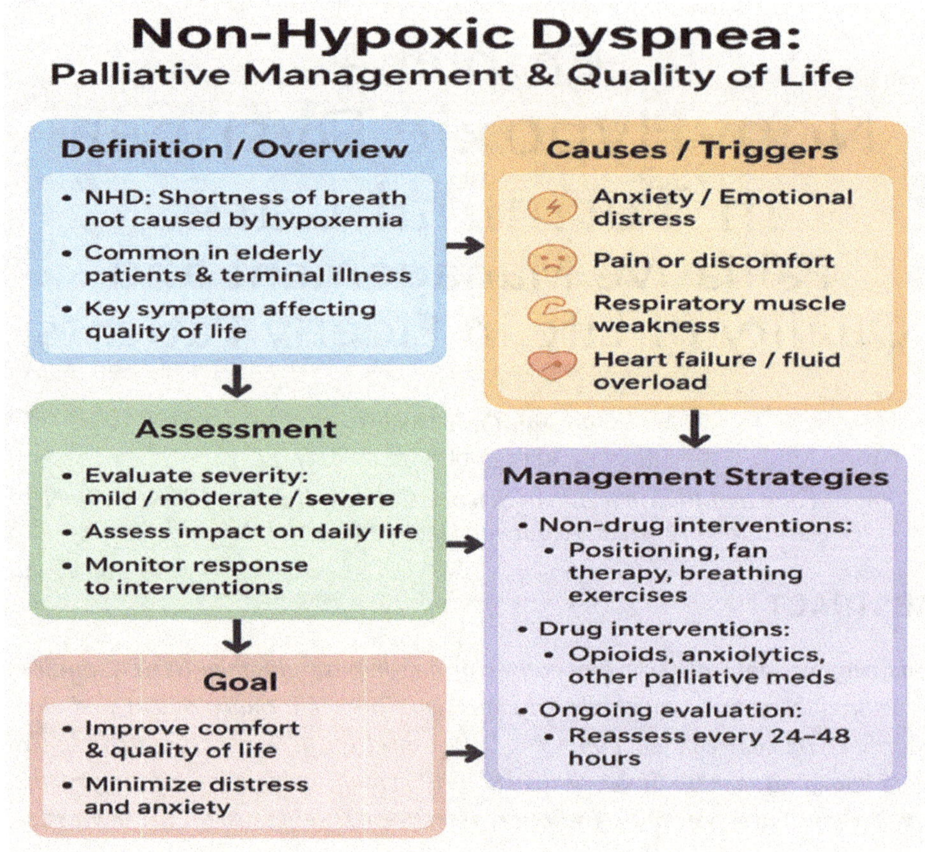

Figure 1 A conceptual schematic abstract of Non-Hypoxic Dyspnea, its definition, common causes and triggers, key assessment criteria, and the core management strategies aimed at improving patient comfort and quality of life.

Dyspnea is one of the most troubling symptoms that palliative care patients have to deal with, especially older patients who are close to death (Hui et al., 2015). Hypoxic dyspnea is widely acknowledged and commonly treated with oxygen supplementation; however, a considerable number of patients experience non-hypoxic dyspnea (NHD), which is marked by breathlessness occurring despite normal oxygen saturation (SpO_2 ≥92%) (Booth et al., 2018). This phenomenon presents a diagnostic and therapeutic challenge, especially in frail, multimorbid elderly patients who already have a significant symptom burden. NHD and hypoxic dyspnea function in markedly different ways and exhibit disparate responses to treatment. It often arises from complex interactions involving central nervous system processing, altered respiratory mechanics, comorbid conditions, and psychological distress, rather than being exclusively due to tissue hypoxia (Parshall et al., 2012). These factors cause the brain to misinterpret signals from the lungs, which keeps the cycle of breathlessness, anxiety, and functional decline going (Banzett & Lansing, 2021).

The burden of NHD in terminal care is substantial. Observational studies indicate that up to 40–70% of elderly patients with advanced cancer, heart failure, chronic lung disease, or neurodegenerative disorders experience NHD in their final months of life (Currow et al., 2009). The symptom not only undermines physical functioning but also causes severe emotional distress, social withdrawal, and a loss of personal dignity. Caregivers often express feelings of helplessness when witnessing "air hunger" in their loved ones, even when oxygen saturation levels are normal, a phenomenon associated with elevated levels of anticipatory grief and post-bereavement distress (Brighton et al., 2019).

For healthcare providers, especially early-career general practitioners and family medicine clinicians, the management of NHD is complicated by three major factors; diagnostic uncertainty, over-reliance on oxygen therapy and lack of standardized management protocols.

Given its multifactorial nature and profound impact on quality of life (QoL), NHD requires a comprehensive, patient-centered approach that combines accurate assessment, individualized symptom control, caregiver support, and compassionate communication. A key research gap in the management of NHD is the lack of structured models to manage NHD in terminal elderly patients. This chapter aims to provide clinicians with the necessary knowledge, diagnostic frameworks, and management models to effectively manage NHD in elderly patients undergoing terminal care.

This chapter presents a narrative review and conceptual framework designed to address the identified clinical and research gaps in NHD management. It is not a report of original research. Our objective is to synthesize current evidence from recent clinical guidelines (e.g., European Association for Palliative Care), systematic reviews, and key observational and interventional studies from 2010-2024 to provide a structured approach for clinicians. Based on this synthesis, we will propose a practical, stepwise model that integrates physiological, pharmacological, and psychosocial strategies to improve the assessment and management of NHD in elderly palliative care patients.

2. LITERATURE REVIEW

Prior to 1996, managing non-hypoxic dyspnea (NHD) required a paradigm shift from a one-size-fits-all approach. Foundational research from 1990 established that different types of dyspnea exist across various cardiopulmonary conditions, with patients able to distinguish between different sensations of breathlessness (Simon et al., 1990). This generated interest into treatments beyond oxygenation. Early studies examined drugs like buspirone for COPD patients (Argyropoulou et al., 1993) and opioids, which proved effective in single-dose trials ("Subcutaneous Morphine," 1993). A crucial 1996 study directly challenged oxygen administration, revealing that for dyspneic cancer patients at rest, oxygen was no more effective than room air (Booth et al., 1996). This was later confirmed by a 2005 systematic review ("A systematic", 2005). By 2009, a prospective analysis revealed no significant variance in opioid response between hypoxic and non-hypoxic palliative care patients ("Use of," 2009), reinforcing that NHD necessitates a therapeutic strategy irrespective of oxygen saturation.

The period 1996–2012 marked the development of evidence for NHD-specific interventions. A randomised pilot study conducted in 1996, showed that counselling and breathing retraining helped lung cancer patients feel better and improved their daily tasks ability ability (Corner et al., 1996). At the same time, the evidence in favour of opioids grew stronger. A 2001 Cochrane review endorsed oral or parenteral opioids for alleviating breathlessness (Jennings et al., 2001), a conclusion corroborated by a 2002 systematic review indicating their superiority over ineffective nebulised opioids (Jennings et al., 2002). A pivotal 2003 study revealed that low-dose, sustained-release oral morphine markedly reduced refractory dyspnea (Abernethy et al., 2003). Increasing acknowledgement of the psychological dimension of dyspnea, notably a documented "vicious cycle" with anxiety (Kemp, 1997), has initiated enquiries into combination therapy. This body of work culminated in the 2012 American Thoracic Society statement, which synthesised findings that dyspnea stimuli activated cortico-limbic areas and that opioids may modulate this perception (Parshall et al., 2012), providing a comprehensive neurophysiological framework for NHD management.

The current approach has solidified into a multimodal, patient-centered paradigm, moving away from oxygen as a default therapy. A trial conducted in 2010, confirmed that non-hypoxic patients with refractory dyspnea benefited nothing from supplemental oxygen ("Refractory breathlessness", 2010), and a 2011 review concluded that its routine application without comprehensive assessment is untenable (Davidson & Johnson, 2011). This shift allowed non-pharmacological strategies to become a main focus, as recommended by guidelines promoting a multidisciplinary approach (Lok, 2016). Airflow stimulation has become an important treatment. A randomised trial in 2020 showed that blowing air on the face with a fan significantly reduced dyspnea (Ting et al., 2020). This builds on a 2017 study that suggested the mechanism is stimulating trigeminal nerve pathways (Puspawati et al., 2017). For patients with aphasia, assessment tools like the Respiratory Distress Observation Scale (RDOS) have been tested and shown to work, making it easier to give this vulnerable group the right care (Campbell et al., 2010). A comprehensive examination of the literature on NHD in the elderly uncovers enduring research deficiencies. Early studies ignored the specific context of frail, multimorbid elderly patients, leaving a gap in understanding the qualitative experience of NHD in conditions like advanced heart failure. A testable hypothesis suggests that elderly patients with heart failure display distinct breathlessness descriptors in contrast to those with COPD, potentially guiding targeted interventions. Later studies showing that opioids work well mostly ignored the higher risks of side effects and polypharmacy in older adults. This opened the door for a trial comparing low-dose morphine with breathing-retraining techniques specifically for this population. More recently, despite strong evidence for fan therapy, its precise neurological mechanisms remain under-explored, and there is a significant lack of research on caregiver-focused educational programs. A hypothesis worth testing is that a structured caregiver program on using fan therapy and managing anxiety can reduce caregiver distress more than standard care. The most significant overarching gap is the scarcity of studies designed for the frail, multimorbid elderly. A pragmatic, multi-arm trial in patients over 75 with NHD is necessary to compare opioid monotherapy, non-pharmacological monotherapy, and combination therapy, using outcomes like quality of life scales, caregiver burden indices, and behavioral dyspnea assessments to provide a comprehensive evaluation.

2.1 Epidemiology and Burden of NHD

Epidemiological studies have constantly shown its high prevalence of NHD, with Hui et al. (2015) reporting that over 50% of patients in acute palliative care units experience significant breathlessness in their final week of life. A large portion of this dyspnea is non-hypoxic in nature. Research by Currow et al. (2009) demonstrated that the trajectory and intensity of dyspnea vary by diagnosis but remain a core symptom across advanced cancer, COPD, heart failure, and interstitial lung disease, with a significant number of patients maintaining severe breathlessness without hypoxemia.

The burden of NHD extends far beyond the physical sensation. It imposes a multifaceted toll on patients' quality of life (QoL), leading to functional impairment, social isolation, and profound psychological distress (Booth et al., 2018). The symptom's intractable nature can lead to a loss of personal dignity and autonomy. This burden also extends to family caregivers, who report extreme helplessness and anxiety when witnessing a loved one's "air hunger" (Brighton et al., 2019). This caregiver distress is a significant factor associated with anticipatory grief and complicated bereavement, highlighting NHD as a critical target for intervention to improve outcomes for both the patient and their support system.

2.2 Pathophysiological Mechanisms: The Evidence Base

A purely pulmonary model of dyspnea has given way to a sophisticated neurophysiological one. Dyspnea is a subjective experience that arises from the interplay of various physiological, psychological, social, and environmental factors, according to the American Thoracic Society's landmark statement (Parshall et al., 2012). A mismatch or neuromechanical dissociation between the brain's respiratory motor command and the incoming afferent feedback from receptors in the lungs, chest wall, and vasculature is thought to be the fundamental mechanism of NHD.

According to recent data, NHD develops when the brain interprets a need for more ventilation that the respiratory system's mechanical response cannot provide (Banzett & Lansing, 2021). This may be caused by a stronger central respiratory drive (for example, metabolic acidosis or anxiety) or by problems with the mechanics of breathing (for example, muscle weakness or ascites). Functional neuroimaging studies have elucidated the central processing of dyspnea, revealing a network that includes the insula, anterior cingulate cortex, and amygdala—areas also associated with pain and emotion (Jolley & Moxham, 2021). This shared neural circuitry establishes a biological foundation for the extensively documented dyspnea-anxiety-dyspnea cycle, wherein fear and panic exacerbate the sensation of breathlessness, subsequently intensifying anxiety.

2.3 Evidence for Assessment Tools

Since dyspnea is inherently subjective, the patient's self-report is the gold standard for assessment. The literature strongly supports the use of validated, patient-reported outcome measures over reliance on physiological signs like oxygen saturation. For rapid clinical assessment, unidimensional scales such as the Numerical Rating Scale (NRS) or the Edmonton Symptom Assessment System (ESAS) are highly practical and sensitive to change (Dudgeon, 2019).

For a more comprehensive evaluation, multidimensional tools capture the full impact of the symptom. The Dyspnea-12 questionnaire, for instance, validly assesses both the physical and affective dimensions of breathlessness and has been shown to be reliable in patients with advanced disease (Yorke et al., 2010). However, Bausewein et al. (2021) note that the choice of tool must be tailored to the clinical context and the patient's functional status, as longer instruments may be burdensome for severely ill individuals. The evidence consistently calls for dyspnea to be assessed as a "fifth vital sign" in palliative care populations to ensure it is identified and treated proactively.

2.4. Efficacy of Management Interventions: A Critical Appraisal

2.4.1 Non-Pharmacological Approaches

Systematic reviews confirm that non-pharmacological therapies are essential for the management of NHD. A seminal randomised controlled trial by Kako et al. (2018) revealed that facial fan therapy significantly alleviates dyspnea, presumably via stimulating the trigeminal nerve, which influences central perception. Evidence from pulmonary rehabilitation supports breathing strategies, such as pursed-lip breathing and timed breathing, which have been successfully adapted for palliative care to enhance patients' sensation of control (Spathis et al., 2017). Moreover, trials of integrated palliative and respiratory care services, such as the one conducted by Higginson et al. (2014), demonstrate that multidisciplinary support, which includes psychoeducation, energy conservation, and carer training, results in substantial reductions in distress for both patients and families.

2.4.2 Pharmacological Management

Opioids are the most evidence-based pharmacological treatment for refractory dyspnea. A Cochrane review concluded that systemic opioids provide a statistically significant and clinically meaningful reduction in breathlessness without causing significant respiratory depression in opioid-naïve patients (Barnes-Harris et al., 2019). This was reinforced by a major RCT by Currow et al. (2020), which found that regular, low-dose sustained-release morphine safely reduced chronic breathlessness in patients with COPD. In contrast, the evidence for benzodiazepines is weak. A Cochrane review by Simon et al. (2016) found no clear benefit for benzodiazepines as first-line treatment for dyspnea, suggesting they may be considered only as an adjunct for co-existing anxiety that is refractory to other interventions.

2.4.3 The Evidence on Oxygen Therapy

The most pivotal evidence regarding NHD management concerns oxygen therapy. A rigorous double-blind, randomized controlled trial by Abernethy et al. (2010) found that palliative oxygen provided no greater benefit than medical air (delivered via nasal cannula) in relieving the sensation of breathlessness in non-hypoxemic patients. Subsequent systematic reviews have consistently upheld this finding, concluding that there is no role for the routine use of oxygen in NHD and that its inappropriate use can cause discomfort and unnecessary cost (Long et al., 2016). Oxygen therapy should therefore be reserved for patients with documented hypoxemia.

2.5. Gaps in Current Knowledge

Even with these improvements, there are still big holes. There aren't many large-scale RCTs that focus specifically on the oldest old (over 85 years) and those with serious cognitive impairment, which are two groups that are very common in terminal care. More research is needed on how to use integrated models effectively in communities and places with few resources (Brighton et al., 2019). We also need to improve our understanding of the best times and doses of opioids for different disease trajectories. Finally, we need to look into new drugs that target the central perception of breathlessness and make standardised protocols that can help doctors, especially in primary care, use this information in their daily work.

3. PATHOPHYSIOLOGY: A CLINICAL PERSPECTIVE

Non-hypoxic dyspnea (NHD) occurs when there is a disconnect between the brain's respiratory drive and the body's mechanical response. The fundamental mechanism is neuromechanical dissociation (Parshall et al., 2012). The brain tells the body to breathe, but a weak respiratory system (cachexia), less elastic lungs, or an increased load (ascites) doesn't respond the way it should. This makes people really want to breathe and work hard (Banzett & Lansing, 2021).

The insula and anterior cingulate cortex are two areas of the brain that deal with this mismatch. They also deal with fear and anxiety (Jolley & Moxham, 2021). The neuroanatomical overlap creates a cycle of dyspnea-anxiety-dyspnea that keeps going: feeling short of breath makes you scared, which makes you more aware of your breathing, which makes you panic and want to breathe more. This is why a person with normal oxygen saturation can feel like they are suffocating, and it explains why treatments like fan therapy and opioids that affect central perception instead of gas exchange are needed.

Figure 2. Key pathophysiological mechanisms on non-hypoxic dyspnea

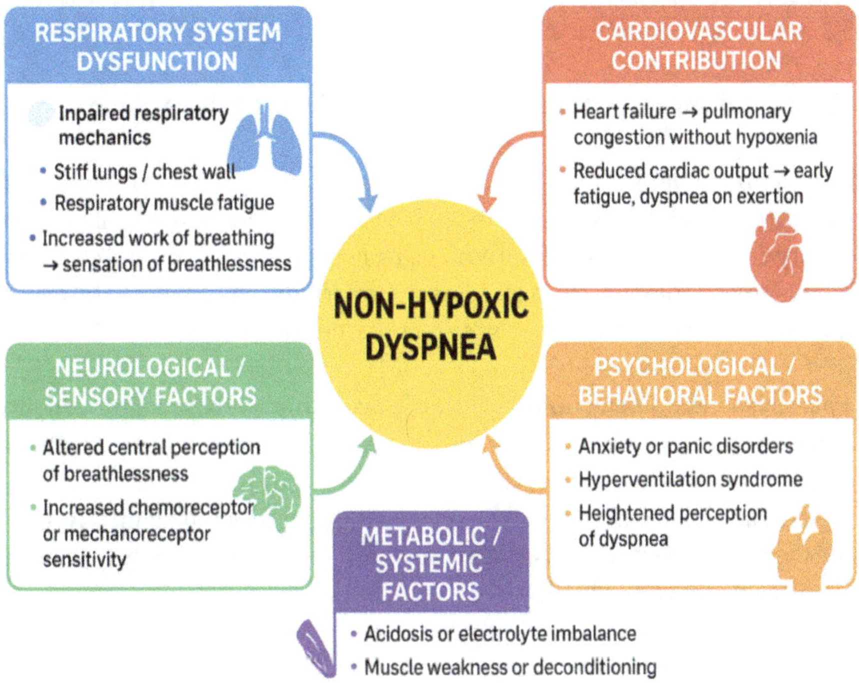

Figure 2 Key Pathophysiological Mechanisms of Non-Hypoxic Dyspnea. The schematic diagram outlines primary contributors across organ systems, including impaired respiratory mechanics, cardiac dysfunction, altered neural perception, systemic factors, and psychological components.

3.1 Mechanisms and Etiology in Geriatric Patients

In older adults, the pathogenesis of NHD include the interplay of age-associated physiological deterioration, comorbid conditions, and cognitive factors.

3.2 Age-Related Physiological Changes

Normal ageing raises the risk of NHD by causing a number of important changes:

Reduced Lung Elastic Recoil: The loss of alveolar elastin fibres makes the lungs less flexible, which makes it harder to exhale (Sharma & Goodwin, 2006).

Increased Chest Wall Stiffness: Calcification of costal cartilage and degeneration of the vertebrae make it harder for the thorax to expand (Janssens, 2005).

Weakness in the respiratory muscles: Sarcopenia causes a 20–30% decline in maximal inspiratory pressure, which makes breathing less efficient (Tolep & Kelsen, 1993).

Decreased Ventilatory Response: Central chemoreceptors exhibit reduced sensitivity to hypercapnia and hypoxia, resulting in altered breathing patterns (Janssens, 2005).

3.3 Comorbidities, Polypharmacy, and Drug Interactions

Multimorbidity heightens NHD risk. Cardiovascular, pulmonary, neurological, and musculoskeletal diseases collectively increase the work of breathing or disrupt respiratory control without necessarily causing hypoxemia (Marengoni et al., 2011).

Polypharmacy complicates management. Prescribing opioids for NHD may have harmful interactions with a patient's current prescription drugs:

1. Pharmacokinetic interactions can result in toxic drug levels, sedation, or delirium when medications such as morphine and benzodiazepines compete for the same liver enzymes.
2. Opioids and other CNS depressants can interact pharmacodynamically, increasing the risk of sedation, falls, cognitive impairment, and respiratory depression (Lauffenburger et al., 2019).

Care can become even more complicated as a result of these interactions, which can set off a "prescribing cascade," in which new medications are prescribed to treat the side effects of others (Rochon & Gurwitz, 2017).

3.4 Neurological Pathways and Dyspnea Perception

A "dyspnea matrix" in the brain processes the sensation:

- Anterior Insula: Combines sensory signals from the respiratory system; too much activity makes breathing feel worse.
- Amygdala: Links dyspnea to fear and anticipatory anxiety (von Leupoldt et al., 2008).
- Anterior Cingulate Cortex: Modulates the emotional and attentional significance of dyspnea.
- Prefrontal Cortex: Governs cognitive appraisal, potentially worsening symptoms through hypervigilance.

This explains the high co-occurrence of NHD and panic symptoms, even without objective respiratory compromise.

3.5 Pathophysiology in Common Terminal Illnesses

- Cancer: Mechanical inhibition of fibrosis or tumor infiltration.
- Chronic Heart Failure: The ventilatory demand is raised by exertional pulmonary congestion.
- COPD: Breathing becomes more difficult due to dynamic hyperinflation caused by air trapping.
- Neurodegenerative diseases: Parkinson's and ALS, for example, impair muscle coordination and central respiratory drive (Parshall et al., 2012).

3.6 Psychological and Systemic Modifiers

The threshold for sensing respiratory discomfort is lowered by anxiety and depression. Muscle fatigue can be brought on by cytokines released by systemic inflammation, which is prevalent in advanced disease (Banzett & Lansing, 2021). By reducing respiratory muscle mass, cachexia exacerbates dyspnea. NHD rarely has a single cause in elderly terminal patients. A multimodal approach to management is required because it is a convergent endpoint of maladaptive neuropsychological processing, specific pathology, and physiological decline.

4. COMPREHENSIVE ASSESSMENT IN PRACTICE

Assessment of NHD must prioritize the patient's subjective experience. In contrast to hypoxic dyspnea, where oxygen saturation easily aids in diagnosis, NHD necessitates meticulous clinical reasoning to differentiate it from various respiratory and non-respiratory etiologies of breathlessness. The goal is to characterize the symptom and identify treatable contributors.

Step 1: Validate and Quantify. Begin by acknowledging the patient's distress. Then, use a simple unidimensional scale such as the 0-10 Numerical Rating Scale (NRS) to establish a baseline (Dudgeon, 2019).

Step 2: Explore the Character and Impact. Ask about triggers, relieving factors, and the functional and affective impact: "How does this breathlessness stop you from doing what is important to you?"

Step 3: Focused Physical Exam and Selective Investigations. The exam aims to identify comorbid factors exacerbating NHD, such as pleural effusions or anemia. Pulse oximetry is used to rule out hypoxemia, confirming the diagnosis of NHD. The key is to avoid over-investigation while remaining alert to potentially manageable contributors.

4.1 Principles of Clinical Assessment

A good NHD assessment should include subjective symptom reporting, objective physiological measures, and an evaluation of functional performance. The primary goal is to characterize the severity and impact of breathlessness and identify contributing factors to guide a targeted management plan (Bausewein et al., 2021).

4.1.1 Patient-Reported Measures

In palliative care, self-report instruments continue to be the gold standard for measuring dyspnea. Validated tools are essential for quantifying symptoms and monitoring response to therapy (Dudgeon, 2019).

1. Unidimensional Scales: These are ideal for rapid clinical assessment. The Numerical Rating Scale (NRS) or Visual Analogue Scale (VAS) quickly capture breathlessness intensity at rest or during activity. This tool is particularly helpful for patients who have low literacy or cognitive impairment. The Modified Borg Scale (0–10) is also useful for measuring perceived exertion and breathlessness at any given time.
2. Multidimensional Tools: For a more comprehensive evaluation, instruments like the Dyspnea-12 Questionnaire capture both the physical sensation and the affective distress (e.g., fear, anxiety) associated with breathlessness, providing a fuller picture of its impact (Yorke et al., 2010).
3. Functional Scales: Activity limitation is evaluated using The Medical Research Council (MRC) Dyspnea Scale (Grades 1–5), which ranges from intense exertion (Grade 1) to the inability to leave the house (Grade 5).

4.1.2 Functional Performance and Clinical Investigation

Functional assessment contextualizes symptom severity but must be adapted for frail patients. While the Six-Minute Walk Test (6MWT) is standardized, it is often impractical; a more relevant alternative is evaluating limitations in Activities of Daily Living (ADLs), such as washing or dressing.

Objective investigations like pulse oximetry and chest imaging are crucial, but their role is primarily to exclude hypoxemia and other reversible causes (e.g., pleural effusion). In NHD, the absence of significant objective findings should direct the clinician's focus toward central perception and respiratory mechanics as the principal factors (Parshall et al., 2012).

4.1.3 Differential Diagnosis and Avoiding Pitfalls

Accurate diagnosis requires differentiating NHD from other common causes of breathlessness in palliative populations. The table below summarizes key distinctions

Table 1. Differentiating NHD from Hypoxic dyspnea and anxiety-related dyspnea

Feature	Non-Hypoxic Dyspnea (NHD)	Hypoxic Dyspnea	Anxiety-Related Dyspnea
SpO_2	Normal (≥92%)	Low (<92%)	Normal
Response to Oxygen	Minimal to none	Improves	Minimal (may improve with placebo/ reassurance)
Response to Opioids/Fan	Often improves	Limited primary effect	Variable; may improve if anxiety is component
Associated Signs	Tachypnea, distress	Cyanosis, hypoxemia	Hyperventilation, tachycardia, panic

Common diagnostic pitfalls must be avoided. These include over-relying on SpO_2 to dismiss breathlessness, misattributing NHD purely to psychological causes, being misled by incidental findings on imaging, and failing to assess patients with cognitive or communication barriers effectively (Johnson et al., 2017).

4.1.4 The Role of Interdisciplinary Assessment

An interdisciplinary approach is paramount. Collaboration among palliative medicine, nursing, physiotherapy, and psychology ensures a holistic evaluation of physical and psychosocial factors, facilitates the prompt initiation of combined interventions, and integrates caregiver education and support from the outset (Higginson et al., 2014).

Clinical Insight: The fundamental diagnostic shift in NHD is moving from the question, "Is the patient hypoxic?" to "Why is the patient short of breath despite normal oxygen levels?" This reframing is critical for early recognition and targeted management of this complex syndrome

5. A MULTIMODAL MANAGEMENT FRAMEWORK

Managing non-hypoxic dyspnea (NHD) in elderly patients at the end of life necessitates multimodal, patient-centered approaches that target both physiological mechanisms and the emotional distress linked to breathlessness. Management follows a stepped-care model, starting with non-pharmacological strategies and adding pharmacological agents as needed. Interventions must commence solely following a systematic evaluation that verifies the absence of hypoxemia and delineates contributing factors. Clinical decisions ought to be informed by the severity of symptoms, their functional implications, and patient preferences.

5.1 Non-Pharmacological Interventions (First-Line)

Mechanism: Directing cool air to the trigeminal nerve area makes it less likely that you will feel short of breath.

- **Fan Therapy:** A handheld fan directed to the cheek provides significant relief by stimulating trigeminal nerve receptors (Kako et al., 2018). Use a handheld fan or a bedside fan that is 6 to 12 inches away from the face during episodes or all the time as needed.
- **Breathing Techniques:** Pursed-lip breathing slows down the breathing rate and keeps the airway pressure high. Diaphragmatic breathing helps with good ventilation and keeps accessory muscles from getting tired. Pursed-lip breathing and diaphragmatic breathing can slow respiratory rate and impart a sense of control (Spathis et al., 2017).
- **Positioning and Body Mechanics**: The high Fowler's position makes the diaphragm move better. Sitting with your arms forward and leaning forward makes it easier to breathe by stabilizing accessory muscles. Lying on your side with your head raised—good for people who are stuck in bed. Activity pacing conserves energy.
- **Psychosocial and Relaxation Techniques:** Guided imagery, mindfulness meditation, and music therapy can lessen the emotional distress part of NHD.

5.2 Pharmacological Management

- **Opioids – First-Line Therapy**

Low-dose systemic opioids mitigate the central perception of dyspnea through μ-opioid receptor modulation in the brainstem, without markedly diminishing respiratory drive when titrated correctly (e.g., morphine 2.5-5 mg orally every 4 hours as needed) (Currow et al., 2020). This reduces the central perception of breathlessness. Numerous randomized controlled trials (RCTs) indicate substantial alleviation of dyspnea with oral morphine in advanced disease, irrespective of hypoxemia.

a) Beginning Protocol:

   i. Elderly people who have never taken opioids: 2.5–5 mg of morphine sulfate by mouth every four hours.
   ii. If you have kidney problems, start with half of the usual dose.

b) Titration: Raise by 25% every 24 to 48 hours, depending on how well the patient feels and how well they can handle it.

c) Monitor: the rate of breathing, the level of sedation, and the adherence to the bowel regimen.

   - **Benzodiazepines (Second-Line):** These should not be first-line for dyspnea itself. They may be considered as a short-term adjunct for refractory anxiety, but must be used cautiously in the elderly (Simon et al., 2016).

5.3 Risks of Inappropriate Opioid Use in the Management of NHD

The use of low-dose opioids for non-hypoxic dyspnea (NHD) in palliative care, while effective, carries significant risks, especially for frail, elderly patients. Inappropriate use can lead to serious adverse effects, primarily involving the central nervous system and gastrointestinal tract. The most formidable risk is respiratory depression, particularly in opioid-naïve patients or those with comorbidities like COPD. Excessive sedation, confusion, and delirium can severely diminish quality of life, while predictable constipation and nausea require proactive management.

- These risks are amplified by polypharmacy and renal impairment. Concomitant use of opioids with other CNS depressants creates a dangerous synergistic effect. Furthermore, in patients with renal disease, morphine metabolites can accumulate, leading to toxicity; guidelines recommend safer alternatives like fentanyl or buprenorphine in such cases.
- Mitigation hinges on a structured protocol: "start low and go slow" with dosing, conduct vigilant monitoring for sedation, implement prophylactic bowel regimens, and perform comprehensive medication reviews. By adhering to these evidence-based strategies, clinicians can safely harness the benefits of opioids to relieve suffering without introducing preventable harm.

5.4 Adjuvant Pharmacotherapy, Psychosocial and Relaxation Techniques

- **Anxiolytics:** Lorazepam 0.5–1 mg SL PRN for acute anxiety-induced dyspnea episodes (avoid regular scheduled dosing to prevent sedation accumulation).

- **Corticosteroids:** Dexamethasone 4–8 mg daily for inflammatory airway obstruction or lymphangitic carcinomatosis.
- **Nebulized agents:** Lidocaine or opioids for episodic dyspnea—consider only if other measures fail.
- Guided imagery, mindfulness meditation, and music therapy can lessen the emotional distress part of NHD.

For patients who are not hypoxemic, supplemental oxygen (oxygen therapy) provides no greater benefit than medical air (Abernethy et al., 2010). Oxygen should be prescribed based on documented hypoxemia ($SpO_2 < 90\%$), not the presence of dyspnea alone.

5.5 Clinical Algorithm for Non-Hypoxic Dyspnea in Terminal Care

Managing non-hypoxic dyspnea (NHD) in terminally ill elderly patients is particularly problematic due to its complex aetiology, variable symptom perception, and common comorbidities. Hypoxic dyspnea is primarily induced by oxygen deficiency, whereas NHD is predominantly attributed to neuromuscular, metabolic, or psychological causes. A standardised clinical algorithm enables healthcare providers methodically check, treat, and check again how patients are reacting. This helps reduce symptoms and enhance quality of life (QoL). The proposed algorithm integrates contemporary evidence-based pharmacological and non-pharmacological interventions, emphasises the significance of interdisciplinary evaluation, and incorporates patient-centered decision-making. The goal is to provide a helpful, step-by-step guide that may be used in many different types of terminal care settings, like oncology, cardiology, and respiratory care units.

Stepwise Clinical Approach

Step 1: Initial Assessment

The first thing to do for someone with dyspnea is to find out what is causing it and how bad it is. This two-pronged approach sets the stage for both making quick decisions and keeping an eye on symptoms over time. Outcomes reported by patients are highly crucial to this process. You can use proven measures like the Numerical Rating Scale (NRS), the Modified Borg Dyspnea Scale, or the Visual Analogue Scale (VAS) to find out how bad and how often you feel short of breath. These steps not only assist patients and doctors talk to one other, but they also let you understand how things evolve over time. A thorough clinical assessment is just as important. This entails a comprehensive medical history and physical examination, emphasising comorbidities such as congestive heart failure, chronic obstructive pulmonary disease, or neurological illnesses, which may exacerbate or induce dyspnea. It is crucial to thoroughly go over prescription profiles to locate medicines that could make breathing problems worse. Any recent decline in functional capacity should be recorded as a potential indicator of disease development. Diagnostic evaluations must be targeted and minimally invasive, aiming to eliminate acute and reversible causes. You may need a chest X-ray or echocardiogram, as well as lab testing for electrolytes, renal function, and B-type natriuretic peptide (BNP). These tools reveal essential information that can assist discern the difference between chronic, non-hypoxic dyspnea and diseases that need prompt treatment. Doctors and nurses also need to look for warning indications. If you suddenly have a lot of trouble breathing, a fever, haemoptysis, or chest pain, you should check for serious illnesses such hypoxaemia, pulmonary embolism, or infection.

Decision Point: If the root cause of dyspnea is determined to be reversible or acute, targeted treatment must be commenced without delay. However, when dyspnea continues without hypoxemia and no reversible cause is found, the care pathway should move on to the next stage of treatment, which should focus on long-term control and symptom relief.

Step 2: Symptom Classification and Risk Stratification

When evaluating non-hypoxic dyspnea (NHD), the emphasis should be on assessing the severity of symptoms and investigating the possible underlying causes. Determining the extent of symptom burden enables clinicians to customize interventions effectively, while recognizing causative factors guarantees that management strategies encompass the complete spectrum of influences on the patient's experience.

There are three main groups of severity levels. People with mild NHD have occasional episodes of shortness of breath that don't make them very uncomfortable, and they usually feel fine when they are resting. Moderate NHD happens when shortness of breath starts to get in the way of daily activities and needs regular monitoring and care. Severe NHD is the most severe level, and it is characterized by constant shortness of breath while at rest, which is often accompanied by significant psychological distress or anxiety. This stratification gives doctors and nurses a way to make clinical decisions and talk to patients and their families.

Along with grading severity, doctors need to think about a lot of other things that could cause or make NHD worse. Neurological disorders, including stroke, Parkinson's disease, or cognitive decline, can modify both the physiological and perceptual aspects of breathlessness. Psychological factors, such as anxiety and depression, are also important because dyspnea may get worse when a person is about to do something hard or stressful. Metabolic disorders make things even more complicated. Conditions like hyperthyroidism, anemia, kidney problems, or electrolyte imbalances can all make the feeling of not being able to breathe worse.

By combining severity grading with an assessment of the cause, doctors can get a full picture of the patient's condition. This makes sure that future management strategies are both focused and broad.

Table 2. Clinical assessment of Non-Hypoxic Dyspnea (NHD): Severity and contributing factors

Severity Level	Definition	Clinical Characteristics	Common Contributing Factors
Mild NHD	Dyspnea occurs intermittently; minimal discomfort	Patient is comfortable at rest; breathlessness limited to exertion	Psychological stress, mild anemia, early metabolic imbalance
Moderate NHD	Dyspnea interferes with daily activities	Requires consistent monitoring and supportive measures; reduced exercise tolerance	Anxiety, depression, neurological conditions (early Parkinson's, mild cognitive impairment)
Severe NHD	Persistent breathlessness, even at rest	Significant distress and/ or anxiety; may impair communication and quality of life	Advanced neurological disease, severe metabolic derangements (renal failure, electrolyte imbalance), progressive anemia

Step 3: Non-Pharmacological Interventions

The main goal of managing dyspnea is to make the patient as comfortable as possible while avoiding both physical and mental triggers. Positioning is very important in this process. Patients should be encouraged to stand or take a semi-Fowler's position, as these positions help the lungs expand and make breathing easier.

Interventions that improve airflow can also help with shortness of breath. For example, pointing a hand-held fan at the patient's face or making sure the room is well-ventilated can help a lot. Certain breathing exercises can also help patients deal with their symptoms. You can get more oxygen and feel less out of breath by breathing through pursed lips and practicing diaphragmatic breathing. It's just as important to make the space around you supportive. Efforts should be made to lessen stressors and create a calm, soothing environment, since stress in the environment can make dyspnea worse. These interventions are even better when they are combined with psychological support. Patients can use cognitive behavioral strategies or relaxation exercises to deal with shortness of breath caused by anxiety, which will make them more comfortable overall.

Last but not least, it is important to check on the patient again in 24 to 48 hours. If the symptoms have not improved or have worsened, further intervention is necessary, and the care plan should progress to the next step in managing persistent dyspnea.

Step 4: Pharmacological Management

The objective of pharmacological management of dyspnea is to utilize evidence-based therapies customized to the severity of symptoms and the patient's comorbid conditions. This method uses opioids as the first line of treatment. Careful titration of low-dose morphine or an equivalent opioid is done to relieve symptoms, especially in patients with kidney or liver problems. Other drugs may be used along with opioids depending on what is causing the shortness of breath. Benzodiazepines can help when anxiety makes breathing problems worse, and low-dose corticosteroids can help when inflammation makes breathing problems worse. Oxygen therapy is not something that is done all the time; it is only done in rare cases of hypoxia.

These drugs are titrated in a careful, step-by-step way. The treatment starts with a low dose, and the patient's response is checked again every 24 to 48 hours. The amount of medicine is changed based on how well it works to relieve symptoms and how well the patient can handle it. If the patient gets enough relief, maintenance therapy continues. If dyspnea continues or if negative effects arise, additional interventions are required, necessitating advancement to the subsequent phase of the management protocol.

Step 5: Interdisciplinary Review and Advanced Planning

The major purpose of multidisciplinary management is to improve patient care by combining expertise from nursing, palliative care, and psychosocial support. One key method is to arrange regular interdisciplinary conferences where healthcare experts, like doctors, nurses, physical therapists, and psychiatrists, work together to talk about tough situations and share ideas. This way of working together makes sure that all the data are used to make care decisions. Another crucial feature is advanced care planning, which makes ensuring that medical treatments fit with the patient's personal objectives, preferences, and cultural values. By taking care of these problems ahead of time, healthcare teams can offer treatment that is both patient-centered and morally right. For severe non-hypoxic dyspnea that doesn't respond to normal therapies, palliative sedation and other escalation methods may be used. But ethics boards need to keep a close eye on these kinds of interventions to ensure sure they are done correctly and in line with both clinical guidelines and the patient's wishes.

5.5.1 Reassessment Loop

Iterative evaluation is a key part of managing dyspnea well. Check the symptoms every 24 to 48 hours to see how bad they are, how they affect your quality of life, and if they could have any bad implications. This constant monitoring lets doctors know if the present drug and non-drug treatments are working. These evaluations ought to guide any requisite adjustments to care plans. Non-pharmacological techniques, such as breathing exercises or positioning, can be used with pharmaceutical treatments, such as opioids or adjuvant medicines, to help with symptoms and make patients more comfortable. It is just as crucial to write down how patients respond in a systematic way. Keeping a systematic record of these observations helps with both continuity of care and making therapeutic decisions in the future. This way, treatment stays focused, effective, and sensitive to the patient's changing needs.

Table 3. Intervention summary

Step	Action	Key Considerations	Reassess
1	Initial Assessment	Exclude acute reversible causes	24h
2	Symptom Classification	Determine severity & contributing factors	24–48h
3	Non-Pharmacological Interventions	Positioning, airflow, breathing, psychological support	24–48h
4	Pharmacological Management	Opioids, adjuvants, titration	24–48h
5	Interdisciplinary Review	Advanced planning, palliative escalation	Ongoing

The suggested clinical protocol offers a systematic, evidence-based approach to managing non-hypoxic dyspnea in elderly dying patients. Healthcare personnel can considerably improve a patient's comfort and quality of life by using a combination of symptom evaluation, non-drug therapy, judicious drug usage, and monitoring from several fields. The algorithm's effectiveness continues to rely on iterative evaluation and patient-centered decision-making. Future validation studies are essential to assess outcomes, enhance stepwise therapies, and ensure applicability across diverse therapeutic settings.

Figure 3. A palliative care management algorithm for non-hypoxic dyspnea

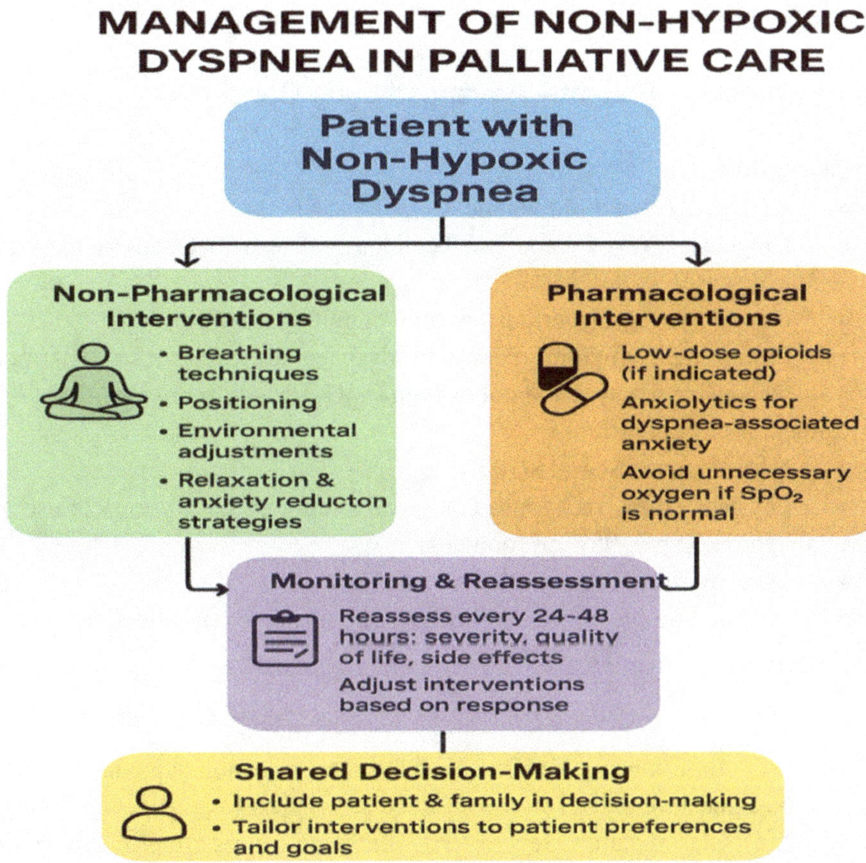

Figure 3 A Palliative Care Management Algorithm for Non-Hypoxic Dyspnea. This schematic outlines a patient-centered approach, from initial assessment through the application of non-pharmacological and pharmacological interventions, emphasizing continuous monitoring and shared decision-making to alleviate suffering and improve quality of life.

5.6 Case Vignettes

Case vignettes offer pragmatic examples of the manifestation of non-hypoxic dyspnea (NHD) in terminally ill patients and illustrate the implementation of the clinical algorithm formulated. Two illustrative cases—one pertaining to oncology and the other, cardiopulmonary issues—underscore the heterogeneity of NHD presentations, the complexities in evaluation, and the necessity for multidisciplinary management approaches. These examples combine drug and non-drug treatments, with a focus on patient-centered care, ongoing evaluation, and improving quality of life.

Case 1: Oncology Patient – Advanced Lung Cancer

Patient Profile:

- Age/Sex: 72-year-old female
- Diagnosis: Stage IV non-small cell lung cancer with extensive metastatic disease
- Comorbidities: Hypertension, mild cognitive impairment
- Presenting Symptom: Persistent dyspnea at rest (NRS 8/10), non-responsive to supplemental oxygen (SpO_2 95% on room air)

Clinical Assessment:

- VAS Dyspnea Score: 8/10
- Physical exam: Tachypnea (28 breaths/min), accessory muscle use, no hypoxia (SpO_2 95% on room air)
- Labs: Within normal limits; no infection
- Imaging: Stable pulmonary metastases; no acute consolidation

Management Using the Algorithm:

Step 1: Assessment: Verified that dyspnea was not hypoxic; recorded baseline severity.

Step 2: Classification: Severe NHD; the main causes are probably neuromuscular and anxiety-related.

Step 3: Non-drug treatments: Semi-Fowler's positioning and bedside fan.

Sitting up straight and using a fan at the bedside
Breathing exercises and ways to relax

Step 4: Pharmacological Interventions:

Started low-dose oral morphine at 2.5 mg every 4 hours and increased it over 48 hrs. Then added lorazepam at 0.5 mg for dyspnea related to anxiety

Step 5: Interdisciplinary Review: Daily rounds by the palliative care team

Keeping in touch with the patient and their family about goals and expectations
Outcome:

- After 48 hours, VAS dyspnea went down to 4/10.
- Better able to join in on conversations and do light activities
- No major negative effects related to opioids were seen

Teaching Points: Case 1

- **Clinical Lessons:**

1. A normal SpO_2 does not rule out severe, treatable dyspnea.
2. Low-dose opioids are first-line pharmacological therapy for NHD, even in opioid-naïve patients.
3. Anxiety is a common amplifier of NHD; combined management of breathlessness and anxiety is often necessary.

- **Common Pitfalls to Avoid:**

1. Continuing ineffective oxygen therapy, which can dry mucous membranes and provide no benefit.
2. Withholding opioids due to unfounded fear of hastening death, thereby allowing preventable suffering.

- **Interdisciplinary Roles:**
    - Physician/Nurse Practitioner: Prescribe and titrate opioids/anxiolytics.
    - Nurse: Administer medications, coach on breathing techniques, and provide continuous symptom assessment.
    - Palliative Care Specialist: Manage complex symptoms and support primary team.
    - Family/Caregiver: Operate fan, provide calming presence, and report symptom changes.

Discussion:

This case exemplifies the multifactorial characteristics of NHD in oncology patients and underscores the necessity of integrating non-pharmacological interventions with meticulously titrated opioids and anxiolytics. Iterative assessment and patient-centered communication helped ease symptoms and keep dignity at the end of life.

Case 2: Cardiopulmonary Patient – Advanced Heart Failure

Patient Profile:

- Age/Sex: 78-year-old male

- Diagnosis: End-stage congestive heart failure (NYHA Class IV)
- Comorbidities: Type 2 diabetes, chronic kidney disease (stage 3)
- Presenting Symptom: Dyspnea at rest, unrelieved by standard oxygen therapy

Clinical Assessment:

- NRS Dyspnea Score: 7/10
- Physical exam: Mild peripheral edema, no hypoxemia (SpO_2 96% on room air)
- Labs: Mild renal impairment, stable electrolytes
- Imaging: Cardiomegaly, no acute pulmonary edema

Management Using the Algorithm:

Step 1: Assessment: ruled out reversible acute causes like infection and pulmonary embolism.

Step 2: Classification: Moderate NHD; contributing factors: cardiac deconditioning and anxiety.

Step 3: Non-drug treatments: Point 1- Semi-Fowler's positioning with pillows. Point 2- Hand-held fan therapy; ways to save energy. Point 3- Guided diaphragmatic breathing exercises.

Step 4: Drug treatments:

2 mg of oral morphine every 6 hours, with careful adjustment of the dose for the kidneys

Thought about taking lorazepam in small doses for anxiety, but was careful because of their age and the fact that they were taking multiple medications.

Step 5: Review by people from different fields:

Teams from cardiology, palliative care, nursing, and physiotherapy worked together

The family talked about care priorities and possible palliative sedation if the patient was not responding to treatment.

Outcome:

After 72 hours, NRS dropped to 3/10

The patient said they felt less anxious and more comfortable sitting up

There was no major hypotension or sedation.

Teaching Points: Case 2

- **Clinical Lessons:**

1. NHD is a major symptom in end-stage heart failure and can be effectively managed with the same principles used in oncology.
2. Renal function must be checked before initiating morphine; consider fentanyl for significant impairment.

3. Fan therapy and positioning are highly effective, low-risk first steps.

- **Common Pitfalls to Avoid:**

1. Failing to adjust the opioid choice or dose for renal function, leading to toxicity.
2. Overlooking simple non-pharmacological measures in favor of complex drug regimens.

- **Interdisciplinary Roles:**
    - **Physician:** Select renal-safe opioids and manage heart failure medications.
    - **Nurse:** Monitor for opioid toxicity (e.g., sedation) and provide family education.
    - **Physiotherapist:** Teach energy conservation and breathing techniques.
    - **Cardiologist:** Advise on optimal management of the underlying cardiac disease alongside palliative goals.

Discussion:

This case highlights the algorithm's effectiveness in patients with substantial comorbidities and polypharmacy. Focusing on non-drug treatments first and then carefully adjusting drug doses later reduced risks and made it easier to control symptoms. Interdisciplinary collaboration facilitated comprehensive care in accordance with patient objectives.

6. IMPACT OF NON-HYPOXIC DYSPNEA ON QUALITY OF LIFE

Non-hypoxic dyspnea (NHD) significantly and variably deteriorates the quality of life (QoL) of elderly patients in terminal care, representing a multifaceted bio-psychosocial challenge that extends beyond physical manifestations, fundamentally transforming life trajectories and imposing substantial burdens on carers.

6.1 Physical and Functional Burden

NHD systematically restricts even the most fundamental activities of daily living (ADLs), resulting in a progressive erosion of independence that significantly impacts patients' autonomy. Clinical observations consistently reveal patients grappling with fundamental activities, including ambulation over short distances, eating, or maintaining uninterrupted conversation. This physical limitation speeds up deconditioning by creating a harmful feedback loop in which less activity leads to muscle and cardiovascular deterioration, which makes the feeling of breathlessness worse. In terminal care settings where comfort and autonomy are paramount, the physical constraints associated with NHD often surpass other symptoms in their effect on daily functioning and perceived quality of life.

6.2 Psychological and Emotional Impact

The distressing sensation of air hunger, despite normal oxygen saturation, elicits profound psychological responses mediated through limbic system circuitry. This neurological engagement causes strong fear responses, which often show up as anxiety disorders, panic attacks, and clinically significant depressive symptoms. The psychological effect works through a number of ways that make it stronger:

- Heightened anxiety due to anticipatory fear, leading patients to engage in avoidance behaviors regarding activities that could trigger dyspnea episodes.
- A depressive burden resulting from the gradual erosion of autonomy and opportunities for social engagement
- Emotional trauma that affects more than just the patients, as caregivers often feel helpless when they see uncontrolled dyspnea episodes.

The psychological aspects of NHD necessitate systematic evaluation and intervention, as unmitigated emotional distress considerably exacerbates the subjective sensation of breathlessness.

6.3 Spiritual and Existential Dimensions

Modern NHD management knows how important it is to link physical breathlessness with existential distress. More and more evidence supports integrated approaches that deal with both physical and spiritual pain. This is because unaddressed existential issues make dyspnea feel worse by making people anxious. A structured spiritual care framework has four main parts:

1. A structured spiritual evaluation employing validated screening enquiries to identify distress and transform ambiguous concerns into explicit clinical objectives.
2. Working together across disciplines makes formal referral paths to board-certified chaplains, with clear differences in roles.
3. Making decisions together about treatment that fits with the patient's goals and values

4. More general outcome measures that include both physical and non-physical indicators of dignity and spiritual well-being

This integrated approach elevates spiritual care from a marginal issue to a fundamental element, producing significant advantages in breaking the cyclical link between existential distress and the interpretation of physical symptoms.

6.4 Social Consequences and Isolation

NHD makes it hard for people to accomplish activities with other people in a lot of different ways. Patients frequently eschew familial gatherings, religious ceremonies, and community functions due to concerns regarding public episodes of dyspnea. People who are more socially disengaged have weaker relationships and a lower sense of self, which makes them feel more alone in both real and mental ways. Patients in their last months have a difficult time because of environmental restrictions, like not being able to walk stairs or use public transport. This renders them physically isolated, which makes their emotional distress worse. The social impacts of NHD are an important area for treatments since keeping social relationships strong can help protect against the emotional effects of deteriorating symptoms.

6.5 Caregiver Burden and Support Needs

When caring for patients with NHD, caregivers face many different kinds of problems, such as:

- Emotional burden: anticipatory grief, constant worry about managing symptoms, and psychological trauma from seeing someone with respiratory distress
- Practical problems: more hours of caregiving, always being on the lookout, and the need to learn clinical skills like how to give opioids and how to position patients.
- Psychological impact: Role strain, sleep disruption, and social isolation arising from intensive care demands.

Structured interventions, such as anticipatory guidance, psychological support, and respite care provision, show that they are very effective at lowering the burden on caregivers and making them more resilient. The establishment of systematic caregiver support programs is a crucial element of holistic NHD management.

6.6 Evidence Base and Patient-Reported Outcomes

Studies utilizing patient-reported outcome measures (PROMs) consistently rank NHD as one of the most distressing terminal symptoms, with an impact analogous to that of severe pain. Key findings from palliative care research include: a significant reduction in quality of life (QoL) scores on standardized measures, such as the EORTC QLQ-C15-PAL, among patients with non-hospice dyspnea (NHD) compared to non-dyspneic counterparts, even after adjusting for comorbidities (Higginson et al., 2013).

- A link between NHD in the last week of life and higher caregiver distress scores during grieving (Ekström et al., 2015)
- Patients often experience significant benefits from even minor symptom relief, allowing them to re-engage in valued activities such as conversation, meal participation, and rest without fear.

Clinical experience consistently shows that NHD relief leads to quick and big improvements in quality of life (QoL), which shows how important it is to manage symptoms aggressively even when the disease is advanced.

7. ETHICAL AND COMMUNICATION FRAMEWORK

7.1 Ethical Foundations in NHD Care

Effective NHD management requires grounding in four essential ethical principles:

1. **Respect for Autonomy:** Upholding older patients' right to make decisions about treatments, including opioid initiation, non-drug therapies, and end-of-life preferences. This requires explaining benefits, risks, and limitations in clear, non-technical language.
2. **Beneficence and Non-maleficence:** Balancing symptom relief against the risks of over-treatment (e.g., unnecessary oxygen) or under-treatment (e.g., opioid hesitancy) through careful titration and continuous monitoring.
3. **Justice:** Addressing disparities in access to effective NHD management, particularly in underserved populations or resource-limited settings where palliative expertise is unavailable.
4. **Dignity:** Acknowledging the whole person by providing care that addresses physical, psychological, and spiritual suffering.

7.2 Communication Principles and Shared Decision-Making

Therapeutic communication begins with empathically acknowledging the distress of breathlessness despite normal oxygen levels. Key strategies include:

- Building trust by validating symptom legitimacy.
- Using shared decision-making to present options with a balanced discussion of impacts on comfort and function.
- Eliciting patient values to align care with personal priorities.
- Documenting agreed-upon plans to ensure consistency across settings and providers.

This approach is vital for navigating trade-offs, such as between symptom control and cognitive preservation, allowing patients to define their preferred balance.

7.3 Cultural and Linguistic Considerations

Cultural competence requires understanding how language and culture shape symptom experience and treatment acceptance. Essential practices are:

- Employing professional interpreters to overcome language barriers.
- Recognizing how cultural beliefs—such as opioid hesitancy or spiritual interpretations of breathlessness—influence care.
- Incorporating culturally significant practices into care plans to enhance comfort and validate identity.
- Acknowledging culturally influenced caregiver needs and experiences.

7.4 Caregiver Education and Support

Caregivers are very important for managing NHD, so they need a lot of training and help. Effective caregiver preparation includes:

- Structured training in early symptom recognition and crisis management
- Mastery of both pharmacological and non-pharmacological intervention techniques
- Access to 24-hour support services for emergency guidance
- Regular assessment of caregiver burden with appropriate respite provision

8. CLINICAL PRACTICE RECOMMENDATIONS

8.1 Standardized Assessment and Protocol Implementation

To manage NHD well, you need to use standardized methods in a planned way:

- Regular use of validated dyspnea assessment tools (Modified Borg Scale, NRS, VAS) in clinical practice
- Clear documentation in electronic health records that separates hypoxic from non-hypoxic dyspnea
- Using step-by-step management protocols that stress non-drug first-line treatments
- Careful titration of opioids with proper monitoring and oversight from multiple disciplines
- Creating clinical decision supports like flowcharts and checklists for different care settings

8.2 Interdisciplinary Collaboration

For NHD management to work, different fields need to work together:

- Regular team rounds with doctors, nurses, rehabilitation specialists, psychologists, and spiritual care providers;
- Early inclusion of palliative care specialists in management planning;
- Clear role definitions and communication pathways between team members;
- Cross-training between palliative specialists and generalists to make sure that protocols are followed in all settings.

8.3 Education and Professional Development

Structured educational strategies are necessary for clinician competence development:

- Full training modules that cover NHD pathophysiology, assessment, and evidence-based interventions
- Interprofessional workshops that cover coordinated symptom management, ethical decision-making, and cultural competence
- Regular updates that include new evidence from major clinical trials and journals

- Simulation-based training that uses scenarios from oncology, cardiopulmonary, and geriatric settings
- The creation of professional learning communities for ongoing skill development

8.4 Policy and Resource Allocation

System-level support is necessary for long-term NHD management:

- Institutional requirements for routine NHD screening and management in terminal care
- Development of safe opioid prescribing guidelines with appropriate monitoring systems
- Fair distribution of resources to make sure that essential equipment (fans, positioning aids) is always available
- Aligning hospital accreditation standards with NHD management protocols
- Advocacy for inclusion of NHD management in national palliative and geriatric care guidelines

8.5 Implementation Framework

There is a set way to follow for successful protocol implementation:

1. Adjusting clinical algorithms to fit the needs of the local population and resources
2. Staff training in stages that includes simulation-based training
3. Ongoing quality improvement using patient-reported outcome measures
4. Making NHD management standards official through policy development
5. Institutional research projects that look at how well protocols work and help improve them

9. CONCLUSION

Non-hypoxic dyspnea (NHD) is a very difficult condition to deal with towards the end of life. It is when a person feels short of breath even though their oxygen saturation is normal. As this chapter has made clear, effectively managing NHD necessitates a fundamental shift from a disease-centered to a person-centred paradigm. The research compiled here leads to one important conclusion: the best care is provided through a standardised, dual-pathway approach that carefully tackles the physical impression of dyspnea while also reducing its existential and spiritual effects.

This approach is put into action through a few main ideas: using systematic assessments with patient-reported outcome measures; managing care in steps that focus on non-drug treatments and carefully adjusted low-dose opioids; and working together across disciplines to include palliative medicine, nursing, psychosocial, and spiritual care. The effectiveness of any clinical algorithm hinges on its integration within a framework of patient-centered and ethical care, founded on shared decision-making, cultural humility, and proactive communication.

Even with these improvements, there are still many chances to be had. Future endeavours should focus on addressing critical research deficiencies, especially in elucidating the specific processes of NHD and assessing the effectiveness of innovative therapies. In clinical practice, it is essential to convert evidence into practice by broadly applying standardised protocols and improving training for frontline physicians. Lastly, policy and innovation must help these efforts by encouraging the creation of new technology and making sure that everyone has equal access to full, respectful treatment. Following these recommendations will help us make sure that NHD management always meets the main purpose of palliative care: to ease suffering and uphold the person's dignity until the very end.

REFERENCES

Abernethy, A. P., Currow, D. C., Frith, P., Fazekas, B. S., McHugh, A., & Bui, C. (2003). Randomised, double blind, placebo controlled trial of sustained release morphine for the management of refractory dyspnea. *BMJ (Clinical Research Ed.)*, *327*(7414), 523–528. DOI: 10.1136/bmj.327.7414.523

Abernethy, A. P., McDonald, C. F., Frith, P. A., Clark, K., Herndon, J. E., Marcello, J., Young, I. H., Bull, J., Wilcock, A., Booth, S., Wheeler, J. L., Tulsky, J. A., Crockett, A. J., & Currow, D. C. (2010). Effect of palliative oxygen versus room air in relief of breathlessness in patients with refractory dyspnea: A double-blind, randomised controlled trial. *Lancet*, *376*(9743), 784–793. DOI: 10.1016/S0140-6736(10)61115-4

American Thoracic Society. (2012). An official American Thoracic Society statement: Update on the mechanisms, assessment, and management of dyspnea. [Note: This reference is formatted with the organizational author and the lead editor] [Parshall] [listed in the in-text citation, as per APA guidelines for edited works.]. *American Journal of Respiratory and Critical Care Medicine*, *185*(4), 435–452. DOI: 10.1164/rccm.201111-2042ST

Argyropoulou, P., Patakas, D., Koukou, A., Vasiliadis, P., & Georgopoulos, D. (1993). Buspirone effect on breathlessness and exercise performance in patients with chronic obstructive pulmonary disease. *Respiration*, *60*(4), 216–220. DOI: 10.1159/000196204

Banzett, R. B., & Lansing, R. W. (2021). Air hunger: A primal sensation and a primary element of dyspnea. *Comprehensive Physiology*, *11*(2), 1449–1483. DOI: 10.1002/cphy.c200001

Barnes-Harris, M., Allcroft, S., & Johnson, M. J. (2019). Opioids for the palliation of refractory breathlessness in adults with advanced disease and terminal illness. *Cochrane Database of Systematic Reviews*, *2019*(6), CD011008. Advance online publication. DOI: 10.1002/14651858.CD011008.pub3

Bausewein, C., Booth, S., & Higginson, I. J. (2021). Measurement of dyspnea in the clinical rather than the research setting. *Current Opinion in Supportive and Palliative Care*, *2*(2), 95–99. DOI: 10.1097/SPC.0b013e3282fec4c5

Booth, S., Kelly, M. J., Cox, N. P., Adams, L., & Guz, A. (1996). Does oxygen help dyspnea in patients with cancer? *American Journal of Respiratory and Critical Care Medicine*, *153*(5), 1515–1518. DOI: 10.1164/ajrccm.153.5.8630592

Booth, S., Moffat, C., Burkin, J., Galbraith, S., & Bausewein, C. (2018). Nonpharmacological interventions for breathlessness. *Current Opinion in Supportive and Palliative Care, 12*(3), 227–235. DOI: 10.1097/SPC.0000000000000362

Brighton, L. J., Miller, S., Farquhar, M., Booth, S., Yi, D., Gao, W., & Maddocks, M. (2019). Holistic services for people with advanced disease and chronic breathlessness: A systematic review and meta-analysis. *Thorax, 74*(3), 270–281. DOI: 10.1136/thoraxjnl-2018-211589

Campbell, M. L., Templin, T., & Walch, J. (2010). A Respiratory Distress Observation Scale for patients unable to self-report dyspnea. *Journal of Palliative Medicine, 13*(3), 285–290. DOI: 10.1089/jpm.2009.0229

Corner, J., Plant, H., A'Hern, R., & Bailey, C. (1996). Non-pharmacological intervention for breathlessness in lung cancer. *Palliative Medicine, 10*(4), 299–305. DOI: 10.1177/026921639601000405

Currow, D. C., Agar, M., & Abernethy, A. P. (2009). Tackling the challenge of breathlessness in advanced disease. *Progress in Palliative Care, 17*(4), 183–189.

Currow, D. C., Ekström, M., & Abernethy, A. P. (2020). Opioids for chronic refractory breathlessness: Patient predictors of beneficial response. *The European Respiratory Journal, 56*(4), 2002021. DOI: 10.1183/13993003.02021-2020

Davidson, P. M., & Johnson, M. J. (2011). The use of palliative oxygen in advanced disease. *Progress in Palliative Care, 19*(2), 66–71.

Dudgeon, D. (2019). Dyspnea, death rattle, and cough. In *Oxford Textbook of Palliative Medicine* (6th ed., pp. 340–355). Oxford University Press.

Ekström, M. P., Abernethy, A. P., & Currow, D. C. (2015). The management of chronic breathlessness in patients with advanced and terminal illness. *BMJ (Clinical Research Ed.), 349*, g7617. DOI: 10.1136/bmj.g7617

Higginson, I. J., Bausewein, C., Reilly, C. C., Gao, W., Gysels, M., Dzingina, M., McCrone, P., Booth, S., & Jolley, C. J. (2014). An integrated palliative and respiratory care service for patients with advanced disease and refractory breathlessness: A randomised controlled trial. *The Lancet. Respiratory Medicine, 2*(12), 979–987. DOI: 10.1016/S2213-2600(14)70226-7

Higginson, I. J., Reilly, C. C., Bausewein, C., Jolley, C. J., & Gysels, M. (2013). The quality of dying and death in a hospital setting for patients with advanced cancer. *Journal of Pain and Symptom Management, 45*(6), 1054–1064. DOI: 10.1016/j.jpainsymman.2012.06.010

Hui, D., dos Santos, R., Chisholm, G., Bansal, S., Souza Crovador, C., & Bruera, E. (2015). Clinical signs of impending death in cancer patients. *The Oncologist, 19*(6), 681–687. DOI: 10.1634/theoncologist.2013-0457

Janssens, J. P. (2005). Aging of the respiratory system: Impact on pulmonary function tests and adaptation to exertion. *Clinics in Chest Medicine, 26*(3), 469–484. DOI: 10.1016/j.ccm.2005.05.004

Jennings, A. L., Davies, A. N., Higgins, J. P., & Broadley, K. (2001). Opioids for the palliation of breathlessness in terminal illness. *Cochrane Database of Systematic Reviews, 2001*(4), CD002066. Advance online publication. DOI: 10.1002/14651858.CD002066

Jennings, A. L., Davies, A. N., Higgins, J. P., Gibbs, J. S., & Broadley, K. E. (2002). A systematic review of the use of opioids in the management of dyspnea. *Thorax, 57*(11), 939–944. DOI: 10.1136/thorax.57.11.939

Johnson, M. J., Bland, J. M., & Currow, D. C. (2017). Breathlessness. In The Oxford Textbook of Palliative Medicine (5th ed., pp. 464-478). Oxford University Press.

Jolley, C. J., & Moxham, J. (2021). The neurophysiology of dyspnea. *Journal of Applied Physiology, 131*(4), 1283–1293. DOI: 10.1152/japplphysiol.00515.2021

Kako, J., Morita, T., Yamaguchi, T., Kobayashi, M., Sekimoto, A., Kinoshita, H., & Ogawa, A. (2018). Fan therapy is effective in relieving dyspnea in patients with terminally ill cancer: A parallel-arm, randomized controlled trial. *Journal of Pain and Symptom Management, 56*(4), 493–500. DOI: 10.1016/j.jpainsymman.2018.07.001

Kemp, C. (1997). *Terminal illness: A guide to nursing care* (2nd ed.). Lippincott.

Lauffenburger, J. C., Robinson, J. G., Oramasionwu, C., & Brookhart, M. A. (2019). Racial/ethnic and gender disparities in the use of high-risk medications among Medicare beneficiaries. *Journal of the American Geriatrics Society, 67*(11), 2296–2302. DOI: 10.1111/jgs.16071

Lok, C. W. (2016). Palliative care in chronic obstructive pulmonary disease. *Journal of Thoracic Disease, 8*(10), E1117–E1121. DOI: 10.21037/jtd.2016.09.43

Long, H., Huang, W., Zheng, P., Li, J., Tao, S., Tang, S., & Zhang, L. (2016). The effectiveness and safety of palliative oxygen therapy for dyspnea in patients with advanced cancer: A meta-analysis. *Oncotarget, 7*(43), 70862–70871. DOI: 10.18632/oncotarget.12234

Marengoni, A., Angleman, S., Melis, R., Mangialasche, F., Karp, A., Garmen, A., Meinow, B., & Fratiglioni, L. (2011). Aging with multimorbidity: A systematic review of the literature. *Ageing Research Reviews, 10*(4), 430–439. DOI: 10.1016/j.arr.2011.03.003

Parshall, M. B., Schwartzstein, R. M., Adams, L., Banzett, R. B., Manning, H. L., Bourbeau, J., Calverley, P. M., Gift, A. G., Harver, A., Lareau, S. C., Mahler, D. A., Meek, P. M., & O'Donnell, D. E. (2012). An official American Thoracic Society statement: Update on the mechanisms, assessment, and management of dyspnea. *American Journal of Respiratory and Critical Care Medicine*, *185*(4), 435–452. DOI: 10.1164/rccm.201111-2042ST

Puspawati, N., Shimizu, Y., & Ishimaru, M. (2017). The effectiveness of fan therapy in reducing dyspnea in patients with chronic obstructive pulmonary disease: A systematic review. *JBI Database of Systematic Reviews and Implementation Reports, 15*(8), 2026–2053. DOI: 10.11124/JBISRIR-2016-003282

Rochon, P. A., & Gurwitz, J. H. (2017). The prescribing cascade revisited. *Lancet, 389*(10081), 1778–1780. DOI: 10.1016/S0140-6736(17)31188-1

Sharma, G., & Goodwin, J. (2006). Effect of aging on respiratory system physiology and immunology. *Clinical Interventions in Aging*, *1*(3), 253–260. DOI: 10.2147/ciia.2006.1.3.253

Simon, P. M., Schwartzstein, R. M., Weiss, J. W., Fencl, V., Teghtsoonian, M., & Weinberger, S. E. (1990). Distinguishable types of dyspnea in patients with shortness of breath. *The American Review of Respiratory Disease*, *142*(5), 1009–1014. DOI: 10.1164/ajrccm/142.5.1009

Simon, S. T., Köskeroglu, P., Gaertner, J., & Voltz, R. (2016). Benzodiazepines for the relief of breathlessness in advanced malignant and non-malignant diseases in adults. *Cochrane Database of Systematic Reviews*, *2016*(10), CD007354. Advance online publication. DOI: 10.1002/14651858.CD007354.pub3

Spathis, A., Booth, S., & Moffat, C. (2017). The breathing, thinking, functioning clinical model: A proposal to facilitate evidence-based breathlessness management in chronic respiratory disease. *NPJ Primary Care Respiratory Medicine*, *27*, 27. DOI: 10.1038/s41533-017-0024-z

Ting, R., Edmonds, P., Higginson, I. J., & Sleeman, K. E. (2020). The use of a handheld fan as a breathlessness intervention in palliative care: A randomized controlled trial. *Journal of Pain and Symptom Management*, *60*(5), 861–868. DOI: 10.1016/j.jpainsymman.2020.06.014

Tolep, K., & Kelsen, S. G. (1993). Effect of aging on respiratory skeletal muscles. *Clinics in Chest Medicine, 14*(3), 363–378.

von Leupoldt, A., Sommer, T., Kegat, S., Baumann, H. J., Klose, H., Dahme, B., & Büchel, C. (2008). The unpleasantness of perceived dyspnea is processed in the anterior insula and amygdala. *American Journal of Respiratory and Critical Care Medicine, 177*(9), 1026–1032. DOI: 10.1164/rccm.200712-1821OC

Yorke, J., Moosavi, S. H., Shuldham, C., & Jones, P. W. (2010). Quantification of dyspnea using descriptors: Development and initial testing of the Dyspnea-12. *Thorax, 65*(1), 21–26. DOI: 10.1136/thx.2009.118521

Chapter 5 Physical Therapy in Palliative and End-of-Life Care for the Elderly in Advanced Chronic End-Stage Diseases: Palliative Care of Physical Therapy for Different Conditions of Elderly Patients

Marwa Mohammed Eleawa
https://orcid.org/0000-0003-1666-2167
Department of Physical Therapy, Applied Science Private University, Amman, Jordan

ABSTRACT

Elderly patients often face advanced chronic illnesses, emphasizing the urgent need for timely access to palliative care (PC). Loss of function is among the most distressing symptoms for patients nearing end of life (EOL). In such contexts, rehabilitation becomes essential for adapting care to changing needs and improving patients' quality of life. The World Health Organization's Rehabilitation initiative and its PC policy framework advocate for the integration of rehabilitation into PC systems globally. These initiatives support functional independence, enabling individuals with incurable conditions to remain socially engaged and self-sufficient despite limited life expectancy. Physical therapy (PT) plays a pivotal role in preserving dignity and independence, and supports emotional well-being through patient education,

DOI: 10.4018/979-8-3373-4099-9.ch005

movement restoration, and interdisciplinary collaboration. This chapter concludes by emphasizing the essential role of PT in palliative and EOL care across a range of serious conditions affecting elderly patients

INTRODUCTION

Serious health-related suffering (SHS) is defined as "pain, suffering, and severe distress associated with life-threatening or life-limiting health conditions and with end of life(EOL) that cannot be alleviated without medical intervention and is potentially responsive to palliative care(PC) (Knaul et al, 2018) Over the past three decades, the global burden of SHS has risen markedly, affecting nearly 73.5 million individuals. Low- and middle-income countries (LMICs) bear a disproportionate share, representing 80% of the global SHS burden and experiencing a rate of increase twice that observed in high-income countries (Knaul et al, 2025). The prevalence of SHS offers a concrete metric for estimating the need for PC services. Understanding the scale and distribution of SHS—across disease types, age groups, and geographic regions—can inform policymakers and healthcare providers as they assess current PC capacities and identify critical gaps in service provision.

The PC is an essential pillar of universal health coverage, and its absence represents a significant barrier to achieving Sustainable Development Goal (SDG): "Ensure healthy lives and promote well-being for all at all ages." By addressing suffering associated with life-limiting illnesses, the PC enhances QOL for both patients and their families—from diagnosis through to EOL (WHO, 2022). This is accomplished through the timely identification, assessment, and management of physical, psychosocial, and spiritual distress.

Globally, an estimated 40 million individuals require a PC each year. However, access remains limited, with only about 14% of global and 35% of regional needs currently met (Knaul et al, 2018) Accurate data on the burden of SHS is vital for assessing population health and evaluating health system performance in the pursuit of universal access to PC(WHO, 2021) Measuring SHS complements traditional metrics such as quality-adjusted life years and disability-adjusted life years, offering a more nuanced understanding of unmet needs (Gutiérrez et al, 2020). Moreover, SHS measurement holds intrinsic value as a global health priority and as a critical component of efforts to achieve the SDG.

Despite its scale and persistence, the burden of SHS—and the corresponding need for PC—remains a solvable challenge. Evidence underscores the urgent need to reduce avoidable suffering through prevention and treatment, while ensuring equitable, comprehensive access to PC, particularly in LMICs(Knaul et al, 2025) . Projections incorporating SHS data suggest that the global burden will nearly double by 2060, with the most significant increases occurring in LMICs, especially in low-income countries, where health systems are least prepared(Sleeman et al., 2019) .

PALLIATIVE CARE AND THE END OF LIFE (EOL)

The PC is a multidisciplinary and holistic approach to healthcare that supports individuals and their families facing the challenges of life-threatening illnesses(WHO, 2023b) . While often associated with hospice or EOL care, PC extends beyond terminal conditions. It encompasses patients who may not have a life-threatening diagnosis and those who continue to receive curative or life-prolonging treatments(Batchelor, 2010).EOL care, by contrast, refers specifically to the phase in which a person's advanced illness is expected to result in death within a short period, with little or no prospect of recovery (Health Quality Ontario, 2014). It prioritizes the enhancement of QOL as a central component in the management of progressive and chronic conditions. This model of care seeks to alleviate suffering through the early identification, precise diagnosis, and comprehensive management of pain and other distressing symptoms—whether physical, psychological, or spiritual in nature (WHO, 2023b).

Evidence indicates that initiating PC services as early as nine months before death can significantly improve caregiver satisfaction, increase the likelihood of dying at home, and enhance patient outcomes—including QOL, symptom control, and overall satisfaction with care (Health Quality Ontario, 2014). Although formal eligibility criteria for PC are uncommon, a projected life expectancy of four to six months is often used as a general guideline for referral (Jordan et al., 2020). Importantly, PC practitioners play a critical role in aligning medical interventions with patients' values and goals, helping them navigate complex treatment decisions within the context of their evolving clinical realities.

As EOL services become an increasingly integral component of healthcare delivery, ensuring the consistent provision of high-quality, compassionate care is essential to safeguarding health and well-being. Given the progressive nature of many conditions requiring EOL care, there is a growing recognition of the need to transition from a curative to a palliative, patient-centred model of care—one that emphasizes comfort, dignity, and QOL over aggressive medical intervention (NHP-CO, 2014). This paradigm shift aligns closely with the principles of PT. Physical therapists are uniquely equipped to adapt their interventions to the evolving needs of individuals across the trajectory of serious illness. Their ability to tailor care is based on functional status, symptom burden, and personal goals, which makes them vital contributors to interdisciplinary PC teams.

This chapter concludes by emphasizing the essential role of Physical therapy (PT) in palliative and EOL care across a range of serious conditions affecting elderly patients. Its contributions span physical, emotional, and social domains, reinforcing its value as an integral component of comprehensive PC.

TEAM-BASED APPROACH TO PALLIATIVE CARE

The PC is fundamentally rooted in a team-based approach that supports both patients and their caregivers. This collaborative model fosters a comprehensive support network, drawing on the diverse expertise of interdisciplinary team members to help patients live as fully and comfortably as possible until EOL. Each delivery of PC involves a wide range of professionals, including physiotherapists, physicians, nurses, support workers, paramedics, pharmacists, and trained volunteers, playing an essential and complementary role in addressing the multifaceted needs of patients and families. Recognizing the value of this integrated model, scholars have conceptualized PC as a triangular partnership involving patients, informal caregivers, and healthcare professionals. This framework emphasizes shared participation and communication, aiming to enhance QOL for both patients and caregivers while also reducing caregiver burden (Belgacem et al., 2013).

PHYSICAL THERAPY AND PALLIATIVE CARE IN AGING

With global populations ageing and morbidity rates rising, the number of individuals living with disabilities and experiencing significant suffering at the EOL is projected to nearly double by 2060 .Recent evidence highlights a high prevalence of hospitalized elderly patients with advanced, end-stage chronic illnesses—a hallmark of geriatric care—who require timely access to PC services (Sganga et al., 2022). To meet this growing need, there is an urgent call for expanding the workforce of geriatricians trained in PC, ensuring equitable access to continuous, coordinated care and evidence-based symptom management. Uncontrolled symptoms and progressive functional decline are common across all life-limiting conditions, particularly in the final months of life (English, 2015). Among these, loss of function is often cited as one of the most distressing experiences for patients with chronic or life-threatening illnesses (Mohammed, 2024) .The intersecting global challenges of population ageing and the rising burden of chronic disease underscore the critical need to scale up high-quality, accessible PC services worldwide.

With advancements in medical treatment, individuals are living longer with life-limiting and disabling multiple chronic conditions. As a result, the global burden of disease is increasingly defined not only by premature mortality but also by the time lived with disability (Stucki, Bickenbach, Gutenbrunner, & Melvin, 2018).For individuals with advanced illness, personal and clinical circumstances can change rapidly. As their condition progresses, so too do their goals, priorities, and functional needs, necessitating regular reassessment and adaptation of care plans (Radbruch, 2020). In this context, rehabilitation plays a vital role in helping patients live as fully and comfortably as possible until EOL, while also supporting families in their caregiving responsibilities.

The World Health Organization's Rehabilitation 2030 initiative underscores the importance of rehabilitation services to address the shifting health demands of an aging global population, characterized by a rising prevalence of both acute and chronic impairments(Montagnini, Javier, & Mitchinson, 2020) .In parallel, there is growing recognition of the value of integrating rehabilitation into PC. The WHO issued a policy framework advocating for the systematic incorporation of rehabilitation within PC services (WHO, 2023). Rehabilitation in this context is designed to enhance quality of survival through a multimodal, person-centered approach that supports functional independence, regardless of life expectancy (Radbruch, 2020). Rehabilitation within PC empowers people with incurable health conditions to actively manage their condition, reduces symptoms and enables individuals to stay independent and socially active. This allows them to enjoy the best possible QOL, right up to the EOL(Montagnini et al., 2020) .This landmark framework affirms the critical role of rehabilitation professionals in PC and offers a strategic foundation that LMICs can leverage to inform and shape national policies aimed at integrating rehabilitation into their PC systems.

PT, through its holistic and patient-centered approach, plays a vital role in addressing common symptoms experienced in PC, including pain, fatigue, and dyspnoea. By enhancing functional capacity, PT supports patients in maintaining or regaining independence and preserving dignity. It also contributes to symptom management—such as alleviating breathlessness and facilitating airway clearance through techniques that address coughing and respiratory discomfort (Mohammed et al., 2023).Restoring movement and function can reduce the risk of secondary complications, promote safe physical activity(PA), and prevent further deterioration. Beyond physical outcomes, physiotherapists play a crucial role in supporting patients' psychological and emotional well-being. Through therapeutic interventions, communication, education, and collaboration with caregivers and interdisciplinary teams, they help patients maintain a sense of dignity and control, even amidst progressive decline. In resource-limited settings, PT may also coordinate with institutional or community-based partners to extend the reach of PC services (Putt et al., 2017).

PHYSICAL THERAPY AND CAREGIVERS OF PATIENTS IN PALLIATIVE CARE

The PT also has an important role in providing families or primary caregivers with the necessary tools (i.e., good body mechanics, the use of different equipment, or assistance in transfer) for the optimal management of patients (Montagnini et al., 2020).PT interventions include strengthening and therapeutic exercises, education for patients and caregivers, balance and fall prevention training, and transfer assistance. Additional techniques frequently used in clinical practice encompass respiratory exercises, ROM activities, endurance training, manual therapy, relaxation techniques, breathing exercises, lymphedema management, and bed mobility support. PT also provide guidance on the use of assistive devices and recommend environmental modifications to facilitate safe and effective performance of daily activities (Mohammed, 2025). Evidence suggests that PT is both feasible and beneficial for most patients receiving PC (Kumar & Jim, 2010). PT interventions can be provided to the patient throughout the different phases of their disease, through dynamic assessments that, adapted to the needs that may arise during the disease process to maximize efficacy by always applying the best tools (Mohammed & Li, 2022).

PALLIATIVE CARE OF PHYSICAL THERAPY IN PATIENTS WITH ADVANCED CANCER

Globally, cancer incidence continues to rise, and advances in treatment have led to improved survival rates. Consequently, a growing number of individuals are living with advanced or incurable cancer. While extended survival represents a clinical success, it also brings a substantial and persistent burden of disease and treatment-related side effects. Many patients experience heightened levels of anxiety and depression, diminished physical function, and increased sedentary behaviour, all of which contribute to a decline in overall QOL(Peddle-McIntyre et al., 2019) . A meta-analysis demonstrated that exercise training significantly improved the six-minute walk distance (6MWD) and had a moderate positive impact on disease-specific global health-related QOL(HRQoL) in individuals with advanced lung cancer, but no significant effects were observed on dyspnoea, anxiety, depression, or lung function (Peddle-McIntyre et al., 2019). Similarly, another Review found that exercise training significantly enhanced functional exercise capacity in patients recovering from lung resection for early-stage non-small cell lung cancer, though it did not yield significant improvements in HRQoL (Cavalheri, Tahirah, Nonoyama, Jenkins, & Hill, 2014).

PA has been shown to significantly enhance both physical and psychological well-being in individuals with advanced cancer, while improved nutritional status is closely associated with better QOL (Albrecht & Taylor, 2012) . Three core interventions—PA, nutritional support, and palliative symptom management—have demonstrated positive effects on patient outcomes (Hall et al., 2019).Each contributes independently to QoL improvement, and their combined use in integrated, multimodal approaches may offer a more comprehensive strategy for addressing the complex needs of patients with advanced disease (Mohammed & Li, 2023). A recent study evaluating multimodal intervention incorporating PA, nutritional support, and palliative symptom management in individuals with advanced lung cancer found the approach to be safe, feasible, and well-tolerated, with a high percentage of recruitment, attendance, and assessment completion, with no intervention-related adverse events reported, and qualitative interviews revealed high levels of participant satisfaction (Ester et al., 2021) As with PA, maintaining body mass index (BMI) and adequate nutritional intake is critical, particularly given that weight stability is a known prognostic factor in advanced lung cancer(ALC). Patients with ALC are especially vulnerable to rapid declines in BMI, underscoring the importance of nutritional interventions (Ester et al., 2021). To further validate these findings, larger, multi-arm-controlled trials are needed to evaluate the specific contributions of nutritional counselling within multimodal interventions on QoL and nutritional outcomes.

A multimodal intervention incorporating PA has shown promise in supporting individuals with ALC. The PA component was individually tailored based on each participant's prior activity level, current physical function, and clinical status. Weekly exercise prescriptions were designed to gradually align with the American College of Sports Medicine (ACSM) Cancer Exercise Guidelines, which recommend 90 minutes of moderate-intensity aerobic exercise (AE) per week, resistance training twice weekly, and flexibility exercises on most days(Ester et al., 2021). Importantly, no adverse events were reported, indicating that, with appropriate professional supervision and individualized planning, patients with ALC can safely engage in structured exercise programs. These findings support the inclusion of ALC patients in general cancer exercise initiatives, provided that interventions are adapted to their specific needs(Ester et al., 2021) .

Cancer-related fatigue (CRF) remains one of the most debilitating and prevalent symptoms experienced by cancer patients across all stages of illness. The CRF is defined as "a distressing, persistent, subjective sense of physical, emotional, and/or cognitive tiredness or exhaustion related to cancer or cancer-related treatment that is not proportional to recent activity and interferes with usual functioning"

(Fleischer, Campbell, & Polo, 2023). Unlike typical fatigue, CRF is not alleviated by rest and can significantly impair daily functioning. Its prevalence varies depending on cancer type, disease stage, and treatment modality, with patients in advanced stages reporting higher levels of fatigue (Al Maqbali et al, 2021). Studies showed that physical exercise is beneficial for the management of CRF in patients with solid tumours (Cormie, Zopf, Zhang, & Schmitz, 2017).Guidelines focusing on CRF in advanced cancer concluded that there is moderate evidence supporting the recommendation of exercise as a core component of fatigue management (Chapman et al., 2022).Effective management of CRF requires a multifaceted approach, in which PT plays a central role. Maintaining PA has been shown to reduce fatigue, enhance functional capacity, and improve overall QOL. Targeted PT interventions can help patients increase activity levels, mitigate fatigue, and preserve independence (Cheville et al., 2013).

Studies in cancer patients have demonstrated the effects of exercise interventions in alleviating fatigue in patients both during and after cancer therapy (Cormie et al., 2017). Physical exercise appears to be safe and is recommended in cancer patients during active treatment with curative intent and in patients with lung cancer undergoing surgery(Ligibel et al., 2022). However, the role of exercise as an intervention for fatigue in advanced cancer is more ambiguous. A recent study in advanced gastrointestinal cancer patients at high risk of developing fatigue reported that the exercise intervention significantly reduced fatigue intensity (Navigante et al., 2022). Another study showed that in patients diagnosed with advanced cancer receiving PC, the therapy took place three times a week for 2 weeks for a 30-minute PT session that included active exercises, myofascial release and proprioceptive neuromuscular facilitation techniques. Results showed that exercise programs caused a significant reduction in fatigue severity and their impact on daily functioning. Moreover, the PT program improved patients' general well-being and reduced the intensity of coexisting symptoms such as pain, drowsiness, lack of appetite and depression with high patients' satisfaction scores (Pyszora, Budzyński, Wójcik, Prokop, & Krajnik, 2017)

PALLIATIVE CARE OF PHYSICAL THERAPY IN END-STAGE RENAL DISEASE (ESRD)

Older adults with ESRD undergoing hemodialysis (HD) are often presented with frailty, impaired mobility, and a higher prevalence of functional disability compared to age-matched individuals in the general population. These limitations are associated with increased mortality risk and frequently hinder the attainment of inpatient rehabilitation goals. A common barrier is the disruption of PT sessions due to scheduling conflicts with off-site dialysis appointments, often documented as "outside clinic visit" absences (Seckinger et al., 2016) Recent evidence suggests that ESRD patients residing in skilled nursing facilities (SNFs) who receive more frequent dialysis (MFD) co-located with rehabilitation services demonstrate significantly higher participation in PT compared to those receiving conventional off-site dialysis. Remarkably, their PT participation rates were comparable to those of non-ESRD SNF residents, despite being more clinically complex, less mobile, and more dependent (Bellin et al., 2023).

SNFs can accommodate frailer, less mobile patients by integrating on-site dialysis services with schedule-coordinated PT, offering significant benefits to both hospitals and patients (Bellin et al., 2023). This model facilitates earlier hospital discharge, potentially reducing inpatient length of stay, while allowing patients to transition out of the acute care environment—thereby minimising exposure to hospital-acquired infections and other iatrogenic complications. Clinical indicators and initial laboratory values of patients receiving on-site more frequent dialysis (Onsite-MFD) reveal that many are discharged from the hospital with substantial clinical compromise and a high burden of disease. The implementation of a centrally supervised care model within SNFs supports the early transfer of these medically complex patients, enabling them to initiate rehabilitation promptly in a more suitable, less intensive care setting (Bellin et al., 2023).

Additional studies have highlighted the broad benefits of MFD, including reduced post-dialysis recovery time and diminished fatigue—factors that are critical for enabling consistent engagement in rehabilitation. One study reported that 99% of patients receiving MFD recovered to their baseline functional status within two hours of post-dialysis, underscoring the potential of this approach to enhance participation in PT and support functional outcomes in this vulnerable population(Bellin et al., 2023; Raimann, 2016) .

Cognitive impairment is highly prevalent among dialysis patients, affecting individuals even at younger ages and across all age groups compared to age-matched individuals in the general population (O'Lone et al., 2016).Many patients begin dialysis with pre-existing cognitive deficits, which often worsen over time and may fluctuate from month to month during treatment(Zhang et al., 2018) Among kidney transplant (KT) candidates, cognitive impairment is also common, with prevalence rates (Gupta et al., 2017) .Emerging evidence supports the role of PA as a promising intervention for preserving cognitive function in this population. A previous study evaluated the effects of a home-based, individualised exercise program on functional and cognitive outcomes in dialysis patients. The intervention included assessments such as the 6MWT and the five-time sit-to-stand test, administered under the supervision of dialysis staff. Results demonstrated significant improvements in self-reported cognitive function and social interaction scores(Manfredini, 2016).The subgroup analyses focusing specifically on older dialysis patients aged

65 years and above revealed that participants in the intervention group maintained stable self-reported cognitive function over time, as measured by the Kidney Disease QOL instrument. In contrast, those in the control group experienced a decline in cognitive function scores on average (Baggetta et al., 2018).

Complementary findings were reported in another study examining the effects of a four-month intradialytic AE cycling program on cerebral blood flow and cognitive performance. Participants in the exercise group demonstrated significant improvements in cognitive function and increased basilar artery blood flow velocity compared to controls. Additionally, a greater proportion of arteries exhibited enhanced flow velocity in the exercise group, suggesting a potential mechanism for cognitive benefit(Stringuetta Belik et al., 2018) . Despite these encouraging short-term outcomes, further research is needed to evaluate the long-term impact of exercise interventions on cognitive health in both dialysis patients and KT candidates and recipients. Understanding whether these cognitive improvements translate into sustained enhancements in QOL and long-term health outcomes remains a critical area for future investigation.

PALLIATIVE CARE OF PHYSICAL THERAPY IN PAIN MANAGEMENT

Pain is among the most distressing and feared symptoms experienced by patients at the EOL, and its effective management is widely recognized as a fundamental component of a dignified and compassionate death(Krikorian, Maldonado, & Pastrana, 2020) . Alleviating pain is therefore a critical priority—not only for patients but also for their families, who often share the emotional burden of witnessing suffering.

Although both cancer and non-cancer patients have substantial PC needs, evidence suggests that the experience and prevalence of pain may differ between these groups(Bandeali, des Ordons, & Sinnarajah, 2019) . A recent systematic review reported that pain was documented in the final week of life in most patients dying from cancer (Hedman et al., 2024) Pain was also common, though to a lesser extent, among individuals with dementia, heart failure, and chronic obstructive pulmonary disease (COPD) . Severe pain was reported in 35% of cancer patients and in 17–21% of those with non-cancer conditions(Hedman et al., 2024) .Importantly, the review found that complete or partial pain relief was achievable in nearly all cases, with only 0.2% of patients receiving no relief at all(Hedman et al., 2024) . These findings underscore the critical importance of timely and tailored pain management strategies in EOL care.

Patients with advanced illnesses frequently experience a range of distressing symptoms, including pain, nausea, vomiting, and psychological distress. As such, the central goal of PC is to enhance QOL by alleviating symptom burden (Jiao & Chow, 2023). In addition to evidence-based conventional treatments, many patients turn to Complementary and Integrative Medicine (CIM) to manage their symptoms and improve well-being (Muecke et al., 2016). Among the various CIM modalities, Music Therapy (MT) has emerged as one of the most widely used interventions. MT has been shown to reduce pain and anxiety and contribute positively to overall QoL in patients with serious illness (Rodgers-Melnick, Rivard, Block, & Dusek, 2023). Most studies support the use of MT as an adjunct to conventional medical care, particularly in the management of pain. However, reductions in pain are often reported as short-term or transient, especially when patients receive only a single MT session(Warth et al., 2014). Furthermore, studies that failed to demonstrate significant effects frequently suffered from methodological limitations, such as small sample sizes or high attrition rates. These findings highlight the need for future research to explore the potential long-term benefits of MT by varying intervention duration and improving study design to minimise attrition bias.

A recent systematic review further identified MT and massage therapy as the complementary modalities with the most promising benefits across several outcome measures—particularly in alleviating pain and enhancing QoL among patients receiving PC at the EOL (Jodie, Anna, & Ursula, 2025).These findings underscore the potential value of integrating complementary medicine (CM) into palliative and hospice care settings. However, continued research is essential to deepen our understanding of CM's role and optimise its application in clinical practice. A recent study demonstrated that over 26 weeks, both acupuncture and massage were linked to significant reductions in pain, as well as improvements in fatigue, insomnia, and overall QOL among patients with advanced cancer(Epstein et al., 2023).

Notably, one study examining a multimodal intervention—including palliative symptom management—reported a clinically meaningful reduction in pain of more than 5% over the course of the intervention(Ester et al., 2021) . Previous studies have investigated the effects of aromatherapy and massage therapy on pain, anxiety, and QOL in patients with advanced cancer. While quantitative outcomes varied, many patients reported subjective improvements, including a heightened sense of well-being, temporary escapism, and emotional respite from the burden of illness (Armstrong et al., 2019).

Musculoskeletal pain is a prevalent and often under-recognized concern at the EOL, particularly among older adults(National Clinical Guideline, 2014) .Despite its frequency, it is frequently underreported and inadequately managed during the EOL, which are most spent in the community—either at home or in care facilities—rather than in hospital settings (Morgan et al., 2019). One reason this area remains underexplored is the predominance of cross-sectional studies on pain prevalence in older adults, which offer limited insight into the progression and trajectory of pain over time(Thomas, 2010). This type of pain arises from a diverse range of musculoskeletal conditions, including osteoarthritis, rheumatoid arthritis, and spinal disorders, each with distinct pathophysiological mechanisms(Thomas, 2010). Future research priorities should include high-quality epidemiological studies to determine the prevalence, natural history, and impact of musculoskeletal pain in the terminal phase of life. Moreover, there is a pressing need for intervention studies that establish an evidence base for effective assessment and management strategies aligned with patient priorities and outcomes (Lillie et al, 2013).

There are notable limitations in the current evidence base regarding the use of opioids for chronic musculoskeletal pain, particularly in older populations, due to concerns about efficacy and adverse effects(McQuay, 2010).While some studies have proposed interventions such as total joint replacement as a potentially effective and systematic strategy for managing musculoskeletal pain in PC settings, such approaches are often impractical. Surgical interventions pose significant logistical and ethical challenges in patients with progressive, life-limiting illnesses, especially given the limited time horizon and the complexity of care transitions near the EOL (Henry & Hayes, 2009).One possible explanation for the scarcity of treatment data in this context is the mismatch between conventional PC tools and the therapeutic approaches typically used for chronic musculoskeletal conditions. This gap underscores the need for tailored, evidence-based strategies that address the unique pain management needs of patients with musculoskeletal disorders in PC and EOL (Lillie et al., 2013) .

PALLIATIVE CARE OF PHYSICAL THERAPY IN THE END STAGE OF OSTEOARTHRITIS (OA)

Aging is accompanied by irreversible degenerative changes, with joint stiffness being highly prevalent among older adults. OA, the most common form of arthritis, and is a leading cause of disability in the elderly population (Peterson & Martin, 2010) . A notable neuromuscular characteristic in ageing individuals is the increased co-activation of agonist and antagonist muscles—defined as the simultaneous contraction of opposing muscle groups. While changes in activation play a beneficial role in joint stabilization and motor learning, its age-related increase is associated with elevated energy expenditure and a heightened risk of falls (Peterson & Martin, 2010) .Over time, these neuromuscular adaptations, coupled with degenerative joint changes, may contribute to the onset and progression of pathological conditions such as OA.

Clinical recommendations for managing knee OA are based on the appropriate application of physical, psychological, and pharmacological therapies. Patients with knee OA commonly present with pain, joint swelling, stiffness, and restricted mobility, primarily due to inflammation of the synovial joint (Diederichs, Berger, & Bartels, 2010).To alleviate pain and enhance physical function, a range of evidence-based PT interventions has been proposed. These include manual therapy, physical agent modalities, bracing and orthotic support, aerobic walking programs, resistance and balance training, home-based exercise regimens, self-management strategies, and weight reduction initiatives (Jamtvedt et al., 2008).While these interventions have demonstrated significant clinical benefits, individuals with end-stage knee OA often continue to experience substantial functional limitations. As a result, many ultimately opt for total knee arthroplasty (TKA) as a definitive intervention to restore mobility and improve QOL(Goh et al., 2019) .

Recent evidence supports the effectiveness of preoperative telerehabilitation in enhancing postoperative outcomes following TKA. In a recent study, patients in the PT and preoperative patient education group participated in a structured 3-week telerehabilitation program consisting of intensive exercise sessions (30 minutes per session, twice daily, five days per week) (An, Ryu, Lyu, Yi, & Lee, 2021). The intervention group demonstrated significant improvements in patient-reported functional outcomes, muscle strength, and knee ROM. Additionally, participants reported lower pain scores six weeks after surgery, indicating the potential of pre-operative telerehabilitation to enhance early recovery in patients with end-stage OA undergoing TKA(An et al., 2021) .Furthermore, another study found that patients referred to home health PT prior to transitioning to outpatient PT exhibited significantly poorer outcomes one-month post-TKA. These included greater declines in stair climb performance, TUG scores, 6MWT, quadriceps and hamstring strength, as well as higher levels of residual knee pain, compared to those referred directly to outpatient PT (Christensen et al., 2020) . These findings suggest that direct referral to outpatient rehabilitation may facilitate a more rapid and effective recovery in the early postoperative period following TKA.

Approximately 25% of individuals with end-stage knee OA report experiencing at least one fall, highlighting the significant fall risk in this population. Research has identified greater low back pain and reduced walking endurance as key factors associated with increased fall incidence among patients with advanced OA (Aljehani, et al 2020). To address this risk, home-based exercise programs have been incorporated into multifactorial intervention strategies tailored to individual needs. These interventions, prescribed by medical specialists, may include falls education, home hazard modification, cardiovascular and visual assessments, medication review, and structured exercise programs. One such program, the Otago Exercise Program (OEP), has been implemented in older adults with OA and coexisting gait and balance impairments. Participants were instructed to perform the exercises three times per week, for approximately 30 minutes per session, over six months. Each participant received an illustrated exercise manual with detailed written instructions and was provided with ankle weights (1–3 kg) tailored to their individual capacity for use during strengthening exercises. Monthly follow-up visits at the hospital were scheduled for the first three months, during which PT assessed progress and adjusted the exercise selection, difficulty level, and ankle weight prescriptions based on individual performance and tolerance (Mat et al., 2017).The OEP aims to enhance postural control and functional stability. While improvements in balance have been observed, current evidence does not indicate a consistent reduction in fall recurrence following the intervention(Mat et al., 2017) .

PALLIATIVE CARE OF PHYSICAL THERAPY IN CASES OF END-STAGE DEMENTIA

Dementia is a chronic decline in one or more areas of cognitive domains sufficient to affect daily life. It is a progressive and disabling disease and is not an inherent aspect of ageing. Dementia of Alzheimer's disease affects 60–80% of all dementia patients and hence is the most common type of dementia("2025 Alzheimer's disease facts and figures," 2025) . Providing support for people with dementia who live at home is an important, yet challenging issue of concern to people with dementia and their families, healthcare providers and policymakers (Dawson, Bowes, Kelly, Velzke, & Ward, 2015).People with dementia have significant difficulties with cognitive function, language and ADLs, and may have behavioural and psychological symptoms of dementia such as apathy, depression, agitation and anxiety (Savva et al., 2009).A study showed 38% of patients died at home, which was their preferred place of care(McLaughlin et al., 2022) . Gaps in the care of patients with dementia are complicated by poor communication during the last years of life (Crowther, Horton, Wilson, & Lloyd-Williams, 2022). The PC showed that end-stage dementia patients are not referred to PC as compared to patients with non-cancer end-stage disease(Schoenherr, Bischoff, Marks, O'Riordan, & Pantilat, 2019) .

Standard advanced directives may be insufficient for individuals with dementia, as the progressive nature of the disease often leads to evolving preferences and a gradual loss of decision-making capacity. As cognitive decline advances, patients may no longer be able to make complex medical or personal decisions, necessitating a careful balance between honouring their autonomy and ensuring appropriate care.

Making informed medical decisions requires intact cognitive functions, particularly attention, executive functioning, and memory (Chang & Bourgeois, 2020). As such, early and ongoing discussions about goals of care, supported by periodic reassessment of capacity, are essential in the management of patients with dementia. Physicians are frequently called upon to assess a patient's capacity across various domains of daily life, including the ability to consent to treatment or adhere to medication regimens(Gasparini, Moro, Amato, Vanacore, & Gambina, 2021). A randomised controlled trial demonstrated that hospitalised patients with late-stage dementia who were referred to PC were significantly more likely to receive comprehensive symptom management, have their spiritual needs addressed (47%), and be enrolled in hospice care (25%) (Chang & Bourgeois, 2020). Furthermore, these patients were more frequently discharged to home or assisted living facilities rather than institutional nursing homes, suggesting that PC involvement may support less restrictive and more person-centered discharge planning(Chang & Bourgeois, 2020). Despite these benefits, many individuals with advanced dementia still do not receive referrals to palliative or hospice services. Several factors have been associated with higher rates of hospice enrollment, including older age, female gender, higher educational attainment, greater cognitive impairment, and more pronounced decline in instrumental ADLs (Gasparini et al., 2021). These disparities highlight the need for more equitable and proactive referral practices to ensure that all eligible patients with advanced dementia have access to appropriate EOL.

Accurate recognition and assessment of pain in individuals with advanced dementia is critical to improving their QOL. Due to communication limitations, pain in this population is often underdiagnosed and undertreated. Several validated tools are available to support clinical assessment, with the most used being the Pain Assessment in Advanced Dementia (PAINAD) scale and the Non-Communicative Patients' Pain Assessment Instrument (NOPPAIN)(Warden, Hurley, & Volicer, 2003) . The PAINAD scale evaluates five behavioural indicators: breathing patterns, negative vocalisations, facial expressions, body language, and consolability (Warden et al., 2003).In contrast, the NOPPAIN tool is based on caregiver observations during routine care, assessing the impact of pain on patient activity, pain intensity, and the location and severity of symptoms. A comprehensive pain management plan should incorporate both pharmacological and non-pharmacological strategies. Non-drug interventions shown to alleviate pain and associated behavioural symptoms in dementia include patient repositioning, music therapy, behavioural interventions, movement-based therapies (e.g., rocking chairs), therapeutic touch, Reiki, personalised bathing routines, heat and relaxation therapies, and pet-assisted therapy(Achterberg, Lautenbacher, Husebo, Erdal, & Herr, 2019) (90). Additionally, therapeutic massage has been identified as a beneficial adjunct to conventional pain management approaches in this population(Kapoor & Orr, 2016) .

NON-PHARMACOLOGICAL MANAGEMENT OF AGITATION IN DEMENTIA: MOVEMENT-BASED THERAPIES

Agitation represents a prevalent and challenging neuropsychiatric manifestation in individuals with dementia, typically presenting as restlessness, repetitive pacing, verbal hostility, or physical aggression. Although pharmacological approaches are commonly employed to manage these symptoms, they are associated with significant adverse effects, including sedation, heightened fall risk, and accelerated cognitive deterioration. In response, movement-based non-pharmacological strategies are increasingly recognized as safer, person-centred alternatives that align with holistic and rehabilitative care principles.

Therapeutic Rationale

Movement-based therapies harness the physiological and psychosocial benefits of physical activity to modulate agitation. These interventions stimulate endorphin release, improve cerebral blood flow, and promote sensory integration, which collectively contribute to mood stabilization and behavioural regulation(Livingston et al., 2014). Moreover, structured movement routines can reduce environmental stressors and foster a sense of autonomy and routine.

Evidence-Based Modalities

-Aerobic Exercise: Engagement in regular low-impact aerobic activities—such as walking, stationary cycling, or chair-based routines—has been linked to measurable reductions in agitation severity among individuals with dementia. Customising these interventions to align with each individual's cognitive status and physical capabilities is essential to promote adherence, optimise therapeutic benefit, and ensure safety.(Choudry, Gould, & Ganti, 2025) .

-Dance and Rhythmic Movement: Music-integrated movement therapies, including dance, engaging preserved procedural memory and emotional responsiveness. These modalities have shown promise in improving affect regulation and reducing agitation episodes(Livingston et al., 2014).

-Tai Chi and Yoga: Mind-body practices that combine slow, deliberate movements with breathing techniques may reduce physiological arousal and enhance self-awareness. Studies suggest these interventions are feasible even in moderate stages of dementia(Choudry et al., 2025).

-Functional Mobility Training: Activities that simulate daily tasks (e.g., transferring, reaching, lifting) help maintain physical function and reduce frustration linked to dependency, which can manifest as agitation(Choudry et al., 2025).

-Multisensory Movement Environments: Incorporating tactile, auditory, and visual stimuli into movement sessions—such as dancing with scarves or walking in nature—can enhance sensory processing and behavioural regulation.

Clinical Considerations, eg

1-Individualisation: Interventions must be adapted to the individual's cognitive stage, physical limitations, and personal preferences to optimise therapeutic outcomes.
2-Safety Protocols: Supervision, environmental modifications, and fall prevention strategies are essential to ensure safety during movement sessions.
3-Interdisciplinary Collaboration: Involvement of physical therapists, occupational therapists, and recreational specialists enhances the design and delivery of movement-based interventions.
4-Outcome Monitoring: Behavioural tracking tools such as the Cohen-Mansfield Agitation Inventory (CMAI) should be employed to assess intervention efficacy and guide adjustments.

Ethical and Cultural Sensitivity

-Therapies should respect cultural norms and individual dignity, avoiding infantilization or coercion. Engaging caregivers in planning and delivery fosters continuity and reinforces therapeutic alliance.

PALLIATIVE CARE OF PHYSICAL THERAPY IN DYSPNEA

Dyspnea is among the most distressing symptoms experienced by patients with advanced illness, particularly at the EOL (Soares et al., 2018). Prior study reported that as death approaches, the prevalence of dyspnea and agitation is comparable between patients dying from dementia and those with terminal cancer (Soares et al., 2018). While self-report remains the gold standard for assessing dyspnea, this method becomes unreliable in individuals with advanced dementia due to impaired communication (Hui et al., 2013). Physiological indicators such as oxygen saturation, heart rate, and respiratory rate show only weak correlations with the subjective experience of dyspnea (Campbell & Templin, 2015). Alternative assessment tools have demonstrated greater reliability in this context. Caregiver assessments and the Edmonton Symptom Assessment Scale are more closely aligned with patients' reported experiences of dyspnea(Crombeen & Lilly, 2020). For non-communicative patients, the Respiratory Distress Observation Scale (RDOS) is a validated tool used by nurses to monitor respiratory distress at the EOL. A score above 3 on the RDOS indicates a need for palliative intervention (Campbell & Templin, 2015)

In managing dyspnea, it is essential to address not only physiological causes but also contributing psychosocial and spiritual factors, including depression, anxiety, interpersonal stressors, and religious concerns. Immediate-release opioids remain the cornerstone of treatment for acute, episodic dyspnea at EOL (Crombeen & Lilly, 2020).Current evidence supports the use of oral and parenteral opioids for symptom relief, while the efficacy of nebulised opioids remains unproven(Kamal, Maguire, Wheeler, Currow, & Abernethy, 2012) .Oxygen therapy can alleviate dyspnea in hypoxemic patients whose pulse oximetry readings fall below 88% while breathing room air. However, patients without hypoxemia do not experience benefits from supplemental oxygen (Campbell, Donesky, Sarkozy, & Reinke, 2021). Directing a fan toward the face is a cost-effective, simple, and safe alternative that does not require a prescription (Kako et al., 2018).This approach may relieve dyspnea by stimulating facial cold receptors, as exposure to cool air on the cheeks has been shown to significantly reduce breathlessness(Chen et al., 2020)

A recent study demonstrated that both Tai Chi (TC) and AE interventions significantly alleviated dyspnea in patients with advanced lung cancer, with sustained benefits observed over time (Takemura et al., 2024). Participants in the TC group engaged in 60-minute sessions twice weekly, while those in the AE group received two 60-minute supervised sessions per week along with home-based exercise guidelines over 16 weeks. Both interventions led to reductions in dyspnea severity, though TC—due to its multi-component nature—produced greater improvements(Takemura et al., 2024).In addition to structured exercise, individuals with severe respiratory illness have reported a range of benefits from breathing techniques, including enhanced confidence, reduced panic, improved disease self-management, and greater control over breathing in daily life (Papp et al, 2018). Breathing exercises—particularly pursed-lip breathing, diaphragmatic breathing, and yoga-based techniques—have shown consistent efficacy in improving breathlessness and HRQOL, especially in patients with COPD and asthma(Burge et al., 2024). These findings support the integration of breathing exercises into symptom management strategies for individuals with serious respiratory conditions.

CHALLENGES OF PALLIATIVE CARE AND PHYSICAL THERAPY

The burden of non-communicable diseases is rising rapidly in LMICs, creating a widening gap between the demand for and availability of PC services(Abu-Odah, 2020) . By 2035, it is projected that nearly two-thirds of all newly diagnosed cancer cases will occur in LMICs (Tefferi, 2015). This trend poses a significant challenge to already strained healthcare systems, many of which lack the organisational infrastructure and financial resources necessary to manage the growing burden of chronic and life-limiting illnesses. The treatment of such conditions in resource-limited settings places considerable pressure on health services and contributes to escalating direct and indirect healthcare costs. These systemic barriers are even more pronounced for supportive services that are not traditionally viewed as central to disease management, such as PT. Ensuring equitable access to such rehabilitative services is essential for delivering holistic, patient-centred PC, particularly in resource-limited settings(Ogundunmade, John, & Chigbo, 2024) .Among the studies reviewed, only half demonstrated statistically significant improvements in PC outcomes, while the other half showed no measurable benefit. Notably, none of the studies addressed enhancements in hospice care experiences (WHO, 2023a). Furthermore, there was limited evidence supporting interventions that improved specific aspects of EOL experience, such as caregiver knowledge, bereavement support, or overall satisfaction with care (WHO, 2023a). These findings underscore the urgent need for targeted, evidence-based strategies to strengthen palliative and hospice care delivery in LMICs.

Most of the existing evidence on rehabilitation within PC originates from high-income countries, where such services are well integrated into health systems and supported by experienced professionals, robust infrastructure, and a culture of formalised home-based care (WHO, 2023a).In contrast, LMICs face distinct challenges in embedding rehabilitation into PC, including limited resources, workforce shortages, and fragmented service delivery. A recent systematic review highlighted the paucity of robust evidence supporting global efforts to improve EOL experiences. Rehabilitation remains underprioritized in many healthcare systems, with limited strategic planning and resource allocation dedicated to its integration, particularly in PC settings(Hui et al., 2013). Several barriers contribute to this gap, including patient perceptions that rehabilitation is burdensome, time-consuming, or ineffective—especially near the EOL. In some cultural contexts, rehabilitation may be viewed as inappropriate or even as offering false hope when curative treatment is no longer the goal (Cheville et al., 2013). A recurring challenge across numerous studies is the high rate of participant attrition. Common reasons for dropout include patient discharge from PT services, clinical deterioration rendering patients too unwell to continue participation, and mortality during PC. These factors frequently led to reduced sample sizes, limiting the statistical power and generalizability of study findings to the broader population of patients receiving rehabilitation in PC settings(K. Putt et al., 2017) .

RECOMMENDATION

Developing strategies to enhance and integrate PC physiotherapy into healthcare systems in resource-constrained/low-income countries is made feasible by this examination of barriers and potential facilitators. A key priority is the incorporation of PC principles into both entry-level and postgraduate PT education. Embedding this content into curricula will help bridge existing knowledge gaps and mitigate personal and professional barriers that may hinder physiotherapists from delivering this specialized care. Additionally, sustained educational initiatives aimed at physiotherapists, patients, and the broader public are essential to raise awareness, shift perceptions, and foster a more supportive environment for the role of PT in PC (Ogundunmade et al., 2024).Expanding PC training for all physiotherapists has the potential to both strengthen the workforce and enhance the quality of care delivered. Establishing a dedicated and specialized career pathway in PC physiotherapy is essential to attract and inspire early-career professionals, positioning the field as a meaningful, secure, and fulfilling career option(Ogundunmade et al., 2024).

To support this development, policymakers should collaborate with regional, national, and international organizations to secure funding for healthcare system improvements that explicitly include PT. This aligns with the recommendations outlined in the WHO Policy Brief on Integrating Rehabilitation into PC Services (WHO, 2023). In LMICs, innovative health financing strategies tailored to local needs are also necessary to ensure sustainable integration of PC services. Recognizing PT as a key stakeholder in national PC policies would facilitate greater inclusion of physiotherapists in interdisciplinary PC teams. Advocacy efforts should also focus on securing health insurance coverage for PC physiotherapy services through stakeholder engagement and policy negotiation. Additionally, expanding the evidence base through robust research in PC physiotherapy will be instrumental in informing policy and guiding implementation(Ogundunmade et al., 2024) . Additionally, improve access in underserved and remote areas.

The establishment of comprehensive PC centres—integrating PT services, particularly at the community level, is essential to improving accessibility and equity in care delivery (Ogundunmade et al., 2024).Such centres would ensure that patients with life-limiting or advanced chronic illnesses receive holistic, multidisciplinary support closer to home. In developing countries, there is an urgent need to increase both financial and logistical investment in the integration of PT within PC services. This includes equipping physiotherapists with the necessary training in core PC competencies and ensuring their active involvement in care planning and delivery. Strengthening the role of physiotherapists in PC will enhance their capacity to contribute meaningfully to improving the QOL for patients across the disease trajectory(Ogundunmade et al., 2024) .

While several studies have explored the role of PT in PC, the descriptions of interventions provided were often limited in detail. Many lacked specific information regarding the types of exercises administered, duration and frequency of sessions, and the nature of patient education delivered(K. Putt et al., 2017). To enhance the utility and reproducibility of future research, it is essential that studies clearly outline the parameters and components of each PT intervention. Moreover, many of the reviewed studies were conducted within multidisciplinary care frameworks, where PT was one of several concurrent interventions. Although this reflects the reality of holistic care in palliative settings, it complicates the ability to isolate the specific effects of PT on patient outcomes. Future research would benefit from study designs that allow for the independent evaluation of PT interventions. Such studies could provide clearer evidence of the unique contributions of PT to symptom management, functional preservation, and QOL in EOL care (K. Putt et al., 2017) .

Enhancing patient engagement and access to rehabilitation in PC requires targeted strategies that prioritize education, accessibility, and person-centered design. Developing and widely disseminating patient education materials can improve understanding of the role and benefits of rehabilitation, while public messaging should emphasise how rehabilitation supports outcomes that matter most to individuals and their families (Bayly et al., 2018; Chowdhury, Brennan, & Gardiner, 2020).Actively involving patients and the public in the co-design of rehabilitation services ensures that programs are responsive to real-world needs and preferences. To overcome common barriers such as distance, transportation, and time constraints, rehabilitation services should be brought closer to patients, whether through community-based delivery, home visits, or tele-rehabilitation platforms. Rehabilitation plans should be tailored to individual needs and capacities, with achievable goals and minimal participation burden to encourage adherence. Additionally, supporting the active involvement of caregivers in the rehabilitation process can enhance continuity of care and reinforce functional gains, particularly in PC contexts where family support is integral (Bayly et al., 2018; Chowdhury et al., 2020) .

Advancing the integration of rehabilitation into PC requires coordinated action across policy, clinical practice, education, and research. National and international consensus statements, policies, clinical guidelines, and practice frameworks should explicitly prioritise this integration to ensure alignment across health systems. Health care planning and budgeting must support the mobilization and efficient allocation of rehabilitation resources, including within PC contexts. Routine data collection within health services should include indicators on the availability, quality, and utilization of rehabilitation, as well as patient functioning, morbidity, and mortality. These data are essential for informed service planning and evaluation. Rehabilitation services should be scaled according to patient needs—considering disease complexity, symptom burden, functional limitations, and the potential for benefit.

To build capacity, professional development programs should be established to equip existing PC providers, including nurses and community health workers, with core rehabilitation competencies. Practice partnerships and interdisciplinary networks can facilitate knowledge exchange and accelerate the implementation of high-quality rehabilitation within PC. Further research is needed to evaluate effective models of rehabilitation in PC, particularly in LMICs. Building existing evidence-based models will help guide scalable and context-appropriate interventions. Additionally, strategies must be developed to address prevailing misconceptions and negative attitudes toward rehabilitation in PC. This includes advocating for the inclusion of rehabilitation in global quality of care assessments and ensuring that awareness efforts among policymakers, healthcare professionals, and the public are culturally sensitive and aligned with local values and beliefs(Abu-Odah, 2020; Jesus, Papadimitriou, Bright, Kayes, & Cott, 2021) Use of trained rehabilitation volunteers to expand the reach of hospice rehabilitation services for individuals with limited access due to geographic or personal constraints (Daniel S. Peterson & Philip E. Martin, 2010).Strengthening strategies that actively involve family members and caregivers—such as inviting them to participate in daily inpatient rounds—has been shown to enhance the frequency and quality of documented goals-of-care discussions (Quigley & McCleskey, 2021).

ETHICAL CONSIDERATIONS IN PHYSICAL THERAPY AT END-OF-LIFE (EOL)

Physical therapy in EOL care requires ethically sensitive decision-making that balances clinical judgment with compassion. Therapists must align interventions with the patient's stage of decline and personal values, emphasizing comfort, dignity, and quality of life over restorative goals. Transparent communication with patients and families is essential to negotiate realistic therapeutic aims—such as pain management, positioning, and meaningful movement—while avoiding overextension or the promotion of unrealistic expectations (Criss et al., 2022).

At the end of life, physical therapists must recognize when interventions become futile—offering limited benefit or imposing undue burden—and collaborate with interdisciplinary teams to align care with palliative principles. Navigating family dynamics is equally critical, as therapists advocate for patient autonomy while mediating expectations and fostering culturally sensitive communication. Additionally, practitioners may face moral distress when asked to deliver non-beneficial care, underscoring the need for institutional support, ethical reflection, and peer consultation to maintain professional integrity and emotional resilience (Criss et al., 2022).

CONCLUSION

Rehabilitation within PC empowers individuals living with incurable health conditions to actively manage their health, mitigate symptoms, and maintain autonomy and social engagement. This support promotes optimal QOL, extending well into the end-of-life (EOL) stage. Despite its proven benefits, rehabilitation remains underprioritized across many healthcare systems. Strategic planning and resource allocation for its integration—particularly in PC contexts—are often insufficient. A significant gap exists in the documentation and implementation of rehabilitation practices in PC, including clear protocols on exercise types, session duration and frequency, and the nature of patient education. Addressing these gaps through expanded PC training for physiotherapists can bolster workforce capacity and enhance the standard of care. Furthermore, establishing a dedicated career pathway in PC physiotherapy is vital for attracting and inspiring early-career professionals, positioning the speciality as a purposeful, stable, and rewarding vocation. In parallel, the development of comprehensive PC centres that integrate physiotherapy—particularly at the community level—is critical to improving accessibility, equity, and overall care delivery.

REFERENCES

2025 Alzheimer's disease facts and figures. (2025). *Alzheimer's & Dementia, 21*(4), e70235. doi:/DOI: 10.1002/alz.70235

Abu-Odah, H. M., Alex Liu, Justina. (2020). Challenges on the provision of palliative care for patients with cancer in low- and middle-income countries: A systematic review of reviews. *BMC Palliative Care, 19*(1), 55–55. DOI: 10.1186/s12904-020-00558-5

Achterberg, W., Lautenbacher, S., Husebo, B., Erdal, A., & Herr, K. (2019). Pain in dementia. *Pain Reports (Baltimore, Md.), 5*(1), e803–e803. DOI: 10.1097/PR9.0000000000000803

Al Maqbali, M., Al Sinani, M., Al Naamani, Z., Al Badi, K., & Tanash, M. I. (2021). Prevalence of Fatigue in Patients With Cancer: A Systematic Review and Meta-Analysis. *Journal of Pain and Symptom Management, 61*(1), 167–189.e114. DOI: 10.1016/j.jpainsymman.2020.07.037

Albrecht, T. A., & Taylor, A. G. (2012). Physical activity in patients with advanced-stage cancer: A systematic review of the literature. *Clinical Journal of Oncology Nursing, 16*(3), 293–300. DOI: 10.1188/12.Cjon.293-300

Aljehani, M. S., Crenshaw, J. R., Rubano, J. J., Dellose, S. M., & Zeni, J. A. (2020). Falling risk in patients with end-stage knee osteoarthritis. *Clinical Rheumatology, 40*(1), 3–9. DOI: 10.1007/s10067-020-05165-6

An, J., Ryu, H.-K., Lyu, S.-J., Yi, H.-J., & Lee, B.-H. (2021). Effects of Preoperative Telerehabilitation on Muscle Strength, Range of Motion, and Functional Outcomes in Candidates for Total Knee Arthroplasty: A Single-Blind Randomized Controlled Trial. *International Journal of Environmental Research and Public Health, 18*(11), 6071. DOI: 10.3390/ijerph18116071

Armstrong, M., Flemming, K., Kupeli, N., Stone, P., Wilkinson, S., & Candy, B. (2019). Aromatherapy, massage and reflexology: A systematic review and thematic synthesis of the perspectives from people with palliative care needs. *Palliative Medicine, 33*(7), 757–769. DOI: 10.1177/0269216319846440

Baggetta, R., D'Arrigo, G., Torino, C., ElHafeez, S. A., Manfredini, F., Mallamaci, F., & Tripepi, G. (2018). Effect of a home based, low intensity, physical exercise program in older adults dialysis patients: A secondary analysis of the EXCITE trial. *BMC Geriatrics, 18*(1). Advance online publication. DOI: 10.1186/s12877-018-0938-5

Bandeali, S., des Ordons, A. R., & Sinnarajah, A. (2019). Comparing the physical, psychological, social, and spiritual needs of patients with non-cancer and cancer diagnoses in a tertiary palliative care setting. *Palliative & Supportive Care, 18*(5), 513–518. DOI: 10.1017/s1478951519001020

Batchelor, N. H. (2010). Palliative or Hospice Care? Understanding the Similarities and Differences. *Rehabilitation Nursing, 35*(2), 60–64. DOI: 10.1002/j.2048-7940.2010.tb00032.x

Bayly, J., Edwards, B. M., Peat, N., Warwick, G., Hennig, I. M., Arora, A., & Maddocks, M. (2018). Developing an integrated rehabilitation model for thoracic cancer services: Views of patients, informal carers and clinicians. *Pilot and Feasibility Studies, 4*, 160. DOI: 10.1186/s40814-018-0350-0

Belgacem, B., Auclair, C., Fedor, M.-C., Brugnon, D., Blanquet, M., Tournilhac, O., & Gerbaud, L. (2013). A caregiver educational program improves quality of life and burden for cancer patients and their caregivers: A randomised clinical trial. *European Journal of Oncology Nursing, 17*(6), 870–876. DOI: 10.1016/j.ejon.2013.04.006

Bellin, E. Y., Markis, W. T., Hellebrand, A. M., Busby, C. M., Wane, K. A., Jordan, C. R., & Kaufman, A. M. (2023). Improved nursing home end-stage renal disease patient participation in physical therapy with onsite, more frequent dialysis. *Hemodialysis International. International Symposium on Home Hemodialysis, 27*(4), 465–474. DOI: 10.1111/hdi.13112

Burge, A. T., Gadowski, A. M., Jones, A., Romero, L., Smallwood, N. E., Ekström, M., & Holland, A. E. (2024). Breathing techniques to reduce symptoms in people with serious respiratory illness: A systematic review. *European Respiratory Review : an Official Journal of the European Respiratory Society, 33*(174), 240012. DOI: 10.1183/16000617.0012-2024

Campbell, M. L., Donesky, D., Sarkozy, A., & Reinke, L. F. (2021). Treatment of Dyspnea in Advanced Disease and at the End of Life. *Journal of Hospice &amp. Palliative Nursing, 23*(5), 406–420. DOI: 10.1097/njh.0000000000000766

Campbell, M. L., & Templin, T. N. (2015). Intensity cut-points for the Respiratory Distress Observation Scale. *Palliative Medicine, 29*(5), 436–442. DOI: 10.1177/0269216314564238

Cavalheri, V., Tahirah, F., Nonoyama, M., Jenkins, S., & Hill, K. (2014). Exercise training for people following lung resection for non-small cell lung cancer – A Cochrane systematic review. *Cancer Treatment Reviews, 40*(4), 585–594. DOI: 10.1016/j.ctrv.2013.11.001

Chang, W.-Z. D., & Bourgeois, M. S. (2020). Effects of Visual Aids for End-of-Life Care on Decisional Capacity of People With Dementia. *American Journal of Speech-Language Pathology*, *29*(1), 185–200. DOI: 10.1044/2019_ajslp-19-0028

Chapman, E. J., Martino, E. D., Edwards, Z., Black, K., Maddocks, M., & Bennett, M. I. (2022). Practice review: Evidence-based and effective management of fatigue in patients with advanced cancer. *Palliative Medicine*, *36*(1), 7–14. DOI: 10.1177/02692163211046754

Chen, Y.-j., Li, X.-x., Ma, H.-k., Zhang, X., Wang, B.-w., Guo, T.-t., & Han, X.-m. (2020). Exercise Training for Improving Patient-Reported Outcomes in Patients With Advanced-Stage Cancer: A Systematic Review and Meta-Analysis. *Journal of Pain and Symptom Management*, *59*(3), 734–749.e710. DOI: 10.1016/j.jpainsymman.2019.09.010

Cheville, A. L., Kollasch, J., Vandenberg, J., Shen, T., Grothey, A., Gamble, G., & Basford, J. R. (2013). A home-based exercise program to improve function, fatigue, and sleep quality in patients with Stage IV lung and colorectal cancer: A randomized controlled trial. *Journal of Pain and Symptom Management*, *45*(5), 811–821. DOI: 10.1016/j.jpainsymman.2012.05.006

Choudry, M., Gould, M., & Ganti, L. (2025). Treatment of agitation in dementia - a systematic review. *International Journal of Emergency Medicine*, *18*(1), 101. DOI: 10.1186/s12245-025-00902-7

Chowdhury, R. A., Brennan, F. P., & Gardiner, M. D. (2020). Cancer Rehabilitation and Palliative Care-Exploring the Synergies. *Journal of Pain and Symptom Management*, *60*(6), 1239–1252. DOI: 10.1016/j.jpainsymman.2020.07.030

Christensen, J. C., Paxton, R. J., Baym, C., Forster, J. E., Dayton, M. R., Hogan, C. A., & Stevens-Lapsley, J. E. (2020). Benefits of direct patient discharge to outpatient physical therapy after total knee arthroplasty. *Disability and Rehabilitation*, *42*(5), 660–666. DOI: 10.1080/09638288.2018.1505968

Cormie, P., Zopf, E. M., Zhang, X., & Schmitz, K. H. (2017). The Impact of Exercise on Cancer Mortality, Recurrence, and Treatment-Related Adverse Effects. *Epidemiologic Reviews*, *39*(1), 71–92. DOI: 10.1093/epirev/mxx007

Criss, M. G., Wingood, M., Staples, W. H., Southard, V., Miller, K. L., Norris, T. L., & Strunk, E. R. (2022). APTA Geriatrics' Guiding Principles for Best Practices in Geriatric Physical Therapy: An Executive Summary. *Journal of Geriatric Physical Therapy*, *45*(2), 70–75. DOI: 10.1519/jpt.0000000000000342

Crombeen, A. M., & Lilly, E. J. (2020). Management of dyspnea in palliative care. *Current Oncology (Toronto, Ont.)*, *27*(3), 142–145. DOI: 10.3747/co.27.6413

Crowther, J., Horton, S., Wilson, K., & Lloyd-Williams, M. (2022). A UK qualitative study of living and dying with dementia in the last year of life. *Palliative Care and Social Practice*, *16*, 26323524221096691–26323524221096691. DOI: 10.1177/26323524221096691

Dawson, A., Bowes, A., Kelly, F., Velzke, K., & Ward, R. (2015). Evidence of what works to support and sustain care at home for people with dementia: A literature review with a systematic approach. *BMC Geriatrics*, *15*, 59. DOI: 10.1186/s12877-015-0053-9

Diederichs, C., Berger, K., & Bartels, D. B. (2010). The Measurement of Multiple Chronic Diseases—A Systematic Review on Existing Multimorbidity Indices. *The Journals of Gerontology. Series A, Biological Sciences and Medical Sciences*, *66A*(3), 301–311. DOI: 10.1093/gerona/glq208

English, A. M. (2015). Physiotherapy in palliative care. In N. Cherny, M. Fallon, S. Kaasa, R. K. Portenoy, & D. C. Currow (Eds.), *Oxford Textbook of Palliative Medicine* (pp. 0): Oxford University Press.

Epstein, A. S., Liou, K. T., Romero, S. A. D., Baser, R. E., Wong, G., Xiao, H., & Mao, J. J. (2023). Acupuncture vs Massage for Pain in Patients Living With Advanced Cancer: The IMPACT Randomized Clinical Trial. *JAMA Network Open*, *6*(11), e2342482. DOI: 10.1001/jamanetworkopen.2023.42482

Ester, M., Culos-Reed, S. N., Abdul-Razzak, A., Daun, J. T., Duchek, D., Francis, G., & Capozzi, L. C. (2021). Feasibility of a multimodal exercise, nutrition, and palliative care intervention in advanced lung cancer. *BMC Cancer*, *21*(1), 159. DOI: 10.1186/s12885-021-07872-y

Fleischer, A., Campbell, C., & Polo, K. M. (2023). Cancer-Related Fatigue (2018-2022). *The American Journal of Occupational Therapy*, *77*(Suppl 1). Advance online publication. DOI: 10.5014/ajot.2023.77S10034

Gasparini, M., Moro, V., Amato, S., Vanacore, N., & Gambina, G. (2021). The evaluation of capacity in dementia: Ethical constraints and best practice. A systematic review. *Annali dell'Istituto Superiore di Sanita*, *57*(3), 212–225. DOI: 10.4415/ann_21_03_04

Goh, S.-L., Persson, M. S. M., Stocks, J., Hou, Y., Welton, N. J., Lin, J., & Zhang, W. (2019). Relative Efficacy of Different Exercises for Pain, Function, Performance and Quality of Life in Knee and Hip Osteoarthritis: Systematic Review and Network Meta-Analysis. *Sports Medicine (Auckland, N.Z.)*, *49*(5), 743–761. DOI: 10.1007/s40279-019-01082-0

Gupta, A., Mahnken, J. D., Johnson, D. K., Thomas, T. S., Subramaniam, D., Polshak, T., & Sarnak, M. J. (2017). Prevalence and correlates of cognitive impairment in kidney transplant recipients. *BMC Nephrology*, *18*(1). Advance online publication. DOI: 10.1186/s12882-017-0570-1

Gutiérrez-Sánchez, D., Gómez-García, R., Cuesta-Vargas, A. I., & Pérez-Cruzado, D. (2020). The suffering measurement instruments in palliative care: A systematic review of psychometric properties. *International Journal of Nursing Studies*, *110*, 103704. DOI: 10.1016/j.ijnurstu.2020.103704

Hall, C. C., Cook, J., Maddocks, M., Skipworth, R. J. E., Fallon, M., & Laird, B. J. (2019). Combined exercise and nutritional rehabilitation in outpatients with incurable cancer: a systematic review. *Supportive care in cancer: official journal of the Multinational Association of Supportive Care in Cancer, 27*(7), 2371-2384. doi:DOI: 10.1007/s00520-019-04749-6

Hedman, C., Fürst, P., Strang, P., Schelin, M. E. C., Lundström, S., & Martinsson, L. (2024). Pain prevalence and pain relief in end-of-life care - a national registry study. *BMC Palliative Care*, *23*(1), 171–171. DOI: 10.1186/s12904-024-01497-1

Henry, C., & Hayes, A. (2009). Promoting high quality care for all at the end of life: Review of NHS National End of Life Care Programme 2004-2007 and implications for primary care. *London Journal of Primary Care*, *2*(2), 96–101. DOI: 10.1080/17571472.2009.11493261

Hui, D., Morgado, M., Vidal, M., Withers, L., Nguyen, Q., Chisholm, G., & Bruera, E. (2013). Dyspnea in hospitalized advanced cancer patients: Subjective and physiologic correlates. *Journal of Palliative Medicine*, *16*(3), 274–280. DOI: 10.1089/jpm.2012.0364

Jamtvedt, G., Dahm, K. T., Christie, A., Moe, R. H., Haavardsholm, E., Holm, I., & Hagen, K. B. (2008). Physical Therapy Interventions for Patients With Osteoarthritis of the Knee: An Overview of Systematic Reviews. *Physical Therapy*, *88*(1), 123–136. DOI: 10.2522/ptj.20070043

Jesus, T., Papadimitriou, C., Bright, F., Kayes, N., & Cott, C. (2021). What Person-Centered Rehabilitation Means in Concept and Practice: The Person-Centered Rehabilitation Model for Adult Physical Rehabilitation Derived from a Scoping Review and Thematic Synthesis. *Archives of Physical Medicine and Rehabilitation, 102*(10), e116. DOI: 10.1016/j.apmr.2021.07.465

Jiao, K., & Chow, A. Y. (2023). The connections of physical and psychosocial symptoms among patients with terminal illnesses: A network analysis. *Palliative Medicine, 37*(1), 120–130. DOI: 10.1177/02692163221128452

Jodie, F., Anna, K., & Ursula, W. (2025). Effectiveness of music therapy, aromatherapy, and massage therapy on patients in palliative care with end-of-life needs: A systematic review. *Journal of Pain and Symptom Management, 69*(1), 102–113. DOI: 10.1016/j.jpainsymman.2024.07.024

Jordan, R. I., Allsop, M. J., ElMokhallalati, Y., Jackson, C. E., Edwards, H. L., Chapman, E. J., & Bennett, M. I. (2020). Duration of palliative care before death in international routine practice: A systematic review and meta-analysis. *BMC Medicine, 18*(1), 368–368. DOI: 10.1186/s12916-020-01829-x

Kako, J., Morita, T., Yamaguchi, T., Kobayashi, M., Sekimoto, A., Kinoshita, H., & Matsushima, E. (2018). Fan Therapy Is Effective in Relieving Dyspnea in Patients With Terminally Ill Cancer: A Parallel-Arm, Randomized Controlled Trial. *Journal of Pain and Symptom Management, 56*(4), 493–500. DOI: 10.1016/j.jpainsymman.2018.07.001

Kamal, A. H., Maguire, J. M., Wheeler, J. L., Currow, D. C., & Abernethy, A. P. (2012). Dyspnea Review for the Palliative Care Professional: Treatment Goals and Therapeutic Options. *Journal of Palliative Medicine, 15*(1), 106–114. DOI: 10.1089/jpm.2011.0110

Kapoor, Y., & Orr, R. (2016). Effect of therapeutic massage on pain in patients with dementia. *Dementia (London), 16*(1), 119–125. DOI: 10.1177/1471301215583391

Knaul, a. (2018). Alleviating the access abyss in palliative care and pain relief-an imperative of universal health coverage: The Lancet Commission report. *Lancet, 391*(10128), 1391–1454. DOI: 10.1016/s0140-6736(17)32513-8

Knaul, a. (2025). The evolution of serious health-related suffering from 1990 to 2021: An update to The Lancet Commission on global access to palliative care and pain relief. *The Lancet. Global Health, 13*(3), e422–e436. DOI: 10.1016/S2214-109X(24)00476-5

Krikorian, A., Maldonado, C., & Pastrana, T. (2020). Patient's Perspectives on the Notion of a Good Death: A Systematic Review of the Literature. *Journal of Pain and Symptom Management, 59*(1), 152–164. DOI: 10.1016/j.jpainsymman.2019.07.033

Kumar, S. P., & Jim, A. (2010). Physical therapy in palliative care: from symptom control to quality of life: a critical review. *Indian Journal of Palliative Care, 16*(3), 138–146. DOI: 10.4103/0973-1075.73670

Ligibel, J. A., Bohlke, K., May, A. M., Clinton, S. K., Demark-Wahnefried, W., Gilchrist, S. C., & Alfano, C. M. (2022). Exercise, Diet, and Weight Management During Cancer Treatment: ASCO Guideline. *Journal of Clinical Oncology, 40*(22), 2491–2507. DOI: 10.1200/jco.22.00687

Lillie, A. K., Read, S., Mallen, C., Croft, P., & McBeth, J. (2013). Musculoskeletal pain in older adults at the end-of-life: A systematic search and critical review of the literature with priorities for future research. *BMC Palliative Care, 12*(1), 27–27. DOI: 10.1186/1472-684X-12-27

Livingston, G., Kelly, L., Lewis-Holmes, E., Baio, G., Morris, S., Patel, N., & Cooper, C. (2014). Non-pharmacological interventions for agitation in dementia: Systematic review of randomised controlled trials. *The British Journal of Psychiatry, 205*(6), 436–442. DOI: 10.1192/bjp.bp.113.141119

Manfredini, a. (2016). Exercise in Patients on Dialysis: A Multicenter, Randomized Clinical Trial. *Journal of the American Society of Nephrology, 28*(4), 1259–1268. DOI: 10.1681/asn.2016030378

Mat, S., Ng, C. T., Tan, P. J., Ramli, N., Fadzli, F., Rozalli, F. I., Tan, M. P. (2017). Effect of Modified Otago Exercises on Postural Balance, Fear of Falling, and Fall Risk in Older Fallers With Knee Osteoarthritis and Impaired Gait and Balance: A Secondary Analysis. *PM&R, 10*(3), 254-262. doi:DOI: 10.1016/j.pmrj.2017.08.405

McLaughlin, D., Hasson, F., Reid, J., Brazil, K., Rutherford, L., Stone, C., & Ballentine, J. (2022). Evaluating a partnership model of hospice enabled dementia care: A three-phased monitoring, focus group and interview study. *Palliative Medicine, 36*(9), 1351–1363. DOI: 10.1177/02692163221116763

McQuay, H. (2010). Drug Treatment of Chronic Pain. In Stannard, C. F., Kalso, E., & Ballantyne, J. (Eds.), *Evidence-Based Chronic Pain Management.*, DOI: 10.1002/9781444314380.ch31

Mohammed, M. (2024). Exercise intervention in frailty, challenges, and recommendations. In *Difficulties and challenges in geriatric health management* (p. 30). IGI Global., DOI: 10.4018/979-8-3693-0675-8.ch007

Mohammed, M. (2025). Rehabilitation and assistive robotics for the elderly and physically challenged. In *Modern technologies in healthcare* (1st ed., p. 20). CRC Press., DOI: 10.1201/9781003481959

Mohammed, M., & Li, J. (2022). Stroke-Related Sarcopenia among Two Different Developing Countries with Diverse Ethnic Backgrounds (Cross-National Study in Egypt and China). *Health Care, 10*(11), 2336. DOI: 10.3390/healthcare10112336

Mohammed, M., & Li, J. (2023). Knowledge mapping and visualization of current sarcopenia and cancer research: A bibliometric analysis. *Beni-Suef University Journal of Basic and Applied Sciences, 12*(1), 51. DOI: 10.1186/s43088-023-00386-5

Mohammed, M., Mehani, S., Aziz, A. A., Mohamed, M. F., & El Nahas, N. (2023). Efficacy of threshold inspiratory muscle trainer versus diaphragmatic plus pursed lip breathing in occupational COPD. *Beni-Suef University Journal of Basic and Applied Sciences, 12*(1), 73. DOI: 10.1186/s43088-023-00409-1

Montagnini, M., Javier, N. M., & Mitchinson, A. (2020). The Role of Rehabilitation in Patients Receiving Hospice and Palliative Care. *Rehabilitation Oncology, 38*(1), 9–21. DOI: 10.1097/01.reo.0000000000000196

Morgan, O. J., Hillstrom, H. J., Ellis, S. J., Golightly, Y. M., Russell, R., Hannan, M. T., & Hillstrom, R. (2019). Osteoarthritis in England: Incidence Trends From National Health Service Hospital Episode Statistics. *ACR Open Rheumatology, 1*(8), 493–498. DOI: 10.1002/acr2.11071

Muecke, R., Paul, M., Conrad, C., Stoll, C., Muenstedt, K., Micke, O., & Huebner, J. (2016). Complementary and Alternative Medicine in Palliative Care: A Comparison of Data From Surveys Among Patients and Professionals. *Integrative Cancer Therapies, 15*(1), 10–16. DOI: 10.1177/1534735415596423

National Clinical Guideline. C. (2014). National Institute for Health and Clinical Excellence: Guidance *Osteoarthritis: Care and Management in Adults*. London: National Institute for Health and Care Excellence (UK)

Navigante, A., Cresta Morgado, P., Daud, M. L., Dos Santos Regis, H., Kolberg, M., Marazzi, C., & De Simone, G. (2022). Physical exercise and fatigue in advanced gastrointestinal cancer during chemotherapy. *BMJ Supportive &amp. Palliative Care, 13*(2), 218–227. DOI: 10.1136/bmjspcare-2021-003516

NHPCO facts and figures on hospice care. 2014. Web site. http://www.nhpco. org/ sites/default/files/public/Statistics_Research/2012_Facts_Fig ures.pdf. Accessed April 15, 2015. (2014). *National Hospice and Palliative Care Organization*. doi:-DOI: 10.1097/01.naj.0000454840.97361.f2

O'Lone, E., Connors, M., Masson, P., Wu, S., Kelly, P. J., Gillespie, D., & Webster, A. C. (2016). Cognition in People With End-Stage Kidney Disease Treated With Hemodialysis: A Systematic Review and Meta-analysis. *American Journal of Kidney Diseases*, *67*(6), 925–935. DOI: 10.1053/j.ajkd.2015.12.028

Ogundunmade, B. G., John, D. O., & Chigbo, N. N. (2024). Ensuring quality of life in palliative care physiotherapy in developing countries. *Frontiers in Rehabilitation Sciences*, *5*, 1331885–1331885. DOI: 10.3389/fresc.2024.1331885

Papp, M. E., Henriques, M., Biguet, G., Wändell, P. E., & Nygren-Bonnier, M. (2018). Experiences of hatha yogic exercises among patients with obstructive pulmonary diseases: A qualitative study. *Journal of Bodywork and Movement Therapies*, *22*(4), 896–903. DOI: 10.1016/j.jbmt.2017.11.001

Peddle-McIntyre, C. J., Singh, F., Thomas, R., Newton, R. U., Galvão, D. A., & Cavalheri, V. (2019). Exercise training for advanced lung cancer. *Cochrane Database of Systematic Reviews*, *2*(2), CD012685–CD012685. DOI: 10.1002/14651858.CD012685.pub2

Peterson, D. S., & Martin, P. E. (2010). Effects of age and walking speed on coactivation and cost of walking in healthy adults. *Gait &amp. Posture*, *31*(3), 355–359. DOI: 10.1016/j.gaitpost.2009.12.005

. *Policy brief on integrating rehabilitation into palliative care services. Copenhagen: Licence: CC BY NC-SA 3.0 IGO (2023).* (2023): World Health Organization Regional Office for Europe. .

Putt, K., Faville, K. A., Lewis, D., McAllister, K., Pietro, M., & Radwan, A. (2017). Role of physical therapy intervention in patients with life-threatening illnesses: A systematic review. *The American Journal of Hospice & Palliative Care*, *34*(2), 186–196.

Pyszora, A., Budzyński, J., Wójcik, A., Prokop, A., & Krajnik, M. (2017). Physiotherapy programme reduces fatigue in patients with advanced cancer receiving palliative care: randomized controlled trial. *Supportive care in cancer: official journal of the Multinational Association of Supportive Care in Cancer*, *25*(9), 2899-2908. doi:DOI: 10.1007/s00520-017-3742-4

Quigley, D. D., & McCleskey, S. G. (2021). Improving Care Experiences for Patients and Caregivers at End of Life: A Systematic Review. *The American Journal of Hospice & Palliative Care*, *38*(1), 84–93. DOI: 10.1177/1049909120931468

Radbruch, a. (2020). Redefining Palliative Care-A New Consensus-Based Definition. *Journal of Pain and Symptom Management*, *60*(4), 754–764. DOI: 10.1016/j.jpainsymman.2020.04.027

Raimann, a. (2016). The Effect of Increased Frequency of Hemodialysis on Volume-Related Outcomes: A Secondary Analysis of the Frequent Hemodialysis Network Trials. *Blood Purification*, *41*(4), 277–286. DOI: 10.1159/000441966

Rodgers-Melnick, S. N., Rivard, R. L., Block, S., & Dusek, J. A. (2023). Effectiveness of music therapy within community hospitals: An EMMPIRE retrospective study. *Pain Reports (Baltimore, Md.)*, *8*(3), e1074. DOI: 10.1097/pr9.0000000000001074

Savva, G. M., Zaccai, J., Matthews, F. E., Davidson, J. E., McKeith, I., & Brayne, C. (2009). Prevalence, correlates and course of behavioural and psychological symptoms of dementia in the population. *The British Journal of Psychiatry*, *194*(3), 212–219. DOI: 10.1192/bjp.bp.108.049619

Schoenherr, L. A., Bischoff, K. E., Marks, A. K., O'Riordan, D. L., & Pantilat, S. Z. (2019). Trends in Hospital-Based Specialty Palliative Care in the United States From 2013 to 2017. *JAMA Network Open*, *2*(12), e1917043–e1917043. DOI: 10.1001/jamanetworkopen.2019.17043

Seckinger, J., Dschietzig, W., Leimenstoll, G., Rob, P. M., Kuhlmann, M. K., Pommer, W., & Schwenger, V. (2016). Morbidity, mortality and quality of life in the ageing haemodialysis population: Results from the ELDERLY study. *Clinical Kidney Journal*, *9*(6), 839–848. DOI: 10.1093/ckj/sfw087

Sganga, F., Salerno, A., Frizza, A., Turriziani, A., Barillaroa, C., & Bernabei, R. (2022). The role of geriatricians in hospital palliative care units for elderly patients affected by end stage diseases. *International Journal of Palliative Nursing*, *28*(5), 202–207. DOI: 10.12968/ijpn.2022.28.5.202

Sleeman, K. E., de Brito, M., Etkind, S., Nkhoma, K., Guo, P., Higginson, I. J., & Harding, R. (2019). The escalating global burden of serious health-related suffering: Projections to 2060 by world regions, age groups, and health conditions. *The Lancet. Global Health*, *7*(7), e883–e892. DOI: 10.1016/S2214-109X(19)30172-X

Soares, L. G. L., Japiassu, A. M., Gomes, L. C., Pereira, R., Peçanha, C., & Goldgaber, T. (2018). Prevalence and intensity of dyspnea, pain, and agitation among people dying with late stage dementia compared with people dying with advanced cancer: A single-center preliminary study in Brazil. *Annals of Palliative Medicine*, *7*(4), 437–443. DOI: 10.21037/apm.2018.05.06

Stringuetta Belik, F., & Oliveira, E Silva, Viviana R., Braga, Gabriel P., Bazan, R., Perez Vogt, B., Costa Teixeira Caramori, J., . . . da Silva Franco, Roberto J. (2018). Influence of Intradialytic Aerobic Training in Cerebral Blood Flow and Cognitive Function in Patients with Chronic Kidney Disease: A Pilot Randomized Controlled Trial. *Nephron*, *140*(1), 9–17. DOI: 10.1159/000490005

Stucki, G., Bickenbach, J., Gutenbrunner, C., & Melvin, J. (2018). Rehabilitation: The health strategy of the 21st century. *Journal of Rehabilitation Medicine*, *50*(4), 309–316. DOI: 10.2340/16501977-2200

Takemura, N., Cheung, D. S. T., Fong, D. Y. T., Hui, D., Lee, A. W. M., Lam, T.-C., & Lin, C.-C. (2024). Tai Chi and Aerobic Exercise on Cancer-Related Dyspnea in Advanced Lung Cancer Patients: A Randomized Clinical Trial. *Journal of Pain and Symptom Management*, *68*(2), 171–179. DOI: 10.1016/j.jpainsymman.2024.04.025

Team-Based Models for End-of-Life Care: An Evidence-Based Analysis. (2014). *Ont Health Technol Assess Ser, 14*(20), 1-49.

Tefferi, a. (2015). In Support of a Patient-Driven Initiative and Petition to Lower the High Price of Cancer Drugs. *Mayo Clinic Proceedings*, *90*(8), 996–1000. DOI: 10.1016/j.mayocp.2015.06.001

Thomas, E. (2010). 185Pain in older people. In P. Croft, F. M. Blyth, & D. van der Windt (Eds.), *Chronic Pain Epidemiology: From Aetiology to Public Health* (pp. 0): Oxford University Press.

Warden, V., Hurley, A., & Volicer, L. (2003). Development and Psychometric Evaluation of the Pain Assessment in Advanced Dementia (PAINAD) Scale. *Journal of the American Medical Directors Association*, *4*(1), 9–15. DOI: 10.1016/s1525-8610(04)70258-3

Warth, M., Kessler, J., Koenig, J., Wormit, A. F., Hillecke, T. K., & Bardenheuer, H. J. (2014). Music therapy to promote psychological and physiological relaxation in palliative care patients: Protocol of a randomized controlled trial. *BMC Palliative Care*, *13*(1), 60. DOI: 10.1186/1472-684x-13-60

WHO. (2021). Assessing the development of palliative care worldwide: a set of actionable indicators. Available at: https://www.who.int/publications/i/item/9789240033351: World Health Organization.

WHO. (2022). World Health Organization *Palliative care fact sheet.* doi:DOI: 10.1097/grh.0000000000000052

WHO. (2023a). Policy brief on integrating rehabilitation into palliative care services. Copenhagen: Licence: CC BY NC-SA 3.0 IGO. *World Health Organization Regional Office for Europe.*

WHO. (2023b). World Health Organisation Palliative Care (2020). Available online at: https://www. who.int/news-room/fact-sheets/detail/palliative-care (assessed October 25, 2023). *World Health Organisation.* doi:DOI: 10.1016/s0266-6138(14)00213-7

Zhang, Y.-h., Yang, Z.-k., Wang, J.-w., Xiong, Z.-y., Liao, J.-l., Hao, L., & Dong, J. (2018). Cognitive Changes in Peritoneal Dialysis Patients: A Multicenter Prospective Cohort Study. *American Journal of Kidney Diseases*, *72*(5), 691–700. DOI: 10.1053/j.ajkd.2018.04.020

APPENDIX

Abbreviations

Serious health-related suffering (SHS)
End of life(EOL)
Low- and middle-income countries (LMICs)
Universal health coverage (UHC)
Palliative care (PC)
Quality-adjusted life years (QALYs)
Sustainable Development Goal (SDG)
World Health Organization's (WHO)
Health related Quality of life (HRQOL)
Physical Activity (PA)
Cancer-related fatigue (CRF)
Physiotherapy (PT)
Quality of life (QOL)
Sustainable Development Goal (SDG)
Body mass index (BMI)
Hemodialysis (HD)
More frequent dialysis (MFD)
Skilled nursing facilities (SNFs)
Complementary and Integrative Medicine (CIM)
Music Therapy (MT)
Osteoarthritis (OA)
Total knee arthroplasty (TKA)
Otago Exercise Program (OEP)
Alzheimer's disease (AD)
Pain Assessment in Advanced Dementia (PAINAD)
Non-Communicative Patients' Pain Assessment Instrument (NOPPAIN)
Respiratory Distress Observation Scale (RDOS)
Tai Chi (TC)
Aerobic exercise (AE)
Non-communicable diseases (NCDs)

Chapter 6

Physical Therapy Modalities in Management of Pressure Ulcers in Elderly: Challenges and Preventive Measures

Marwa Mohammed Eleawa
https://orcid.org/0000-0003-1666-2167
Department of Physical Therapy, Applied Science Private University, Amman, Jordan

ABSTRACT

Pressure ulcers (PUs) pose a significant health concern, especially among frail older adults. Effective management of PUs necessitates a coordinated, multidisciplinary approach. Despite significant advancements in medical technology, a universally effective, accessible, and adaptable treatment option that addresses the varied needs of individuals with PUs remains elusive. This persistent gap has led researchers to explore novel and unconventional therapeutic avenues, including those rooted in the field of physical therapy. Within this collaborative framework, physiotherapeutic modalities present promising opportunities as integral components of comprehensive, interprofessional wound care strategies. This chapter presents in brief the surgical management of PUs in the elderly, in addition to a cohesive framework for integrating physiotherapy-based interventions with conventional medical management to optimise healing outcomes. It underscores the pivotal role of caregiver education and the implementation of individualised preventive strategies tailored to each patient's unique needs.

DOI: 10.4018/979-8-3373-4099-9.ch006

INTRODUCTION

Pressure ulcers (PUs), also referred to as pressure injuries, bed sores, decubitus ulcers, or pressure sores, are localized areas of tissue damage involving the skin and underlying structures. They typically result from sustained mechanical forces such as pressure, shear, or friction (Panel., 2009) . These lesions are not only painful and debilitating but are also linked to increased morbidity and mortality (Panel., 2009). Their management imposes a substantial burden on healthcare systems—requiring considerable staff time, resources, and financial investment (Brown, 2003).

The PUs are most prevalent among individuals with severe illness or neurological impairments, such as those with spinal cord injuries or significant immobility, including patients using prostheses, orthopedic braces, or plaster casts(Marwa Mohammed, 2024).Additional risk factors include compromised nutritional status, particularly in the elderly, which further exacerbates vulnerability (M. Mohammed & Li, 2022).

PUs are also linked to increased infection rates, including serious complications such as osteomyelitis (Panel., 2009). These ulcers are commonly observed across diverse care settings, including acute hospital wards, nursing homes, and home-based care—especially among patients with profound disabilities. Epidemiological data indicate that approximately 60–70% of all reported PUs occur in adults aged 65 and older, with geriatric ward patients showing an incidence rate ranging from 8% to 20%(Campbell & Parish, 2010) .

PUs are classified into four stages according to the guidelines established by the European Pressure Ulcer Advisory Panel (EPUAP) and the National Pressure Ulcer Advisory Panel (NPUAP)(Panel., 2009) :

- **Grade 1:** Characterized by intact skin with persistent discoloration—commonly presenting as non-blanchable erythema or localized blue, purple, or black pigmentation over bony prominences. Additional signs may include localized warmth, edema, induration, or pain. In individuals with darker skin tones, blanching may not be visible, necessitating careful clinical assessment.
- **Grade 2:** Involves partial-thickness skin loss affecting the epidermis and/or dermis. Lesions typically appear as shallow, open ulcers with a red-pink wound bed and no slough. Alternatively, they may present as intact or ruptured blisters containing serous or serosanguinous fluid.
- **Grade 3:** Represents full-thickness tissue loss with necrosis or damage to subcutaneous tissue, not extending through the fascia or exposing bone, tendon, or joint capsule. Subcutaneous fat may be visible, and slough or undermining may be present. Ulcer depth varies with anatomical site—shallow in regions with minimal adipose tissue (e.g., nose, ear, occiput, malleolus), but

potentially deeper in areas of greater adiposity. Bones, tendons, and muscles remain concealed.

- **Grade 4:** Involves full-thickness skin and tissue loss with extensive destruction extending to muscle, bone, tendon, or joint capsule. Ulcers may penetrate supporting structures, increasing the risk of osteomyelitis or osteitis. Depth is location-dependent, and exposed bone or muscle is either visible or palpable.

PUs ASSESSMENT

A comprehensive skin assessment for identifying PUs involve a systematic head-to-toe inspection, with particular focus on bony prominences. This process integrates both visual and tactile evaluation—visually identifying discoloration and tactually detecting abnormal tissue characteristics such as bogginess or increased firmness. When the individual can communicate, reported pain in specific areas further informs the assessment(Kottner et al., 2019).

In addition to visual and tactile skin assessments, clinicians utilize standardized tools like the Braden Scale to evaluate a patient's susceptibility to PUs. These instruments assess both intrinsic and extrinsic risk factors that contribute to PUs formation. Regular skin and risk assessments are essential and should be tailored to the care setting—whether hospital, long-term care, outpatient clinic, or home environment. In institutional settings such as hospitals and long-term care facilities, assessments are typically conducted upon admission, daily, during clinical deterioration, and at discharge(Kottner et al., 2019).

In outpatient settings, skin and risk assessments are conducted at every visit to proactively identify any signs of pressure-related damage. These routine evaluations support early detection and enable the implementation of timely, individualized prevention strategies based on each patient's risk profile(Kottner et al., 2019).

COMPLICATIONS OF PUs

Chronic wounds are frequently linked to age-related conditions such as arteriosclerosis, venous insufficiency, hypertension, diabetes, and other metabolic disorders(Marwa Mohammed & Li, 2023). Increasingly, older adults are also at risk due to postoperative complications and prolonged immobilization, which can precipitate pressure injuries (Han & Ceilley, 2017).

Prevalence rates for PUs range widely—from 8.8% to 53.2% with incidence rates reported between 7% and 71.6%(Q. H. Zhang et al., 2013) . These wounds are defined by impaired healing dynamics and delayed tissue regeneration, often leading to persistent anatomical and functional disruptions in the skin(Järbrink et al., 2017) . They significantly hinder recovery and disrupt the normal phases of wound healing(WH), rendering them refractory to standard therapeutic approaches(Frykberg & Banks, 2015).

With global population ageing and evolving disease patterns, PUs remain a widespread and persistent challenge in nursing care worldwide(Lei et al., 2025) . Affected individuals frequently endure pain, exudate, malodor, and other distressing symptoms that severely compromise their QOL. Chronic wounds are particularly debilitating, often leading to loss of independence, functional decline, and the need for institutional care. In severe cases, they may contribute to premature mortality (Gould et al., 2015; Raeder, Jachan, Müller-Werdan, & Lahmann, 2020).

The burden of chronic wounds is amplified in older adults, both clinically and economically. Estimates suggest that medical expenses and productivity losses related to these conditions exceed $10 billion annually—much of which is attributed to wound care in patients over 65 years (Gould et al., 2015).PUs, in particular, act as conduits for infection, delay recovery, and necessitate prolonged nursing care(-Graves, Birrell, & Whitby, 2005) . Their chronic nature often demands long-term management, further impairing patient autonomy and placing strain on healthcare systems. Altogether, the multifaceted consequences of pressure injuries, including increased morbidity, extended hospitalization, and elevated mortality—highlight the urgent need for effective prevention and timely intervention. Addressing PUs not only enhances patient outcomes but also reduces healthcare expenditure and mitigates the risk of complications.

PUs commonly develop over bony prominences such as the heels, hips, buttocks, and sacrum. The sacral region is particularly reporting a prevalence rate of 30.7%. The trochanter also represents a high-risk area, ranking as the third most frequent location for PUs with an overall prevalence of 7%, following the heels and sacral/coccygeal regions(Q. Zhang, Sun, & Yue, 2015).

Acute hospitalization, particularly among patients with impaired physical mobility, is recognized as a significant risk factor for the development of PUs(Järbrink et al., 2017) . Where prolonged mechanical loading impairs local circulation. This compromised blood flow leads to ischemia, cellular necrosis, and eventual tissue breakdown, resulting in open wounds that are often slow to heal—and in some cases, may never fully resolve (Q. Zhang et al., 2015). This intense or prolonged pressure and shear may lead to skin breakdown extending beyond the superficial layers to involve deeper anatomical structures such as muscle fascia, tendons, and bone.

Additional contributory factors, including poor nutritional status, unfavorable microclimatic conditions, compromised circulation, and underlying comorbidities, further exacerbate the risk of PUs development and progression(Gamston, 2019).

Prevention remains a critical component of care due to the chronic and debilitating nature of these lesions.

From a clinical governance perspective, the occurrence of PUs are considered a negative indicator of healthcare quality and is widely regarded as a preventable adverse event(Machado, Viana, & Sbruzzi, 2017) . Managing chronic wounds—such as those resulting from PUs —requires a coordinated, multifactorial therapeutic approach aimed at tissue regeneration and repair. Central to this process is the enhancement of re-epithelialization, achieved through interventions that align with evidence-based wound care frameworks. The systematic evaluation and treatment of chronic wounds continue to rely on the TIME principles: Tissue management, Inflammation and infection control, Moisture balance, and Edge of wound assessment (Harries, Bosanquet, & Harding, 2016). This structured methodology underpins effective clinical decision-making and supports tailored interventions within multidisciplinary care teams.

Effective PUs management requires a coordinated, multidisciplinary approach, typically involving physicians, nurses, podiatrists, certified diabetes educators, dietitians, orthotists or prosthetists, and specialized physiotherapists (Kloth, 2009). Within this framework, physiotherapeutic modalities offer promising potential as part of comprehensive, interprofessional wound care strategies(Heerschap, Nicholas, & Whitehead, 2019) .Despite notable advancements in medical technology over recent decades, there remains not universally effective, accessible, and versatile treatment option that addresses the diverse needs of all patients with PUs—particularly those without contraindications (Dreyfus et al, 2018). This gap has prompted researchers to explore innovative and unconventional interventions, including those within the field of physical therapy(Polak et al., 2017) .

International clinical guidelines increasingly advocate for the use of physical therapies in the management of chronic PUs. These modalities can accelerate WH, reduce the risk of complications, and support preventive strategies. This chapter outlines the surgical management of pressure sores in addition to the integration of physiotherapy-based interventions alongside medical management to enhance healing outcomes, while also emphasising the importance of caregiver education and patient-specific preventive measures.

THE NORMAL PHASES OF WH

WH represents a fundamental physiological response to tissue injury, characterized by a highly coordinated and multifaceted biological process. Rather than a linear event, it entails a dynamic interplay among diverse cellular populations, cytokines, signaling mediators, and vascular components. The initial phase involves vasoconstriction and platelet aggregation, which act to arrest hemorrhage. Subsequently, neutrophils are among the first inflammatory cells to infiltrate the wound site, initiating a cascade of immune responses. These cells secrete a repertoire of cytokines and mediators that facilitate key reparative mechanisms, including angiogenesis, thrombosis, and reepithelialization. Concurrently, fibroblasts contribute to tissue remodeling by depositing extracellular matrix components that provide structural scaffolding for regeneration(Ozgok Kangal & Kopitnik, 2025).

The inflammatory phase initiates the wound healing process and is marked by hemostasis, chemotactic signaling, and enhanced vascular permeability. These mechanisms collectively serve to minimize further tissue damage, facilitate wound closure, eliminate cellular debris and microbial contaminants, and promote the migration of reparative cells. This phase typically spans several days(Coger et al., 2019). The subsequent proliferative phase is defined by the development of granulation tissue, reepithelialization, and neovascularization, and may extend over several weeks. Finally, during the maturation and remodeling phase, the wound undergoes structural refinement and achieves optimal tensile strength as tissue integrity is restored(Bowden, Byrne, Maini, & Moulton, 2016).

CHALLENGES IN WH

Chronic wounds are generally expected to achieve complete healing within three months, provided they demonstrate a minimum 50% reduction in surface area by the fourth week post-onset(Frykberg & Banks, 2015). Deviations from this trajectory—particularly in the absence of identifiable comorbidities—necessitate prompt reassessment and consideration of advanced therapeutic interventions. Among the emerging technologies in wound care are bioengineered allogeneic cellular constructs, stem cell-based therapies, xenogeneic cellular matrices, and targeted growth factor applications(Frykberg & Banks, 2015). The implementation of these advanced modalities should be guided by robust clinical evidence and is typically reserved for cases that fail to progress along the expected healing continuum.

Chronic wound infections can significantly impede the healing process. Their management is inherently complex and necessitates a multidisciplinary approach. Differentiating between a chronic uninfected wound and one that is infected remains a clinical challenge, particularly due to the presence of atypical signs. These may include exacerbated pain, friable granulation tissue, delayed healing beyond expected timelines, wound dehiscence, and malodour—features that may be difficult to detect by non-specialist personnel(Gardner, Frantz, & Doebbeling, 2001). Inappropriate or delayed intervention is common and must be meticulously avoided to reduce the risk of infection-related complications and suboptimal outcomes.

SURGICAL MANAGEMENT OF PUs

The development of PUs among adults in acute care hospital settings has been linked to a range of contributing factors, including mechanical forces such as pressure, shear, and friction; physiological and clinical conditions such as moisture, infection, ischemia, anaemia, hypoalbuminemia, diabetes mellitus, and incontinence; as well as demographic and functional vulnerabilities, notably male gender, sensory perception loss, and age-related frailty(Fisher, Wells, & Harrison, 2004).

Conservative treatment modalities are generally insufficient for stage III and IV of PUs, necessitating surgical intervention—most notably flap reconstruction performed by plastic surgeons(Fisher et al., 2004) . Success depends on the availability of resources at all levels, a multidisciplinary approach including surgeons, internist, dietitians, dedicated and well-trained nurses, primary care physicians, and nursing home caregivers, because without these, surgery is likely to fail due to inadequate postoperative care and support, increasing the likelihood of ulcer recurrence(Soban, Kim, Yuan, & Miltner, 2017). Comprehensive care encompasses thorough wound management, targeted optimisation across disciplines, and proactive family education to support long-term outcomes.

Surgical reconstruction, when integrated with patient rehabilitation and educational initiatives, has been shown to significantly reduce the postoperative recurrence of PUs (Fisher et al., 2004). The foundational surgical principles for managing these wounds include thorough excision of all devitalized tissue and coverage of the defect with a durable, well-vascularized tissue flap, typically achieved through plastic surgical techniques. Local flaps remain the preferred option for coverage and may include musculocutaneous, fasciocutaneous, or perforator flaps, applied in configurations such as rotation, advancement, or island flaps (Chiang, Wang, & Tzeng, 2018).

In cases involving extensive tissue loss, negative pressure wound therapy (NPWT) may be employed following adequate debridement to optimise wound bed preparation. Within our series, V–Y advancement flaps were most frequently utilised for sacral PUs due to their simplicity and adaptability to a wide range of defect sizes(C. Y. Chen et al., 2020).

For elderly patients presenting with multiple PUs, previous studies have favoured surgical strategies characterised by reduced operative time, minimal intraoperative bleeding, and shortened anaesthesia duration(C. Y. Chen et al., 2020) . Consequently, a multistage surgical approach is often required. Given the laxity of aged skin, delayed primary closure performed in layered fashion can effectively eliminate dead space while minimizing tension and the risk of wound dehiscence(Chiang et al., 2018).

Primary closure may be considered a straightforward option for pressure sore defects measuring less than 16 cm^2. However, plastic surgeons are generally advised against employing this technique for resurfacing PUs due to its historically high complication rates. In a previous study, the dehiscence rate following primary closure reached 34%(Fisher et al., 2004). Among documented cases, primary closure was applied in 24.6% of wounds, with minor complications—defined as partial dehiscence followed by secondary healing—occurring in 5.9%, and major complications—total dehiscence—reported in 14.7%. Notably, these outcomes exceeded initial expectations, suggesting that with appropriate patient selection and wound assessment, primary closure may be viable in select cases(C. Y. Chen et al., 2020).

The predominance of elderly patients with pressure sores contributes to prolonged wound healing times, which may explain the elevated complication rates compared to general surgical procedures. Larger defects typically require more extensive flap coverage, which increases wound tension and may compromise perfusion. The relatively diminished vascular supply in larger flaps is a likely contributor to the higher incidence of complications observed in these cases. For elderly patients presenting with multiple PUs, treatment protocols prioritize minimal operative time, reduced intraoperative bleeding, and lower complication rates. Importantly, postoperative outcomes are enhanced by controlling systemic infection, which not only improves patient QOL but also reduces caregiver burden.

Despite this, surgical management can fail. There are two cases: failures after the first surgery (due to lack of healing) and distant recurrences after a period of complete healing. Older age might be responsible for delayed wound healing and was suggested to be a risk factor for the occurrence of PUs(Tsai et al., 2023)

PHYSICAL THERAPY MODALITIES FOR WOUND TREATMENT

A-Extracorporeal shock wave therapy (ESWT)

Contemporary wound care represents the current gold standard in managing chronic wounds; however, its efficacy can be further augmented through the integration of biophysical modalities (Sopel et al., 2024). Among these, **ESWT** has emerged as a promising adjunctive treatment. ESWT utilizes mechanical energy generated by acoustic waves to elicit targeted biological responses within affected tissues (Sopel et al., 2024).

ESWT represents a valuable adjunct to conventional wound care, offering a noninvasive and well-tolerated option that can accelerate healing trajectories in older, immobilized patients with chronic wounds. The primary mechanism involves the induction of mechanical stress, which stimulates cellular activity through mechanotransduction. This process is thought to activate key signaling pathways, resulting in elevated production of growth factors, cytokines, and other mediators critical to tissue repair and regeneration. ESWT may also play a role in modulating inflammatory responses, promoting neovascularization, and enhancing cellular proliferation at wound sites(Sopel et al., 2024).

By facilitating these physiological processes, ESWT contributes meaningfully to tissue healing for the treatment of chronic wounds (Sopel et al., 2024) . Emerging evidence supports the efficacy of ESWT in promoting the healing of chronic skin ulcerations, particularly in patients with severe physical disabilities (Larking et al., 2010). Recent clinical findings indicate that a single application of radial ESWT—administered at 300 + 100 shocks/cm^2, with a pressure of 2.5 bar, pulse energy of 0.15 mJ/mm^2, and frequency of 5 Hz—can produce notable immediate improvements in older adults with chronic wounds. Planimetric parameters, including wound area, length, and width, demonstrated measurable reductions following just one session, underscoring the modality's therapeutic potential (Dymarek et al., 2024).The ESWT procedure was conducted using a radial applicator under strictly sterile conditions. A sterile ultrasound gel was first applied directly to the wound surface and its edges, followed by placement of a polyurethane film as a protective barrier. A second layer of ultrasound gel was then added atop the film to ensure optimal contact between the applicator head and underlying tissues. Treatment was initiated at the wound margins, progressing carefully toward the center, with meticulous attention to technique and avoidance of contact with bony structures. Notably, the intervention was performed without local anesthesia and elicited no pain during administration(Dymarek et al., 2024).

To date, clinical research on ESWT for wound management remains limited. Existing randomized controlled trials have primarily investigated ESWT's efficacy in treating diabetic foot ulcers (DFUs)(Galiano, Snyder, Mayer, Rogers, & Alvarez, 2019; Jeppesen, Yderstraede, Rasmussen, Hanna, & Lund, 2016; Snyder, Galiano, Mayer, Rogers, & Alvarez, 2018) , with only isolated studies addressing venous leg ulcers (VLUs)(Dolibog et al., 2018) and PUs (Larking et al., 2010). While preliminary findings suggest potential benefits, current evidence is insufficient to warrant widespread clinical adoption of ESWT for chronic wounds. Studies emphasize the need for further investigation, including rigorously designed clinical trials to evaluate ESWT's biophysical mechanisms and to establish a standardized protocol for its application in chronic wound care (Dymarek et al., 2024).

B-Photodynamic Therapy (PDT)

Photobiomodulation (PBM)is defined by its application of low-intensity electromagnetic radiation, where the therapeutic effects are mediated by light-induced cellular responses rather than thermal mechanisms. PBM encompasses non-ionizing wavelengths ranging from red to infrared (600–1000 nm), which penetrate the skin at varying depths and activate cellular processes that foster tissue regeneration (Silva et al, 2025). The modality influences a variety of inflammatory and enzymatic pathways, modulating key biomarkers and accelerating wound repair. Clinically, this translates to shortened healing durations, improved inflammatory control, and reduced pain perception (Silva et al., 2025).

A specialized subset of PBM employs coherent, monochromatic laser light to elicit therapeutic responses. This technique—commonly referred to as Low-Level Light Therapy (LLLT)—is used adjunctively in managing pressure injuries through PBM and/or photodynamic therapy (PDT) (Machado et al., 2017).

The PDT is regarded as a safe and minimally invasive modality for enhancing WH. Its ease of application and topical versatility make it a valuable adjunctive approach, particularly when repeated treatments are necessary. Despite its therapeutic promise, discomfort during sessions remains a notable limitation, and further research is warranted to establish standardized treatment protocols (Bacci & Kang, 2022).

PDT initiates acute inflammatory responses that stimulate endogenous repair mechanisms. This process leads to elevated levels of neutrophils, tumor necrosis factor-alpha (TNF-α), and interleukin-6 (IL-6), which contribute to the early phases of tissue regeneration(Li et al., 2022) . In addition, PDT promotes neovascularization through vascular endothelial growth factor (VEGF) activity, facilitating the remodeling and restoration of damaged tissues. **PDT**, in contrast, combines PBM with a photosensitizing agent to initiate photochemical reactions that generate reactive oxygen species (ROS)—such as singlet oxygen. These reactions exert antimicrobial effects, targeting bacterial and fungal pathogens at the site of infection through irreversible damage to microbial cell membranes (Maj et al, 2025).

PDT involves the targeted irradiation of a photosensitizing agent using a specific light source to initiate photochemical reactions within the affected tissue. This process generates ROS, such as oxygen radicals, which damage subcellular organelles, activate signaling pathways, and ultimately induce cell death. Building upon this principle, photodynamic antimicrobial chemotherapy (PACT) has emerged as a novel approach for eradicating pathogenic bacteria. PACT is characterized by its broad-spectrum antimicrobial activity, high safety profile, and resistance-independent mechanism of action(Wang et al., 2014).

A previous study utilizing polyethylenimine–chlorin e6 (PEI–ce6) as the photosensitizer, in combination with incoherent red-light irradiation, demonstrated accelerated healing in cutaneous infections caused by Staphylococcus aureus, reducing WH time by an average of 8.6 days compared to controls(Wang et al., 2014). Similarly, the application of Phellodendron liquid in conjunction with diode laser irradiation exhibited notable bactericidal effects against PUs with mixed bacterial infections. This combination enhanced wound resolution by stimulating epidermal growth factor (EGF) expression in granulation tissue, facilitating early repair and promoting the formation of viable tissue suitable for grafting or flap closure. Despite encouraging preliminary results, photodynamic antimicrobial therapy for infected pressure injuries remains in the early stages of clinical application. Comprehensive studies with larger cohorts and extended follow-up are necessary to validate its safety, therapeutic efficacy, and cost-effectiveness(Wang et al., 2014).

The LLLT utilizes amplified light at low radiation power to produce a range of biochemical, bioelectric, and bioenergetic effects. These therapeutic responses contribute to enhanced microcirculation, analgesia, anti-inflammatory and anti-edematous actions, and ultimately promote WH (desJardins-Park, Foster, & Longaker, 2018). LLLT activates endogenous repair mechanisms by modulating key signaling molecules, including the TGF-β family, platelet-derived growth factors, interleukins (IL-6, IL-13, IL-15), and matrix metalloproteinases (MMPs), all of which are integral to the WH cascade. Notably, TGF-β plays a pivotal role in fibroblast proliferation and extracellular matrix remodeling(desJardins-Park et al., 2018) .

The application of LLLT presents several practical advantages: it is simple to administer, capable of covering large treatment areas, compatible with wearable technologies, and offers potential for self-administration. Moreover, it is relatively cost-effective compared to other therapeutic modalities. However, a major limitation remains its requirement for frequent, near-daily sessions to achieve optimal clinical outcomes (Heiskanen & Hamblin, 2018).

The LLLT has gained prominence, particularly using near-infrared (NIR, 800–900 nm) and red light (600–700 nm) wavelengths. Notably, wavelengths around 658 nm at a dose of 4 J/cm^2 have demonstrated significant therapeutic effects in PUs management, while higher single wavelengths have shown limited efficacy. Moreover, studies employing cluster probes in PUs treatment revealed no substantial clinical advantage (Machado et al., 2017). A single-blind randomized trial involving patients with PUs examined LLLT across four groups: 940 nm, 808 nm, 658 nm, and sham laser therapy. Sessions were conducted daily (five days per week) over a one-month period. Digital planimetry assessed WH progress at baseline, post-treatment, and at one and three-month follow-ups. Strikingly, only the 658 nm wavelength produced statistically significant improvements in wound dimensions and healing trajectory. In contrast, the more commonly used wavelengths of 940 nm and 808 nm did not yield superior outcomes compared to sham treatment (Machado et al., 2017). While LLLT has demonstrated reductions in ulcer surface area when compared with standard care or placebo, some investigations report minimal influence on complete wound closure (Iordanou et al, 2002). These findings underscore the need for wavelength-specific treatment protocols and further validation in clinical practice.

Recent reviews indicate that laser wavelengths of 650 nm, 660 nm, and 880 nm demonstrate promising therapeutic potential in reducing the initial size of pressure injuries and promoting WH(Glass, 2021; Kuffler, 2015) . A randomized, placebo-controlled interventional trial involving participants—receiving laser therapy three times per week over eight weeks (totaling 24 sessions)—revealed a statistically significant reduction in lesion parameters. Notably, the group treated with red LED exhibited the most accelerated healing rates, underscoring the influence of specific wavelengths on clinical outcomes(Baracho et al., 2021) . Furthermore, infrared light therapy at 637 nm was associated with markedly improved healing rates compared to control groups (Percival, Francolini, & Donelli, 2015). These findings suggest that the selection of wavelength plays a critical role in optimizing therapeutic responses and should be tailored to the individual clinical presentation. Given the variability in response across wavelengths and modalities, there is a pressing need for further research to establish standardized protocols and clinical guidelines.

A recent study investigated the efficacy of laser therapy in a cohort of patients presenting chronic PUs-related wounds. Laser treatment was administered at a dosage of 4 J/cm^2 over one month. Inclusion criteria comprised wounds staged II, III, or IV according to the EPUAP/NPUAP classification system, with wound areas ranging from 0.5 to 50 cm^2, a duration of 6 to 24 months, and localization in the sacral and pelvic regions. The findings revealed that irradiation at 658 nm significantly promoted WH, attributed to both anti-inflammatory effects and enhanced angiogenesis, proliferation, and tissue remodeling(Taradaj et al., 2018). These therapeutic outcomes were reflected in systemic reductions in pro-inflammatory cytokines—most notably interleukins and TNF-α—suggesting a facilitated transition from inflammation to proliferation. Histopathological analysis of wound biopsies further confirmed decreased TNF-α activity after two weeks of irradiation, coinciding with initiation of granulation and remodeling processes(Palmieri, Vadalà, & Laurino, 2020; Taradaj et al., 2018).Additionally, elevated expression of VEGF during the initial two weeks indicated robust angiogenic stimulation. This response tapered and stabilized as healing progressed. The TGF-β1 activity also peaked under 658 nm exposure, reinforcing its role in cellular proliferation(Taradaj et al., 2018). Conversely, laser wavelengths of 940 nm and 808 nm failed to elicit comparable biological responses or healing outcomes, underscoring the wavelength-specific efficacy of 658 nm in PUs management (Taradaj et al., 2018).

C-Visible Polarized Light Therapy (VPLT)

It has emerged as a supportive modality in the management of WH. The therapeutic device emits polychromatic, incoherent, and polarized light that mimics natural sunlight—without ultraviolet radiation—making it a safe, low-energy intervention. The polarized nature of the light enhances tissue penetration, particularly on flat surfaces, which may contribute to its biological effects. Although the molecular mechanisms underlying VPLT remain incompletely understood, preliminary evidence suggests its potential in promoting healing in chronic wounds(Taha et al., 2022).

Improvements observed in clinical settings highlight its promise as an adjunctive treatment. Nevertheless, further research is warranted to elucidate its cellular actions and establish standardized protocols for widespread clinical implementation.

D-Electrical stimulation (ES)

Electrical stimulation (ES) is recognized as a safe, accessible, and cost-effective modality with minimal adverse effects in wound management. During WH, endogenous bioelectric fields (EBFs) are naturally generated by epidermal cells through Na^+/K^+-ATPase activity. These EBFs regulate key cellular functions, including migration, proliferation, differentiation, and gene expression(Rajendran, Challen, Wright, & Hardy, 2021) .ES can replicate these physiological processes, enhancing the cellular dynamics essential for chronic wound (CW) repair (Rajendran et al., 2021).

Various forms of ES are available—including direct current, alternating current, and pulsed current—applied via mono- or bipolar electrodes. Not all modalities are beneficial across all healing phases; for instance, alternating current appears most effective during the early inflammatory stage(Aleksandrowicz et al, 2021) . Despite growing interest, standardized clinical protocols for ES remain limited, warranting further investigation(Koel & Houghton, 2014).

In practice, ES is typically administered as a complementary therapy alongside conventional wound care. Electrodes are positioned circumferentially around the wound, with treatment sessions lasting from 45 minutes to several hours, often repeated weekly over extended periods(Aleksandrowicz et al., 2021) . However, its time-intensive nature and logistical demands may restrict widespread use. Given these considerations, ES is best suited for carefully selected patients with chronic wounds who are at elevated risk for delayed healing (Koel & Houghton, 2014).

A recent systematic review demonstrated strong support for the use of ES therapy in managing various chronic wound types, with efficacy in treating PUs(Rajendran et al., 2021). Several randomized trials have investigated the efficacy of high-voltage monophasic pulsed current (HVMPC) in treating chronic wounds, including VLUs, PUs, and DFUs. Across these studies, HVMPC demonstrated consistent benefits in promoting WH. The therapeutic protocol typically involved twin-peak monophasic pulses with pulse durations of either 50 μs or 100 μs, and a standard frequency of 100 pulses per second (pps). The applied current was sub-threshold, eliciting sensory responses without inducing motor effects(Polak et al., 2016).

In the reviewed studies, HVMPC was applied to PUs for approximately 5.3 hours daily, typically administered overnight. The device was programmed to deliver 40 minutes of stimulation followed by a 20-minute rest cycle over an 8-hour period, continued for a minimum of three months or until complete wound closure (Rajendran et al., 2021). Current clinical guidelines recommend ES for the management of stage II to IV PUs(Gould et al., 2016; Panel, 2014). However, these guidelines lack specificity regarding stimulation parameters—such as current type, duration, frequency, and amplitude—likely due to insufficient empirical evidence. This ambiguity places the burden of protocol selection on the treating therapist, potentially contributing to the limited clinical adoption of ES in PUs management(Koel & Houghton, 2014).Nonetheless, available evidence supports the effectiveness of ES in promoting WH, with moderate-level data indicating that HVMPC yields superior outcomes compared to direct current (DC) modalities (Kawasaki et al., 2014). These findings suggest that standardizing ES parameters could enhance clinical implementation and optimize therapeutic efficacy in PUs care.

In comparative clinical studies, the weekly reduction in wound surface area was 12.39% for HVMPC combined with standard wound care (SWC), versus 6.96% for SWC alone or SWC with sham HVMPC. The net therapeutic benefit attributed to HVMPC was 5.4% per week—representing a 78% improvement relative to SWC alone or sham stimulation protocols. Evidence from Level 1, 2, and 4 studies consistently demonstrates that HVMPC in conjunction with SWC significantly enhances healing outcomes in stage II–IV PUs. Specifically, Level 1 studies confirm that HVMPC contributes to marked reductions in wound size, increases the likelihood of complete healing, and substantially mitigates the risk of deterioration. HVMPC has also demonstrated a favorable safety profile, with rare adverse effects reported(Girgis & Duarte, 2018) .

Treatment setups generally placed the active electrode directly over the wound site, while the dispersive electrode was positioned on healthy skin at a distance of 15–30 cm(Franek et al., 2012) . Electrode polarity varied across studies: some maintained either cathodal or anodal stimulation throughout the course of treatment, while others alternated polarity. For example, certain protocols-initiated therapy with cathodal stimulation, reversing polarity on a weekly basis, or transitioned from cathode (during the first 1–3 weeks) to anode stimulation in subsequent weeks(Franek et al., 2012) [58]. Session durations ranged between 45 and 60 minutes, typically administered once daily, five to seven times per week (Franek et al., 2012).

Mechanistically, HVMPC stimulates fibroblast proliferation near the cathode, enhances keratinocyte activity, promotes collagen synthesis, augments local blood flow, and exerts antibacterial effects. These outcomes are further supported by the galvanotaxis theory, which explains cellular migration in response to electric charge: fibroblasts and keratinocytes migrate toward the cathode, while the anode attracts macrophages, neutrophils, epithelial cells, and slower-moving fibroblasts (Girgis & Duarte, 2018).

E-Ultrasound therapy (UT)

It utilizes sound waves to produce both thermal and non-thermal effects within biological tissues. When applied intensively, UT elevates tissue temperatures to approximately 40 °C, resulting in enhanced vascular perfusion, cellular proliferation, collagen synthesis, and tissue regeneration. Additionally, UT exerts anti-inflammatory effects that contribute to the WH process. On-thermal mechanisms of UT include acoustic streaming and cavitation, which induce particle displacement and generate localized microenvironmental gases (Palmieri et al., 2020). Cavitation plays a critical role in wound cleansing by disrupting necrotic tissue while preserving surrounding healthy structures (Palmieri et al., 2020).

Wound care applications utilize ultrasound in two main frequency ranges: low-frequency ultrasound(LFU) (22.5–40 kHz) and high-frequency ultrasound (HFUS; 1–3 MHz)(Polak et al., 2014). HFUS at 3 MHz has been shown to increase expression of alpha-smooth muscle actin (α-SMA) and transforming growth factor-beta 1 (TGF-β1) in dermal fibroblasts. This frequency is absorbed more superficially than 1 MHz, which aligns with the positioning of fibroblasts at the surface of tissue culture substrates(Olyaie, Rad, Elahifar, Garkaz, & Mahsa, 2013) . Sonication duration generally ranges from 1–5 minutes per square centimeter of wound or periwound area. Some protocols recommend limiting each session to a maximum of 10 minutes irrespective of wound size, although empirical justification for this limit is lacking. HFUS treatments are administered one to five times weekly (Olyaie et al., 2013).

A recent clinical study explored the effects of high-frequency ultrasound (HFUS) and HVMPC in elderly patients with PUs. Participants aged 60–95 years with Category II, III, or IV ulcers were randomly assigned to one of three intervention arms: (1) using SWC, involving supportive and topical treatments; (2) SWC + HFUS administered at 1 MHz, 0.5 W/cm^2, 20% duty cycle, and 1–3 minutes/cm^2; or (3) SWC + HVMPC delivered at 154 μs pulse duration, 100 pps, 100 V, and 250 μC/sec, for 50 minutes per session. Both adjunct modalities were applied once daily, five times per week (Polak et al., 2016). Results showed that the percentage reduction in PUs surface area was significantly greater in the SWC + HFUS and SWC + HVMPC groups compared to the SWC-only control group. Additionally, the HVMPC group achieved a notably higher proportion of ulcers that reduced in size by at least 50%, approaching clinical significance compared to controls. However, no statistically significant differences were observed between the HFUS and HVMPC groups regarding overall treatment outcomes. Importantly, no adverse clinical effects were reported during the study period (Polak et al., 2016).

The LFU has demonstrated efficacy in WH and is commonly employed in the management of leg ulcers (LU). LFU is typically applied directly to the periwound skin for 5–10 minutes per session, commencing within 2–5 days of injury. A topical coupling gel is used to ensure optimal transmission between the skin and the applicator(Palmieri et al., 2020) .

CHALLENGES OF BED SORE HEALING

Unfortunately, the development of PUs is influenced by a range of risk factors, broadly categorized into intrinsic and extrinsic domains. Intrinsic factors reflect an individual's physiological status and tolerance levels—including existing skin integrity, perfusion deficits, comorbid conditions such as diabetes, elevated humidity exposure, and low serum albumin levels(Marwa Mohammed, Mehani, Aziz, Mohamed, & El Nahas, 2023). Extrinsic contributors involve mechanical and behavioural components, such as immobility and diminished sensory perception or response capabilities(Coleman et al., 2014).

Management of PUs focuses on promoting natural wound healing by relieving pressure, performing debridement, managing colonization or infection, providing nutritional support, and implementing strategies to prevent recurrence(Kruger, Pires, Ngann, Sterling, & Rubayi, 2013) . Pain and discomfort should be controlled by analgesics. Whenever possible, the patient should be moved from the bed to a chair, and physical therapy should be consulted for assistance with ambulation and/or exercise (Al Aboud & Manna, 2025). Prolonged bed rest can lead to a range of other serious complications. Immobility causes muscle weakness and atrophy, especially in the legs and back. This can impair mobility and make recovery more difficult once the person can move again(Al Aboud & Manna, 2025) .Additionally, joint stiffness and the development of contractures can occur, further limiting the range of motion. Another major concern is the development of deep vein thrombosis, as immobility slows blood circulation and can lead to the formation of blood clots, especially in the lower extremities

PREVENTING PUs IN ADULTS

According to the National Pressure Injury Advisory Panel, European Pressure Ulcer Advisory Panel, and Pan Pacific Pressure Injury Alliance (2025), several best practices have been strongly supported for the prevention of pressure injuries(National Pressure Injury Advisory Panel, 2025):

Nutrition Screening

Robust evidence affirms that conducting nutrition screening for individuals at risk of pressure injury is recommended as good clinical practice.

Repositioning Protocols

Independent of the type of full-body pressure redistribution surface utilized, it is considered good practice to reposition at-risk individuals regularly. Repositioning intervals may be adjusted based on the redistribution capacity of the support surface and the individual's clinical response. Nonetheless, no support surface can entirely substitute for repositioning.

Full-Body Support Surfaces

Healthcare organizations are advised to maintain access to a range of full-body support surfaces suited to diverse clinical needs. These surfaces should be inventoried, stored, and used in strict adherence to manufacturer guidelines.

Prevention in Seated Individuals

When selecting seating systems or wheelchairs for pressure redistribution and shear reduction, it is recommended to evaluate the following:

- The individual's overall risk of pressure injuries
- Independence, mobility, and activity requirements
- Body dimensions, shape, and weight distribution
- Posture, deformity, and asymmetry and their impact on pressure distribution
- Need for advanced features (e.g., dynamic weight shifting)
- Personal preferences and care goals

Heel Pressure Injury Prevention

Elevating the heels of individuals at risk, ensuring that the heels remain off the support surface, is recognized as a beneficial preventative measure.

CLINICAL ASSESSMENT AND REPOSITIONING STRATEGIES

Effective PUs prevention in elderly patients relies immensely on comprehensive skin assessments and evidence-based repositioning protocols. Skin evaluations should incorporate patient-reported pain or discomfort and involve inspection of areas prone to pressure for signs of compromised integrity. Key indicators include discoloration, variations in skin temperature, firmness, and moisture—especially in cases of incontinence, edema, or dry and inflamed tissue (Panel., 2009).

Repositioning remains a cornerstone of PUs prevention. Adults identified as at risk should be encouraged to adjust their position regularly, preferably every six hours. For people unable to reposition independently, assistance should be provided, with appropriate equipment employed as necessary. The frequency and method of repositioning should be documented to ensure consistency and accountability(Panel., 2009) .

Among preventive measures, repositioning has generated considerable debate regarding optimal intervals for efficacy. Research indicates that no significant differences exist between repositioning every 2–3 hours versus every 4 hours, suggesting the need for individualized approaches. Additional strategies include avoiding vigorous skin massage, ensuring adequate nutritional and hydration support, utilizing pressure-relieving surfaces, and applying protective barrier creams—all of which align with best practice guidelines for PUs prevention(Panel., 2009) .

A recent study investigating the physiological responses to sustained pressure revealed that the sacral and trochanteric skin of healthy volunteers exhibited only a modest rise in local temperature following two hours of direct pressure—specifically, from 35.34 °C to 36.72 °C—though this change was statistically significant for sacral regions(Lupiáñez-Pérez et al., 2021) (45). Tissue perfusion and oxygen saturation (SaO_2) in the trochanteric area also increased under pressure; however, these changes did not reach statistical significance. These findings underscore the importance of accounting for anatomical variability when developing individualized repositioning protocols. Variations in biomechanical and biological responses across pressure-prone regions suggest that repositioning strategies should be tailored to specific anatomical sites to optimize PUs prevention.

SUPPORT SURFACES IN PUs PREVENTION AND MANAGEMENT

Support surfaces—including specialized beds, mattresses, overlays, and cushions—play a critical role in pressure redistribution by cushioning vulnerable anatomical areas and minimizing localized tissue stress. These surfaces are designed to either mould to the patient's body, distributing weight across a broader contact area, or mechanically alter pressure points to reduce exposure duration.

Support surfaces are broadly categorized into two types:

- **Constant Low-Pressure (CLP) Devices**: These conformable surfaces aim to disperse pressure uniformly by adapting to the patient's shape. Examples include:
  - Standard and alternative foam mattresses (e.g., convoluted or cubed foam overlays)
  - Gel-, fibre-, air-, water-, and bead-filled mattresses
  - Sheepskins

These materials are generally classified as low-technology (low-tech) solutions, offering basic but effective pressure redistribution.

- **Alternating Pressure (AP) Devices**: These systems cyclically adjust internal pressure beneath the patient, thereby reducing the duration of applied mechanical stress at any given site.

Additionally, **high-specification CLP devices** integrate advanced engineering features for enhanced clinical benefit:

- **Air-fluidized beds**, which circulate warm air through fine ceramic beads beneath a permeable sheet to maximize pressure dispersion
- **Low-air-loss beds**, composed of air sacs that emit warmed air for microclimate control and uniform support

These technologies are considered high-tech CLP systems, offering greater therapeutic efficacy in complex or high-risk clinical scenarios(McInnes et al., 2015; Marwa Mohammed, 2025).

SUPPLEMENTARY SUPPORT SURFACES IN PRESSURE INJURY PREVENTION

In addition to standard support systems, several specialized surfaces are employed to aid in the prevention and management of pressure injuries. Turning beds and frames, for instance, facilitate patient repositioning either manually or through motorized tilting mechanisms, supporting individuals with limited mobility. Operating table overlays function similarly to low-tech constant low-pressure (CLP) surfaces by distributing pressure during surgical procedures.

Wheelchair cushions serve dual roles: conforming cushions expand the contact area to reduce interface pressure, while mechanical variants—such as alternating-pressure systems—cyclically modify the pressure landscape to minimize sustained stress. Similarly, limb protectors encompass various pads and cushions designed to shield bony prominences from excessive pressure.

Alternating-pressure (AP) devices operate via cyclical inflation and deflation of air-filled cells, generating variable interface pressures between the body and the support surface. These are available in multiple formats, including cushions, mattress overlays, and single- or multi-layer mattress replacements. Given their dynamic functionality and complexity, AP devices are classified as high-tech support surfaces.

Additional options such as turning/tilting beds, net beds, and specialized frames automate repositioning in patients unable to move independently(McInnes et al., 2015) . Clinical findings indicate that individuals placed on standard foam mattresses face a higher risk of developing PUs compared to those using high-specification foam mattresses. Moreover, the use of sheepskin overlays has been linked to a reduced incidence of pressure injuries. Although alternating-pressure mattresses may offer greater cost-efficiency than AP overlays, current evidence remains inconclusive regarding the relative effectiveness of high-specification CLP versus AP surfaces in ulcer prevention. Therefore, further rigorous, comparative studies are warranted to guide clinical decision-making and optimize patient outcomes(McInnes et al., 2015) .

THE ROLE AND SUPPORT NEEDS OF FAMILY CAREGIVERS IN PRESSURE ULCERS MANAGEMENT

Family caregivers serve as a cornerstone of home-based care, contributing significantly to rehabilitation, nutritional support, emotional wellbeing, and wound management. Their active participation plays a pivotal role in influencing WH outcomes and improving patients' overall quality of life (Adelman, Tmanova, Delgado, Dion, & Lachs, 2014). However, despite their importance, many caregivers—particularly those without prior experience—face challenges related to limited knowledge, inadequate care skills, and insufficient ability to recognize early warning signs of pressure injuries(Latimer et al., 2019) . These gaps can lead to delayed intervention, neglect of long-term wound care, and exacerbation of ulcer severity.

Inappropriate care practices, such as infrequent repositioning and suboptimal wound hygiene, continue to be observed among family caregivers. Addressing these issues requires structured educational initiatives that equip caregivers of disabled older adults with the competencies necessary to identify pressure injuries and respond appropriately. The inclusion of case-based teaching methods may further enhance learning outcomes.

To foster greater accessibility to specialised guidance and support, community-driven efforts should be mobilised to disseminate knowledge through diverse media platforms, including new digital channels and instructional video content. Such approaches can strengthen caregiver capacity and reduce reliance on institutional care by encouraging early detection and informed home-based management(Y. Chen et al., 2025) .

CONCLUSION

Physiotherapeutic modalities are emerging as valuable contributors to integrative and collaborative wound care approaches. Evidence suggests their potential to enhance healing rates, reduce complications, and support preventative strategies. Nonetheless, the existing body of research is insufficient, underscoring the urgency for further inquiry. Specifically, well-designed clinical trials are needed to elucidate the biophysical mechanisms of Extracorporeal Shockwave Therapy (ESWT) and to establish standardized protocols for its application in chronic wound management. To substantiate the safety, efficacy, and cost-effectiveness of ESWT, longitudinal investigations incorporating substantial sample sizes and prolonged follow-up periods are essential.

Similarly, Low-Level Laser Therapy (LLLT) presents variability in patient response across wavelengths and delivery methods. Therefore, further research is warranted to formulate consistent protocols and clinical guidelines. In the context of PUs, current findings emphasize the need to standardize electrical stimulation (ES) parameters to optimize clinical integration and treatment outcomes. When implemented effectively, these modalities may empower caregivers, facilitate early detection, and promote informed home-based care—ultimately alleviating reliance on institutional services.

REFERENCES

Adelman, R. D., Tmanova, L. L., Delgado, D., Dion, S., & Lachs, M. S. (2014). Caregiver burden: A clinical review. *Journal of the American Medical Association, 311*(10), 1052–1060. DOI: 10.1001/jama.2014.304 PMID: 24618967

Al Aboud, A. M., & Manna, B. (2025). Wound Pressure Injury Management(Archived). In *StatPearls*. Treasure Island (FL) ineligible companies. Disclosure: Biagio Manna declares no relevant financial relationships with ineligible companies.: StatPearls Publishing

Aleksandrowicz, H., Owczarczyk-Saczonek, A., & Placek, W. (2021). Venous Leg Ulcers: Advanced Therapies and New Technologies. *Biomedicines, 9*(11). Advance online publication. DOI: 10.3390/biomedicines9111569 PMID: 34829797

Baracho, V. D. S., Chaves, M. E. A., Huebner, R., Oliveira, M. X., Ferreira, P., & Lucas, T. C. (2021). Phototherapy (cluster multi-diode 630 nm and 940 nm) on the healing of pressure injury: A pilot study. *Journal of Vascular Nursing: Official Publication of the Society for Peripheral Vascular Nursing, 39*(3), 67–75. DOI: 10.1016/j.jvn.2021.06.002 PMID: 34507703

Bowden, L. G., Byrne, H. M., Maini, P. K., & Moulton, D. E. (2016). A morphoelastic model for dermal wound closure. *Biomechanics and Modeling in Mechanobiology, 15*(3), 663–681. DOI: 10.1007/s10237-015-0716-7 PMID: 26264498

Brown, G. (2003). Long-term outcomes of full-thickness pressure ulcers: Healing and mortality. *Ostomy/Wound Management, 49*(10), 42–50. PMID: 14652420

Campbell, C., & Parish, L. C. (2010). The decubitus ulcer: Facts and controversies. *Clinics in Dermatology, 28*(5), 527–532. DOI: 10.1016/j.clindermatol.2010.03.010 PMID: 20797513

Chen, C. Y., Chiang, I. H., Ou, K. L., Chiu, Y. L., Liu, H. H., Chang, C. K., & Tzeng, Y. S. (2020). Surgical treatment and strategy in patients with pressure sores: A single-surgeon experience. *Medicine, 99*(44), e23022. DOI: 10.1097/md.0000000000023022 PMID: 33126386

Chen, Y., Cai, T., Le, P., Zhang, L., Chen, Y., Wu, L., & Lu, Y. (2025). Family caregivers' perceptions and challenges in the care of pressure injuries in daily life: A qualitative study. *BMC Geriatrics, 25*(1), 490. DOI: 10.1186/s12877-025-06114-1 PMID: 40610938

Chiang, I. H., Wang, C. H., & Tzeng, Y. S. (2018). Surgical treatment and strategy in patients with multiple pressure sores. *International Wound Journal, 15*(6), 900–908. DOI: 10.1111/iwj.12942 PMID: 29956467

Coger, V., Million, N., Rehbock, C., Sures, B., Nachev, M., Barcikowski, S., & Vogt, P. M. (2019). Tissue Concentrations of Zinc, Iron, Copper, and Magnesium During the Phases of Full Thickness Wound Healing in a Rodent Model. *Biological Trace Element Research, 191*(1), 167–176. DOI: 10.1007/s12011-018-1600-y PMID: 30552609

Coleman, S., Nixon, J., Keen, J., Wilson, L., McGinnis, E., Dealey, C., & Nelson, E. A. (2014). A new pressure ulcer conceptual framework. *Journal of Advanced Nursing, 70*(10), 2222–2234. DOI: 10.1111/jan.12405 PMID: 24684197

desJardins-Park, H. E., Foster, D. S., & Longaker, M. T. (2018). Fibroblasts and Wound Healing: An Update. *Regenerative Medicine, 13*(5), 491–495. DOI: 10.2217/rme-2018-0073 PMID: 30062921

Dolibog, P., Dolibog, P., Franek, A., Brzezińska-Wcisło, L., Arasiewicz, H., Wróbel, B., & Błaszczak, E. (2018). Randomized, controlled clinical pilot study of venous leg ulcers treated with using two types of shockwave therapy. *International Journal of Medical Sciences, 15*(12), 1275–1285. DOI: 10.7150/ijms.26614 PMID: 30275753

Dreyfus, J., Gayle, J., Trueman, P., Delhougne, G., & Siddiqui, A. (2018). Assessment of Risk Factors Associated With Hospital-Acquired Pressure Injuries and Impact on Health Care Utilization and Cost Outcomes in US Hospitals. *American Journal of Medical Quality, 33*(4), 348–358. DOI: 10.1177/1062860617746741 PMID: 29262690

Dymarek, R., Kuberka, I., Walewicz, K., Taradaj, J., Rosińczuk, J., & Sopel, M. (2024). Is Shock Wave Application Effective on Various Chronic Wounds in the Geriatric Population? Preliminary Clinical Study. *Clinical Interventions in Aging, 19*, 665–679. DOI: 10.2147/cia.S448298 PMID: 38706636

Fisher, A. R., Wells, G., & Harrison, M. B. (2004). Factors associated with pressure ulcers in adults in acute care hospitals. *Holistic Nursing Practice, 18*(5), 242–253. DOI: 10.1097/00004650-200409000-00007 PMID: 15497604

Franek, A., Kostur, R., Polak, A., Taradaj, J., Szlachta, Z., Blaszczak, E., & Kucio, C. (2012). Using high-voltage electrical stimulation in the treatment of recalcitrant pressure ulcers: Results of a randomized, controlled clinical study. *Ostomy/Wound Management, 58*(3), 30–44. PMID: 22391955

Frykberg, R. G., & Banks, J. (2015). Challenges in the Treatment of Chronic Wounds. *Advances in Wound Care (New Rochelle, N.Y.), 4*(9), 560–582. DOI: 10.1089/wound.2015.0635 PMID: 26339534

Galiano, R., Snyder, R., Mayer, P., Rogers, L. C., & Alvarez, O. (2019). Focused shockwave therapy in diabetic foot ulcers: Secondary endpoints of two multicentre randomised controlled trials. *Journal of Wound Care, 28*(6), 383–395. DOI: 10.12968/jowc.2019.28.6.383 PMID: 31166864

Gamston, J. (2019). Pressure induced skin and soft tissue injury in the emergency department. *Emergency Medicine Journal: EMJ, 36*(10), 631–634. DOI: 10.1136/emermed-2018-207807 PMID: 31311786

Gardner, S. E., Frantz, R. A., & Doebbeling, B. N. (2001). The validity of the clinical signs and symptoms used to identify localized chronic wound infection. *Wound Repair and Regeneration, 9*(3), 178–186. DOI: 10.1046/j.1524-475x.2001.00178.x PMID: 11472613

Girgis, B., & Duarte, J. A. (2018). High Voltage Monophasic Pulsed Current (HVMPC) for stage II-IV pressure ulcer healing. A systematic review and meta-analysis. *Journal of Tissue Viability, 27*(4), 274–284. DOI: 10.1016/j.jtv.2018.08.003 PMID: 30177421

Glass, G. E. (2021). Photobiomodulation: The Clinical Applications of Low-Level Light Therapy. *Aesthetic Surgery Journal, 41*(6), 723–738. DOI: 10.1093/asj/sjab025 PMID: 33471046

Gould, L., Abadir, P., Brem, H., Carter, M., Conner-Kerr, T., Davidson, J., & Schmader, K. (2015). Chronic wound repair and healing in older adults: Current status and future research. *Wound Repair and Regeneration, 23*(1), 1–13. DOI: 10.1111/wrr.12245 PMID: 25486905

Gould, L., Stuntz, M., Giovannelli, M., Ahmad, A., Aslam, R., Mullen-Fortino, M., & Gordillo, G. M. (2016). Wound Healing Society 2015 update on guidelines for pressure ulcers. *Wound Repair and Regeneration, 24*(1), 145–162. DOI: 10.1111/wrr.12396 PMID: 26683529

Graves, N., Birrell, F., & Whitby, M. (2005). Effect of pressure ulcers on length of hospital stay. *Infection Control and Hospital Epidemiology, 26*(3), 293–297. DOI: 10.1086/502542 PMID: 15796283

Han, G., & Ceilley, R. (2017). Chronic Wound Healing: A Review of Current Management and Treatments. *Advances in Therapy, 34*(3), 599–610. DOI: 10.1007/s12325-017-0478-y PMID: 28108895

Harries, R. L., Bosanquet, D. C., & Harding, K. G. (2016). Wound bed preparation: TIME for an update. *Int Wound J, 13 Suppl 3*(Suppl 3), 8-14. doi:DOI: 10.1111/iwj.12662

Heerschap, C., Nicholas, A., & Whitehead, M. (2019). Wound management: Investigating the interprofessional decision-making process. *International Wound Journal, 16*(1), 233–242. DOI: 10.1111/iwj.13017 PMID: 30393966

Heiskanen, V., & Hamblin, M. R. (2018). Photobiomodulation: Lasers vs. light emitting diodes? *Photochemical & Photobiological Sciences, 17*(8), 1003–1017. DOI: 10.1039/c8pp90049c PMID: 30044464

Iordanou, P., Baltopoulos, G., Giannakopoulou, M., Bellou, P., & Ktenas, E. (2002). Effect of polarized light in the healing process of pressure ulcers. *International Journal of Nursing Practice, 8*(1), 49–55. DOI: 10.1046/j.1440-172x.2002.00338.x PMID: 11831427

Järbrink, K., Ni, G., Sönnergren, H., Schmidtchen, A., Pang, C., Bajpai, R., & Car, J. (2017). The humanistic and economic burden of chronic wounds: A protocol for a systematic review. *Systematic Reviews, 6*(1), 15. DOI: 10.1186/s13643-016-0400-8 PMID: 28118847

Jeppesen, S. M., Yderstraede, K. B., Rasmussen, B. S., Hanna, M., & Lund, L. (2016). Extracorporeal shockwave therapy in the treatment of chronic diabetic foot ulcers: A prospective randomised trial. *Journal of Wound Care, 25*(11), 641–649. DOI: 10.12968/jowc.2016.25.11.641 PMID: 27827284

Kang, K., & Bacci, S. (2022). Photodynamic Therapy. *Biomedicines, 10*, 2701. DOI: 10.3390/biomedicines10112701

Kawasaki, L., Mushahwar, V. K., Ho, C., Dukelow, S. P., Chan, L. L., & Chan, K. M. (2014). The mechanisms and evidence of efficacy of electrical stimulation for healing of pressure ulcer: A systematic review. *Wound Repair and Regeneration, 22*(2), 161–173. DOI: 10.1111/wrr.12134 PMID: 24372691

Kloth, L. C. (2009). The role of physical therapy in wound management - part one. *The Journal of the American College of Certified Wound Specialists, 1*(1), 4–5. DOI: 10.1016/j.jcws.2008.08.001 PMID: 24527101

Koel, G., & Houghton, P. E. (2014). Electrostimulation: Current Status, Strength of Evidence Guidelines, and Meta-Analysis. *Advances in Wound Care (New Rochelle, N.Y.), 3*(2), 118–126. DOI: 10.1089/wound.2013.0448 PMID: 24761352

Kottner, J., Cuddigan, J., Carville, K., Balzer, K., Berlowitz, D., Law, S., & Haesler, E. (2019). Prevention and treatment of pressure ulcers/injuries: The protocol for the second update of the international Clinical Practice Guideline 2019. *Journal of Tissue Viability*, *28*(2), 51–58. DOI: 10.1016/j.jtv.2019.01.001 PMID: 30658878

Kruger, E. A., Pires, M., Ngann, Y., Sterling, M., & Rubayi, S. (2013). Comprehensive management of pressure ulcers in spinal cord injury: Current concepts and future trends. *The Journal of Spinal Cord Medicine*, *36*(6), 572–585. DOI: 10.1179/2045772313y.0000000093 PMID: 24090179

Kuffler, D. P. (2015). Improving the ability to eliminate wounds and pressure ulcers. *Wound Repair and Regeneration*, *23*(3), 312–317. DOI: 10.1111/wrr.12284 PMID: 25801293

Larking, A. M., Duport, S., Clinton, M., Hardy, M., & Andrews, K. (2010). Randomized control of extracorporeal shock wave therapy versus placebo for chronic decubitus ulceration. *Clinical Rehabilitation*, *24*(3), 222–229. DOI: 10.1177/0269215509346083 PMID: 20156981

Latimer, S., Chaboyer, W., Thalib, L., McInnes, E., Bucknall, T., & Gillespie, B. M. (2019). Pressure injury prevalence and predictors among older adults in the first 36 hours of hospitalisation. *Journal of Clinical Nursing*, *28*(21-22), 4119–4127. DOI: 10.1111/jocn.14967 PMID: 31216388

Lei, H., Zhong, K., Chen, Z., Li, P., Chen, J., Li, H., & Zhou, J. (2025). Global Burden of Pressure Ulcer and Contributing Factors from 1990 to 2021: A Systematic Analysis with Forecasts to 2035. *Advances in Wound Care (New Rochelle, N.Y.)*. Advance online publication. DOI: 10.1089/wound.2025.0021 PMID: 40272818

Li, L., Yang, Y., Yang, Z., Zheng, M., Luo, G., He, W., & Yin, R. (2022). Effects of ALA-PDT on the macrophages in wound healing and its related mechanisms in vivo and in vitro. *Photodiagnosis and Photodynamic Therapy*, *38*, 102816. DOI: 10.1016/j.pdpdt.2022.102816 PMID: 35378277

Lupiáñez-Pérez, I., Gómez-González, A. J., Marfil-Gómez, R. M., Morales-Asencio, J. M., García-Mayor, S., León-Campos, Á., & Morilla-Herrera, J. C. (2021). Tissue temperature, flux and oxygen of sacral and trochanteric area under pressure of healthy subjects: A quasi-experimental study. *Journal of Tissue Viability*, *30*(2), 207–215. DOI: 10.1016/j.jtv.2021.01.006 PMID: 33487523

Machado, R. S., Viana, S., & Sbruzzi, G. (2017). Low-level laser therapy in the treatment of pressure ulcers: Systematic review. *Lasers in Medical Science*, *32*(4), 937–944. DOI: 10.1007/s10103-017-2150-9 PMID: 28116536

Maj, A., Kusiak, A., Garbacz, K., Cichońska, D., & Świetlik, D. (2025). Photodynamic therapy in non-surgical treatment of periodontitis. *Scientific Reports, 15*(1), 5903. DOI: 10.1038/s41598-025-89563-3 PMID: 39966437

McInnes, E., Jammali-Blasi, A., Bell-Syer, S. E., Dumville, J. C., Middleton, V., & Cullum, N. (2015). Support surfaces for pressure ulcer prevention. *Cochrane Database of Systematic Reviews, 2015*(9), Cd001735. DOI: 10.1002/14651858.CD001735.pub5 PMID: 26333288

Mohammed, M. (2024). Exercise intervention in frailty, challenges, and recommendations. In *Difficulties and challenges in geriatric health management* (p. 30). IGI Global., DOI: 10.4018/979-8-3693-0675-8.ch007

Mohammed, M. (2025). Rehabilitation and assistive robotics for the elderly and physically challenged. In *Modern technologies in healthcare* (1st ed., p. 20). CRC., DOI: 10.1201/9781003481959

Mohammed, M., & Li, J. (2022). Stroke-Related Sarcopenia among Two Different Developing Countries with Diverse Ethnic Backgrounds (Cross-National Study in Egypt and China). *Healthcare (Basel), 10*(11). Advance online publication. DOI: 10.3390/healthcare10112336 PMID: 36421660

Mohammed, M., & Li, J. (2023). Knowledge mapping and visualization of current sarcopenia and cancer research: A bibliometric analysis. *Beni-Suef University Journal of Basic and Applied Sciences, 12*(1), 51. DOI: 10.1186/s43088-023-00386-5

Mohammed, M., Mehani, S., Aziz, A. A., Mohamed, M. F., & El Nahas, N. (2023). Efficacy of threshold inspiratory muscle trainer versus diaphragmatic plus pursed lip breathing in occupational COPD. *Beni-Suef University Journal of Basic and Applied Sciences, 12*(1), 73. DOI: 10.1186/s43088-023-00409-1

National Pressure Injury Advisory Panel. E. P. U. A. P. a. P. P. P. I. A. (2025). Prevention and Treatment of Pressure Ulcers/Injuries: Quick Reference Guide. *The International Guideline: Fourth Edition.*

Olyaie, M., Rad, F. S., Elahifar, M. A., Garkaz, A., & Mahsa, G. (2013). High-frequency and noncontact low-frequency ultrasound therapy for venous leg ulcer treatment: A randomized, controlled study. *Ostomy/Wound Management, 59*(8), 14–20. PMID: 23934374

Ozgok Kangal, M. K., & Kopitnik, N. L. (2025). Physiology, Wound Healing. In *StatPearls*. Treasure Island (FL) ineligible companies. Disclosure: Nancy Kopitnik declares no relevant financial relationships with ineligible companies.: StatPearls Publishing Copyright © 2025, StatPearls Publishing LLC.

Palmieri, B., Vadalà, M., & Laurino, C. (2020). Electromedical devices in wound healing management: A narrative review. *Journal of Wound Care, 29*(7), 408–418. DOI: 10.12968/jowc.2020.29.7.408 PMID: 32654604

Panel, N. P. U. A. (2014). *National Pressure Ulcer Advisory Panel, European Pressure Ulcer Advisory Panel and Pan Pacific Pressure Injury*. Cambridge Media.

Panel., E. P. U. A. P. a. N. P. U. A. (2009). Prevention and treatment of pressure ulcers: quick reference guide. *Washington DC: National Pressure Ulcer Advisory Panel, 2009.*

Percival, S. L., Francolini, I., & Donelli, G. (2015). Low-level laser therapy as an antimicrobial and antibiofilm technology and its relevance to wound healing. *Future Microbiology, 10*(2), 255–272. DOI: 10.2217/fmb.14.109 PMID: 25689537

Polak, A., Franek, A., Blaszczak, E., Nawrat-Szoltysik, A., Taradaj, J., Wiercigroch, L., & Juras, G. (2014). A prospective, randomized, controlled, clinical study to evaluate the efficacy of high-frequency ultrasound in the treatment of Stage II and Stage III pressure ulcers in geriatric patients. *Ostomy/Wound Management, 60*(8), 16–28. PMID: 25105475

Polak, A., Kloth, L. C., Blaszczak, E., Taradaj, J., Nawrat-Szoltysik, A., Ickowicz, T., & Kucio, C. (2017). The Efficacy of Pressure Ulcer Treatment With Cathodal and Cathodal-Anodal High-Voltage Monophasic Pulsed Current: A Prospective, Randomized, Controlled Clinical Trial. *Physical Therapy, 97*(8), 777–789. DOI: 10.1093/ptj/pzx052 PMID: 28789467

Polak, A., Taradaj, J., Nawrat-Szoltysik, A., Stania, M., Dolibog, P., Blaszczak, E., & Kucio, C. (2016). Reduction of pressure ulcer size with high-voltage pulsed current and high-frequency ultrasound: A randomised trial. *Journal of Wound Care, 25*(12), 742–754. DOI: 10.12968/jowc.2016.25.12.742 PMID: 27974012

Raeder, K., Jachan, D. E., Müller-Werdan, U., & Lahmann, N. A. (2020). Prevalence and risk factors of chronic wounds in nursing homes in Germany: A Cross-Sectional Study. *International Wound Journal, 17*(5), 1128–1134. DOI: 10.1111/iwj.13486 PMID: 32815303

Rajendran, S. B., Challen, K., Wright, K. L., & Hardy, J. G. (2021). Electrical Stimulation to Enhance Wound Healing. *Journal of Functional Biomaterials, 12*(2). Advance online publication. DOI: 10.3390/jfb12020040 PMID: 34205317

Silva, A. M. D., Silva, G. M., Martins, J. C., Bavaresco, T., & Echevarría-Guanilo, M. E. (2025). Photobiomodulation and photodynamic therapy in the treatment of pressure injuries: A scoping review. *Revista Latino-Americana de Enfermagem, 33*, e4488. DOI: 10.1590/1518-8345.7495.4488 PMID: 39969041

Snyder, R., Galiano, R., Mayer, P., Rogers, L. C., & Alvarez, O. (2018). Diabetic foot ulcer treatment with focused shockwave therapy: Two multicentre, prospective, controlled, double-blinded, randomised phase III clinical trials. *Journal of Wound Care, 27*(12), 822–836. DOI: 10.12968/jowc.2018.27.12.822 PMID: 30557108

Soban, L. M., Kim, L., Yuan, A. H., & Miltner, R. S. (2017). Organisational strategies to implement hospital pressure ulcer prevention programmes: Findings from a national survey. *Journal of Nursing Management, 25*(6), 457–467. DOI: 10.1111/jonm.12416 PMID: 27487972

Sopel, M., Kuberka, I., Szczuka, I., Taradaj, J., Rosińczuk, J., & Dymarek, R. (2024). Can Shockwave Treatment Elicit a Molecular Response to Enhance Clinical Outcomes in Pressure Ulcers? The SHOck Waves in wouNds Project. *Biomedicines, 12*(2). Advance online publication. DOI: 10.3390/biomedicines12020359 PMID: 38397961

Taha, M. M., El-Nagar, M. M., Elrefaey, B. H., Elkholy, R. M., Ali, O. I., Alkhamees, N., & Felaya, E. E. E. (2022). Effect of Polarized Light Therapy (Bioptron) on Wound Healing and Microbiota in Diabetic Foot Ulcer: A Randomized Controlled Trial. *Photobiomodulation, Photomedicine, and Laser Surgery, 40*(12), 792–799. DOI: 10.1089/photob.2021.0175 PMID: 36315226

Taradaj, J., Shay, B., Dymarek, R., Sopel, M., Walewicz, K., Beeckman, D., & Rosińczuk, J. (2018). Effect of laser therapy on expression of angio- and fibrogenic factors, and cytokine concentrations during the healing process of human pressure ulcers. *International Journal of Medical Sciences, 15*(11), 1105–1112. DOI: 10.7150/ijms.25651 PMID: 30123047

Tsai, Y. J., Lin, C. H., Yen, Y. H., Wu, C. C., Carvajal, C., Molte, N. F., & Hsieh, C. H. (2023). Risk factors for pressure ulcer recurrence following surgical reconstruction: A cross-sectional retrospective analysis. *Frontiers in Surgery, 10*, 970681. DOI: 10.3389/fsurg.2023.970681 PMID: 36936658

Wang, C., Huang, S., Zhu, T., Sun, X., Zou, Y., & Wang, Y. (2014). [Efficacy of photodynamic antimicrobial therapy for wound flora and wound healing of pressure sore with pathogen infection]. *Zhonghua Yi Xue Za Zhi, 94*(31), 2455–2459. PMID: 25400056

Zhang, Q., Sun, Z., & Yue, J. (2015). Massage therapy for preventing pressure ulcers. *Cochrane Database of Systematic Reviews, 2015*(6), Cd010518. DOI: 10.1002/14651858.CD010518.pub2 PMID: 26081072

Zhang, Q. H., Sun, Z. R., Yue, J. H., Ren, X., Qiu, L. B., Lv, X. L., & Du, W. (2013). Traditional Chinese medicine for pressure ulcer: A meta-analysis. *International Wound Journal, 10*(2), 221–231. DOI: 10.1111/j.1742-481X.2012.00969.x PMID: 22512889

APPENDIX

Abbreviation

Pressure Ulcers (PUs)
European Pressure Ulcer Advisory Panel (EPUAP)
National Pressure Ulcer Advisory Panel (NPUAP)
Wound Healing (WH)
Extracorporeal Shock Wave Therapy (ESWT)
Diabetic Foot Ulcers (DFUs)
Venous Leg Ulcers (VLUs)
Low-Level Light Therapy (LLLT)
Photodynamic Therapy (PDT)
Photobiomodulation (PBM)
Tumor Necrosis Factor-Alpha (TNF-α)
Interleukin-6 (IL-6)
Vascular Endothelial Growth Factor (VEGF)
Reactive Oxygen Species (ROS)
Photodynamic Antimicrobial Chemotherapy (PACT)
Polyethylenimine–Chlorin E6 (PEI–ce6)
Epidermal Growth Factor (EGF)
Matrix Metalloproteinases (MMPs)
Near-Infrared (NIR)
Visible Polarized Light Therapy (VPLT)
Electrical stimulation (ES)
Endogenous Bioelectric Fields (EBFs)
Chronic Wound (CW)
Direct Current (DC)
High-Voltage Monophasic Pulsed Current (HVMPC)
Pulses Per Second (pps)
Standard Wound Care (SWC)
Ultrasound therapy (UT)
Low-Frequency Ultrasound (LFU)
Oxygen Saturation (SaO_2)
Constant Low-Pressure (CLP)
Alternating Pressure (AP)
Allow-Technology (low-tech).

Chapter 7
Integrating AI-Powered Wearables Into Palliative Care Management for Elderly Patients

Temitope Emmanuel Komolafe
https://orcid.org/0000-0003-4161-0158
Shanghai University of Medicine and Health Sciences, China

Blessing Funmi Komolafe
Shanghai University of Medicine and Health Sciences, China

Liang Zhou
Jiading District Central Hospital, Shanghai University of Medicine and Health Sciences, China

Adegbola Oyedotun Adeniji
https://orcid.org/0009-0004-6637-7094
Federal Medical Centre, Owo, Nigeria

Wenlong Zhao
Shanghai University of Medicine and Health Sciences, China

Tao Wu
Shanghai University of Medicine and Health Sciences, China

ABSTRACT

The increase in population of elderly people across the world is presenting a dauting challenge for palliative cares because elderly people are often encountered health challenges and other chronic diseases. This chapter delves into integration of artificial intelligence (AI)-powered wearable devices into elderly palliative cares. These advanced technologies allow proper monitoring of patient vital signs, track symptoms and adopt predictive analysis to prove patient's outcome. (AI)-powered wearable can monitor disease progression, allow remote monitoring which promote patient autonomy especially at home or hospices settings. We presented a comprehensive framework that include diagnostic and therapeutic advantages, case studies and other

DOI: 10.4018/979-8-3373-4099-9.ch007

ethical issues such data privacy and informed consent. This chapter also present challenges such users' acceptability, we also mentioned other real-world applications such as CardioMEMS, Control-IQ, Sepsis Watch and the rest. We conclude the chapter by providing guidelines and recommendation to sharpen future research

1.0 INTRODUCTION

1.1 Overview of Aging and Terminal Care Challenges

The population of elderly people is increasing at alarming rate, which is posing great challenges to the healthcare systems. According to the world's population prospects, the world's population is projected to rise to 10.3 billion in the mid-2080 according to projection (UN, 2022). The number of people with age of 65years and above will exceed the number of children under the age of 18years by 2080. In that direction, the population of people above 80years of age will also exceed the infants (UN,2022). This paradigm shift is largely fueled by low-rate fertility in some developed and developing countries of the world like China, Japan, South Korea, Italy and Spain, which ultimately mount pressure on the healthcare and social care systems. As aged-people population continue to increase, there will be high demand for sustainable healthcare services prompting a significantly shift in healthcare management service to include social protections and amenities for caregivers (Khan et al., 2024).

According to World Health Organization (WHO) projection of 2050, the population of elderly of 60years and above will increase from 12% to 22% (WHO, 2024). The shift in this demographic representation poses a major threat, because older people are highly susceptible to chronic diseases, mental health challenges and disabilities which require a sustainable healthcare system (WHO, 2024). This poses a great demand on the healthcare systems and other social services likewise for terminal care (Gianfredi et al., 2025). Also, other non-communicable diseases like cardiovascular disease, diabetes and cancer are prevalent in elderly people, this has caused more burden healthcare systems (AIHW, 2021). Adverse drug reaction from continuous use of medications to monitor elderly patients, malnutrition, all these further put additional strains on healthcare resources (Atella et al., 2019).

This would result into high demand for terminal and long-term healthcare services, putting great pressure on already existing healthcare systems and other social support services. Terminal as popularly referred to as end-of-life care is also greatly affected by this demographic shift, because the elderly people are always affected and they need model that can seamlessly integrate physical, phycological and social support services (Arimany-Manso et al., 2025). However, there exist a great gap in palliative care services, as many elderly people prefer to aggressive treatments in hospitals but die at home, this creates a disconnect the healthcare they desired and the one they received. In recent time, there is increase in this caregiver gaps, as most family members are not available to provide informer care as result of reduction in birthrate in most advanced countries. The paid caregivers are always overworked, combined systemic barriers like ageism have negatively impact quality of healthcare services and also the resources (Logevity, 2021).

To address challenges associated with terminal care, we need an integrated and comprehensive policy solutions that focus more accessibility, equity and dignity of older people. This can be achieved by investing in palliative healthcare facilities, improve welfare of caregiver support staffs and promote elderly voice in our society. We strongly believe that AI adoption into various domain can transform terminal care using an innovative and personalized healthcare solutions.

1.1.1 The Role of AI Technology in Enhancing Palliative Care

The adoption of advanced technologies like AI-powered wearables devices is a game changer for elderly palliative care management. The primary goal of palliative care is to manage pain, to improve quality of life and proper support to patient with life-threatening health challenges (Anagnostou, 2017). The recent wave of smart wearables that consist of biosensors and AI software has revolutionized this area (Shajari et al., 2023). These devices monitor vital signs like heart rate, respiratory rate, oxygen saturation, physical activities and even sleep patterns for early detection of critical health issues (Chan et al., 2022). These devices analyse this physiological data using AI-algorithm to enable real-time intervention, and this will prevent unnecessary hospitalization and enhance comfortability of patients (Health Management, 2024).

Furthermore, AI-powered wearables promote patient-centered care by improving autonomous interactions between patients, caregivers and healthcare experts (Mahajan et al., 2025). In real-life applications, wearables can give caregivers notice when the symptoms soar higher which trigger faster response for autonomous control. Some of these devices also use voice assistance technology and emotion-tracking functions in order to integrate emotional support and helping clinicians to solve health issues like mental and anxiety even depression commonly to elderly people (Liu et al., 2024). Moreover, these technologies can also be technically incorporate cognitive perspectives making them available to elderly populations. In wearables, acquired data can be synergistically adopted into electronic health records (EHRs) enhancing progression in care service delivery and multidisciplinary collaboration (Bonfiglio, 2025).

In this era where healthcare systems are pressured as results of increasing elderly population, AI-enabled wearables can offer a scalable and cost-effective solutions that can be adopted into palliative healthcare management. Despite the potential solution, using such devices must come with addressing ethical concerns, privacy and equity concerns. In such application, maintaining data security, getting informed consent, and preventing algorithms bias are vital criterial for responsible application of this AI-Technologies. Moreso, we must strive to synergies this digital bridge in both in low- and middle-income countries to ensure mutual benefits for elderly across the globe (UN, 2023). As these technologies continue to advance, AI-enabled wearables give a critical tool for delivering anticipatory palliative cares for elderly people worldwide with emotional instinct into such design. Figure 1 presents a smart dashboard for intelligent intensive care units (eICU).

Figure 1. 5G-enabled smart electronic intensive care unit (eICU) adapted with AI for patient health data management. The dashboard shows real-time monitoring interface from a 5G-based intelligent ICU. This deploys some vital signs and also shows anatomic visualization electrocardiography monitoring, lab test trends, mortality risk prediction comparison using APACHE, SOFA. This support multi-center data integration and facilitates data-driven decision-making in critical care settings

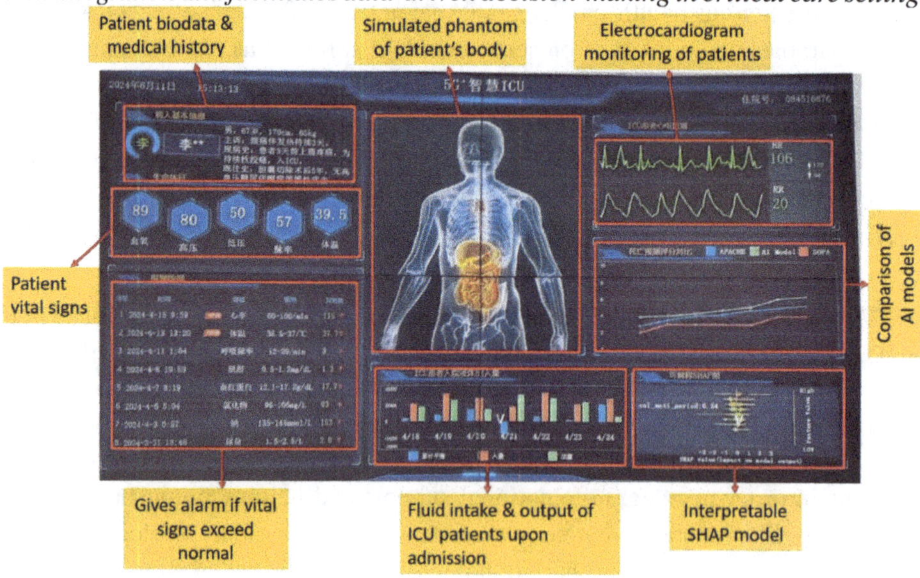

Collaborative Research Centre, Shanghai University of Medicine & Health Sciences

2.0 CLINICAL PROFILE OF ELDERLY PATIENTS IN PALLIATIVE CARE

2.1 Common Clinical Conditions of Elderly Patients

In elderly patients, there is prevalence of a complex blending of clinical conditions that significantly impact their quality of life and healthcare need (Kumlin et al., 2020). The more people grow old, there is increase in likelihood of developing chronic and degenerative diseases (Sun and Li, 2023). Among the most prevalent conditions are cardiovascular diseases like hypertension, cardiovascular diseases, diabetes mellitus, chronic respiratory disorders such as chronic obstructive pulmonary disease (COPD), and musculoskeletal challenges like arthritis and osteoporosis (Petries et al., 2018). Figure 2 shows some common clinical conditions experienced by elderly patient. Neurodegenerative disorders like Alzheimer's disease and other forms of dementia are also common, which affect the cognitive function of patients (Ramachandran et al., 2021). Mostly, older adults suffer from multimorbidity i.e. when a patient suffers from two or more chronic diseases, this tends to complicate treatment procedures which ultimately increase the risk of hospitalizations, medication errors, and reduce patient functionality (Ren et al., 2023). These conditions often progress stealthily and thus require long-term monitoring and sustainable management, which places significant pressure on caregivers and health systems.

In addition to chronic physical illnesses, elderly individuals frequently present with geriatric syndromes such as frailty, falls, incontinence, delirium, and pressure ulcers (Cicerchia et al., 2010). These syndromes result from the cumulative effect of age-related physiological decline and are often underdiagnosed due to their non-specific presentation (Li et al., 2021). Mental health issues, particularly depression and anxiety, are also prevalent, yet remain underreported due to social stigma or misinterpretation as normal aging. Sensory impairments like hearing loss and vision decline which lead to isolation and quality of life reduction. As related to the palliative care, these conditions require targeted management strategies that focus on patient comfortability, functionality, and dignity instead of therapeutic values. Embedding such AI-powered wearables technology provide powerful and sustainable solutions (Kuebler et al., 2024). By continuously monitoring vital signs, activity levels, sleep patterns, and even emotional states, these technologies can provide early detection of disease deterioration to enhanced personalized care, and facilitate timely interventions to improve patient outcomes and easing caregiver burden.

Figure 2. Common clinical conditions among elderly patients. This diagram presents prevalent clinical conditions in elderly patients. Effective planning and management depend on examinations of these critical conditions outlined in the figure

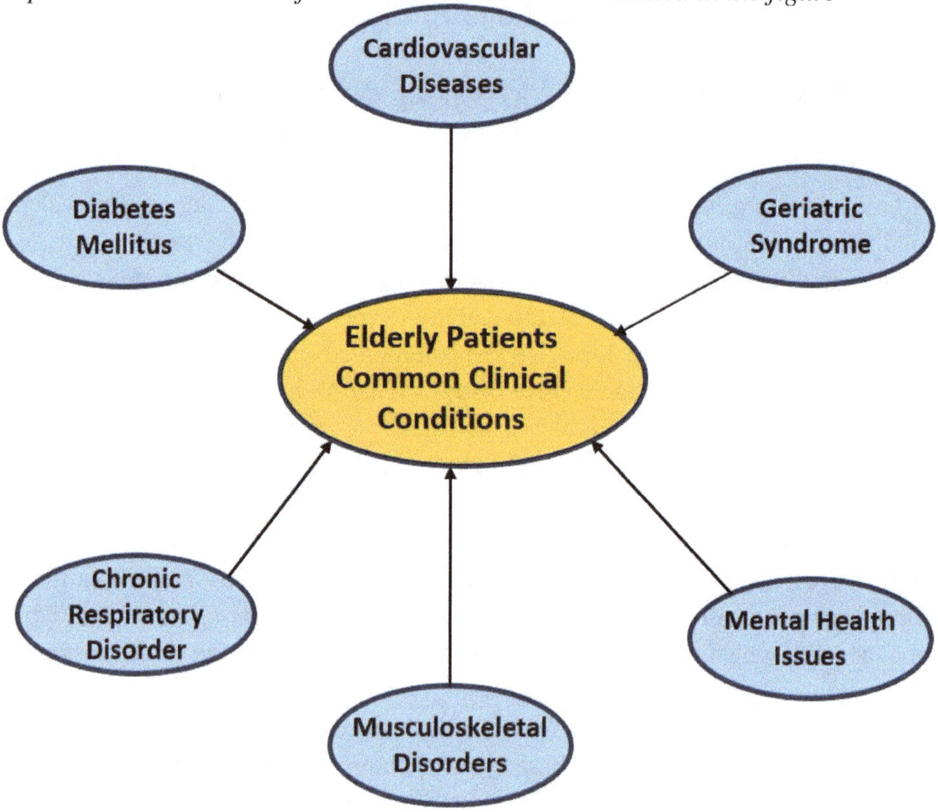

Palliative care for elderly is often accompanied by wide range of diagnostic and therapeutic issues as result of multi-comorbidity, physiological changes due age and other symptoms (Roller-Wirnsberger et al., 2020). Communication barriers, cognitive decline and sensory impairment make detection of distress more challenging (Sutin et al., 2018). Let look for instance, detection of arthritis pain from pain caused by cancer requires persistence monitoring (Funabashi et al., 2022). Traditional care methods depend on phasal clinical evaluations, which may not caption early warning sign of disease worsening.

Taking a very common example from previous experience, an old man nearly 70 years old had cancer, living in under-developed countries of the world without modern facilities, before he received an accurate diagnosis, it might be too late because the cancer will have metastasized to surrounding internal organs and the man may die early. Assuming such patient was privilege of assessing modern facilities with good diagnostic accuracy, such condition might be detected early, commenced early treatment which might definitely prolonged the lifespan of such an individual.

In general, reporting of early symptoms are not commonly reported in elderly patients, as this can warrant accurate treatment due to timely response (Bertolazzi et al. 2024).

Embedding AI-enabled wearable technology into palliative care is capable of eliminating these challenges. Sensors fixed with wearables attached to patients monitor vital signs like heartrate, oxygen saturation level, body temperature, sleep pattens and other physical activities (Helmer et al. 2025). When this sensor works with AI, the acquired data can be monitored and processed in real-time to detect any tiny changes physiological changes before the symptom's surfaces, this will ensure early interventions and personalized care. For example, predictive models can alert clinicians to increased risks of respiratory failure detection or sepsis monitoring (Zhou et al., 2024; Zhou et al., 2025) which allow intervention therapeutic without waiting for the next clinical appointment, for more details on this see Figure 3.

Figure 3. The role of AI technology in enhancing palliative care. This framework shows how AI-enabled wearable devices can enhance palliative cares in elderly populace

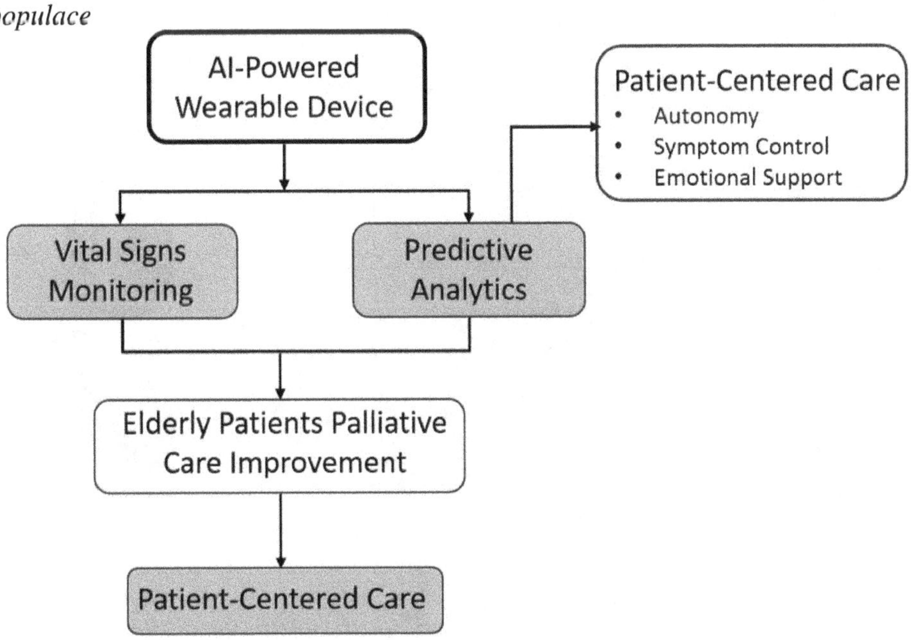

The treatments or therapeutic benefits of AI-enabled wearables enables doctors to monitor how patients are responding to prescribed medication, identifying side effects and dose optimization. The real-time feedback gotten reduced error committed by trial and error in systems management in palliative care (Mahajan et al., 2024). Likewise, AI-enabled wearables can be used as supporting care-giver to monitor patient symptoms while preserving quality of life by synchronizing clinical actions physiological realities and preference of patients. The integration of such technology shows the novel and effective means to manage diagnostic and therapeutic health issues in palliative cares (Awad et al., 2021), drifting from reactive approach to proactive method.

Figure 4. AI Wearable Devices for physiological measurement in elderly patients. This figure illustrates how AI-enabled devices can be used to monitor male patient. These devices help in predictive and personalized healthcare management for chronic disease

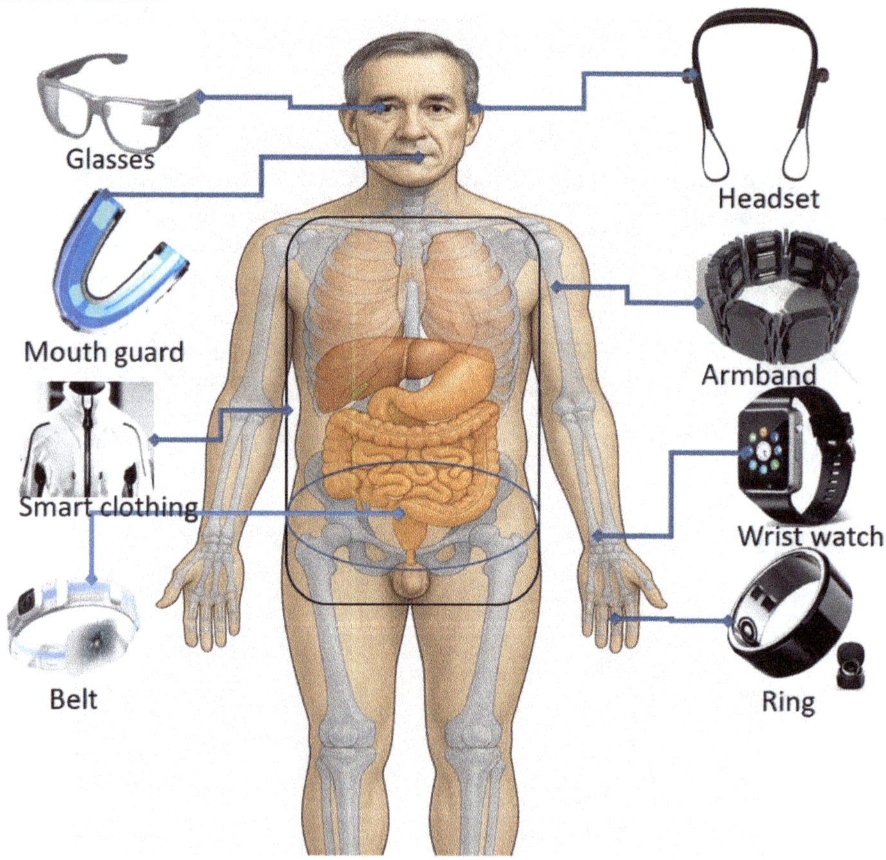

3.0 AI-Powered Wearables: Capabilities and Use Cases

3.1 Description of Wearable AI Wearable Devices and Application

Wearable devices is a transformative tool in healthcare that have revolutionized the system, especially in area of monitoring and management of chronic diseases in palliative cares for elderly patients. They are lightweights, non-invasive and comes in different forms like smartwatches, smart clothing's even implantable monitors (Bonfiglio, 2025). Wearables are equipped with various sensors that take physiological and others like behavioral data like heat rate, respiratory, oxygen saturation sleep quality pattern, electrodermal activity (Assaad et al., 2025). This continuous and passive data collection very important in palliative care especially when patients experience sudden changes in health status for timely and personalized intervention (Kamal et al., 2012). Figure 4 shows example of wearable technology for monitoring physiological changes in elderly patients.

The adoption of AI significantly improves how these wearables device's function, it also ensures real-time data analysis and decision making (Nahavandi, et al., 2022). These AI process large amount of data collected, analyze the structure of data to detect patterns and use this trend to make decision, some of these intrinsic trends are not noted by people. For example, machine learning (ML) a subset of AI can detect early sign of sepsis, cardiac arrest or other respiratory disease even before the onset of any sign, this will allow prompt and quick intervention (Ramani et al., 2021). These predictive abilities are essential ingredients in early intervention palliative care scenarios which improve quality of life and reduce emergency admission. The ability of AI to predicts is very important in palliative care management, which helps in early intervention to improve the life's quality and prevent unnecessary hospitalization (Murphree et al.,2021). It also helps in designing a personalized care. Gaining insight from patient history and perspective and compare with the large data acquired from patients. AI tools can be adopted in targeted intervention that goes with condition of patients and want they wanted (Ghanem et al.,2024). This process will adjust patient medication, variation in physical activities or giving alert to the caregivers when the slight changes in physiological signs which can be from stress or any discomfort.

The devices that use natural language processing (NLP) models are designed for translations, for instance interpreting voice commands or patients' symptoms to make interaction seamlessly for elderly patients (Lazzaroni et al., 2024). In summary, the hybrid of wearable devices and AI models provide a paradigm shift in elderly palliative care, useful at home and in hospitals. The hybrid systems did not only promote continuous health management but also support both clinical and personalized care delivery. As these technologies' advances, we expect to notice great improvement in comfort level, quality of life for wearables which improve elderly patient's palliative care. See Figure 5 for more general application of AI-enabled wearables.

Figure 5. Functional application of AI-enabled wearables. This diagram depicts various areas that AI-enabled wearables can be adopted

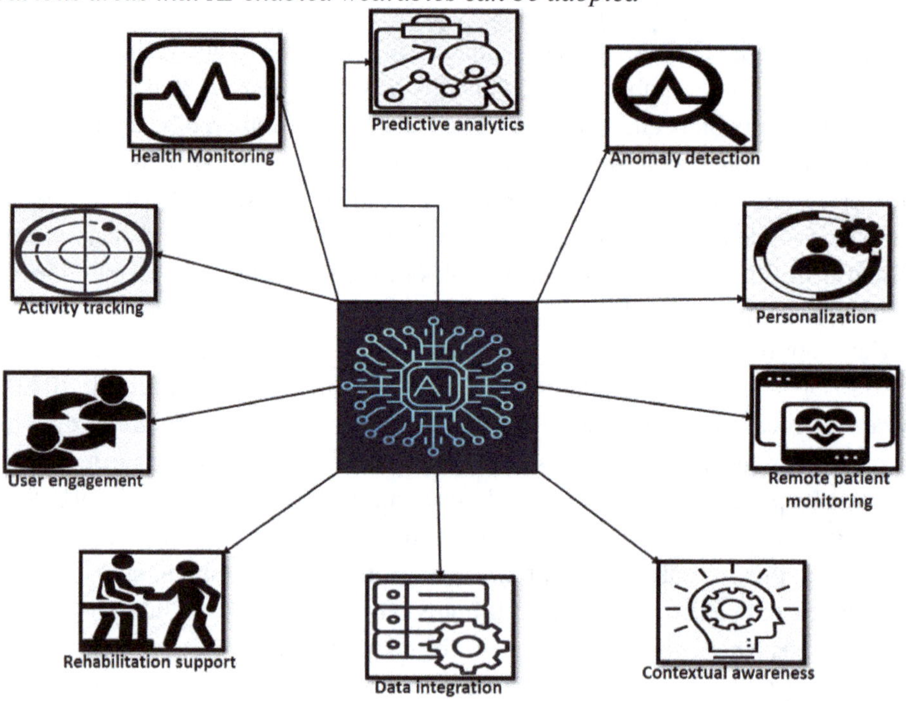

3.2 Current Applications of AI in Chronic and Acute Care

Artificial Intelligence (AI) is greatly turning tables in healthcare industry, particularly in the management of chronic and acute diseases. In chronic disease management, AI-enabled devices are vital tools for long-term disease management by predicting how disease progresses and given optimal dose regime for proper elderly patience compliance (Dong et al., 2025).

Let's look at this example, management of diabetes, AI algorithms will analyze glucose levels in the blood, and feeding habits and physical activities, these data are gathered and the output recommend insulin medication dosages suitable and other dietary recommendation for the elderly patients. In similar application, AI algorithms can monitor hypertension and heart failure by predicting excessive breathing that help prevent emergency admission of patients (Chaikijurajai et al., 2020).

In acute care scenarios, AI applications are developed to apply for fast diagnosis and quick decision making. AI-enabled devices in emergency rooms and intensive care units (ICU) can analyze vast amount of data in real-time to predict early warning signs for sepsis, cardiac arrest or other respiratory sickness (Pinsky et al., 2024). In prediction of disease, these devices can flag critical changes in parameters like heart rate, oxygen saturation level suitable for clinical timely action. AI-enabled imaging can be adopted into stroke management, in which AI algorithm interpreted computed tomography (CT) scan and magnetic resonance imaging (MRI) scan for both detection and prediction of severity of ischemic strokes (Gobinath et al., 2025). This guides the administration of therapy and effective management.

Furthermore, natural language processing (NLP) is effective at extracting relevant clinically information from electronic health records (EHRs), which reduced doctor's workload for effective diagnostic task. In both acute and chronic care management, tools like AI chatbots, virtual assistants are proving patient with 24 hours a day health guidance Open MedScience. (2024, December 6). These tools are very important for elderly patients who have difficulty in walking or cognitive challenges to maintain continuous engagement with healthcare reducing dependence on healthcare assistance. For more information on AI application for chronic and acute disease management, see Figure 6.

When this device is synchronized with wearable technologies, AI becomes even more potent providing real-time continuous monitoring when compared to traditional clinical settings. This synergy provides a solid model that can overcome shortcomings of chronic and acute care to pride early detection, enhanced personalized treatment and ensures continuity in healthcare workflow (Chen et al., 2025). In summary, application of AI is redesigning a new course for healthcare management, making it more predictive, preventive and patients centered which are vital for elderly care management.

Figure 6. Recent applications of AI in management of chronic and acute disease. In chronic care, AI is applied for prediction of disease progression, wearable monitoring and treatment planning, while in acute care it supports fast diagnosis and prediction.

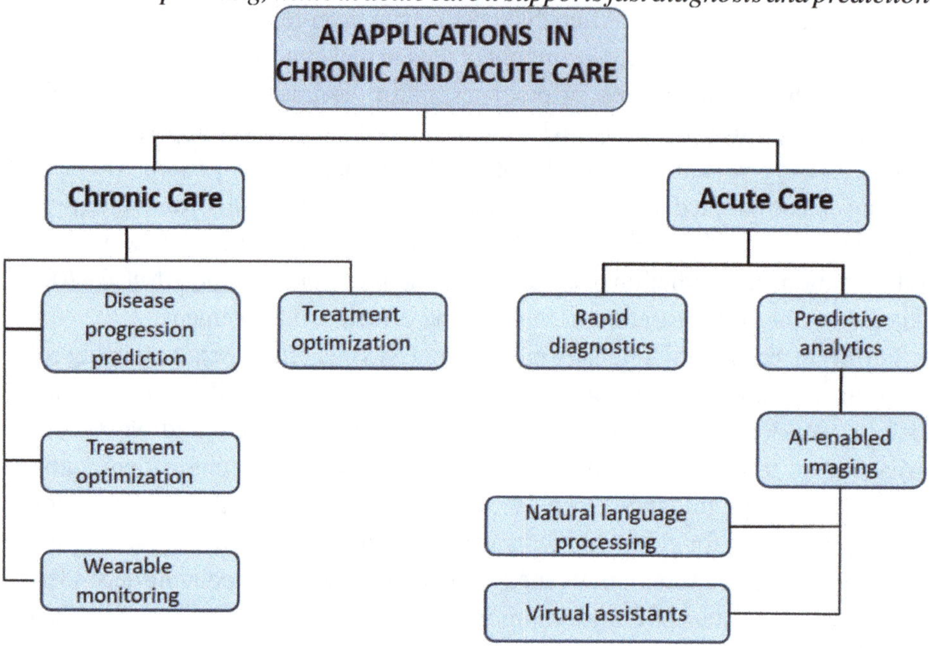

3.3 Case studies on the AI Application in Chronic and Acute Disease Management

The practical case studies of artificial intelligence (AI) in both chronic and acute clinical disease management as shown by real-world case studies which demonstrate the outcome improvement in elderly care. In chronic disease management, typical example is the AI-powered platform for management of heart failures. The "Guardian" system developed by CardioMEMS (Abraham et al., 2016) permit remote monitoring pulmonary pressure in the artery with specially designed implantable sensors. The data received is processed by AI algorithms that can predict in advance the onset of psychological failure, for early intervention of clinicians and prevent hospital re-admission. With this development, the quality of life is improved because it needs to reduce the number of elderly patients that depend on emergency care especially those with chronic diseases like heart failure (Radhoe et al., 2023).

In the management of diabetes, AI-enabled wearables like continuous glucose monitoring (CGM) system embedded with "Control-IQ" algorithm developed by Tandem Diabetes are pathfinders for insulin drug delivery (Habif et al., 2020). Apart from real-time monitoring, it also predicts of insulin absorption and dose adjustment. A recent clinical trial studies with elderly patients with Type 1 diabetes has shown that these embedded systems improve time-range system and simultaneously easing the burden of manual intervention, this great improvement have found potential application for geriatric diabetes management while such is difficult because of cognitive compliance. Figure 7 highlight cases for the AI application in both chronic and acute disease management.

Application of AI in acute diseases management have demonstrated a remarkable breakthrough, for example using AI-enable device for decision support system for the emergency departments (ED) in hospitals to predict sepsis. "Sepsis watch" system was developed by the Johns Hopkins Hospital, this device embeds vital signs, laboratory data and electronic health records (EHRs) to flag patients with high risk of sepsis with 1hour of onset (Adams et al.,2022). When this device gives alarm, it will remind healthcare personnel to quickly administer antibiotics to such patient, thus increasing the survival rates. The same principle also works for AI-enabled platform called "Viz.ai", this platform was developed to fast-track diagnosis of stroke, this works by analyzing all the brain scan images, the output give alert to healthcare personnel to carry out surgical intervention or administer drug like thrombolytics.

All the few cases mentioned above have shown the potential of AI-enabled devices which incorporated real-time physiological data from clinical data or wearable devices. In palliative care management, we could deploy such system to monitor symptoms escalation, pain management, which can be adapted by multi-disciplinary team of experts working in the healthcare management. Their approach will helps minimizing suffering, maintain dignity of elderly patients. As AI begin to evolve in coming years, their integration into both chronic and acute care management provides a pathway towards a more holistic, responsive and personalized healthcare service delivery.

Figure 7. Case study on application of AI in chronic and acute disease management. In chronic scenarios, CardiMEMS and Control-IQ improves heart failure and diabetes care. In acute Sepsis Watch and ViZ.ai support early detection and timely intervention necessary.

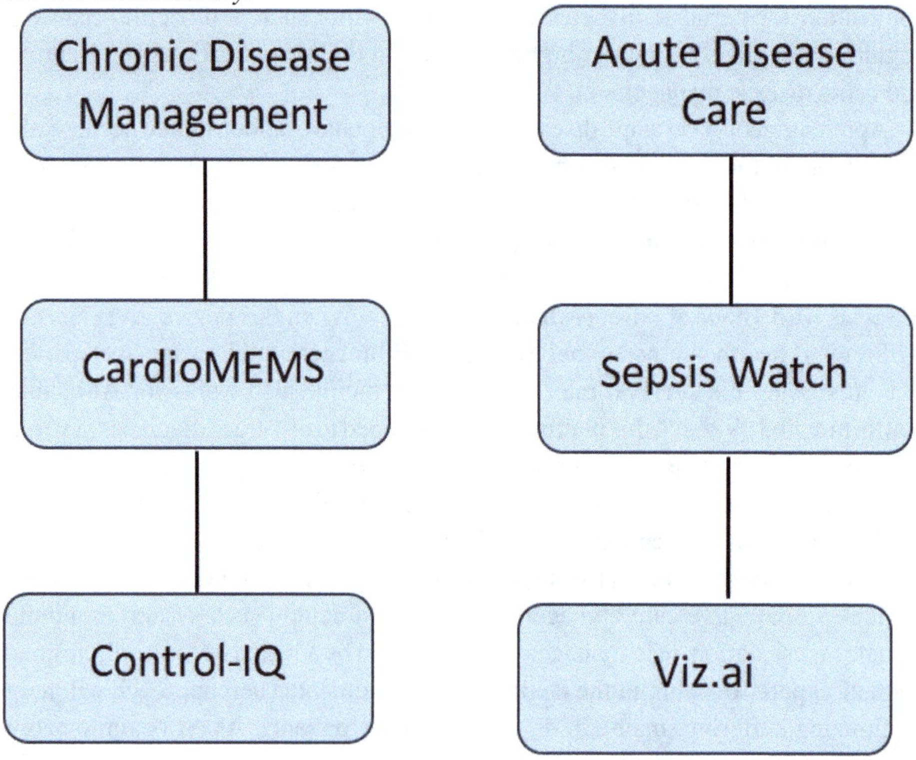

3.4 Case Summary of Rhino-Orbital-Cerebral Mucormycosis in an Elderly Diabetic Patient

This is case study of 67 years old female with diabetes and hypertension, who presented post-COVID pandemic with the following progressive symptoms, that include right-sided headache, nasal congestion, mucopurulent nasal discharge and hyposmia. This was initially managed by our neurology department team and later referred to Ear, Nose, and Throat (ENT) in 2022. Imaging relieved results sphenoethmoidal lesion over the olfactory groove, skull base and orbital apex which connotes invasive. Over 3 months, her condition rapidly deteriorated, with worsening visual symptoms, orbital proptosis, and neurological deficits and loss of consciousness.

Repeated CT scans showed erosion of the right maxillary posterior with pterygopalatine fossa. Biopsy was done under anesthesia from the maxillary antrum and sphenoid sinus revealed greyish-black tissue with areas of necrosis. Histopathology examination confirmed mucormycosis through fungal staining. A diagnosis of rhino-orbital-cerebral mucormycosis (ROCM) was established. See CT image of ROCM.

Because of the delicate nature of the patient' illness, surgical intervention was delayed while attempt was made to stabilize her. She was placed on liposomal Amphotericin B and placed on supportive care. She was not referred to higher hospital facilities because of socio-economic states, while the treatment was going on, her condition worsened due to intra-cranial involvement and died following ICU admission.

The ROCM is rapidly progressive angioinvasive fungal infection often experienced by elderly patients as result of deteriorated immune system. The case above emphasizes need for early diagnosis, multidisciplinary care and timely intervention. For future care application, designing a wearable that monitor early symptoms and monitor symptoms deterioration for elderly patients at high risk.

Figure 8. Axial cranial CT showing rhino-orbital-cerebral mucormycosis in a diabetic patient. Non-contrast axial cranial CT demonstrating asymmetrical opacification and soft tissue swelling of the right orbit, suggestive of orbital involvement. The image shows hyperdense areas consistent with sinus wall involvement, indicative of invasive fungal sinusitis extending to the orbital and possibly intracranial compartments

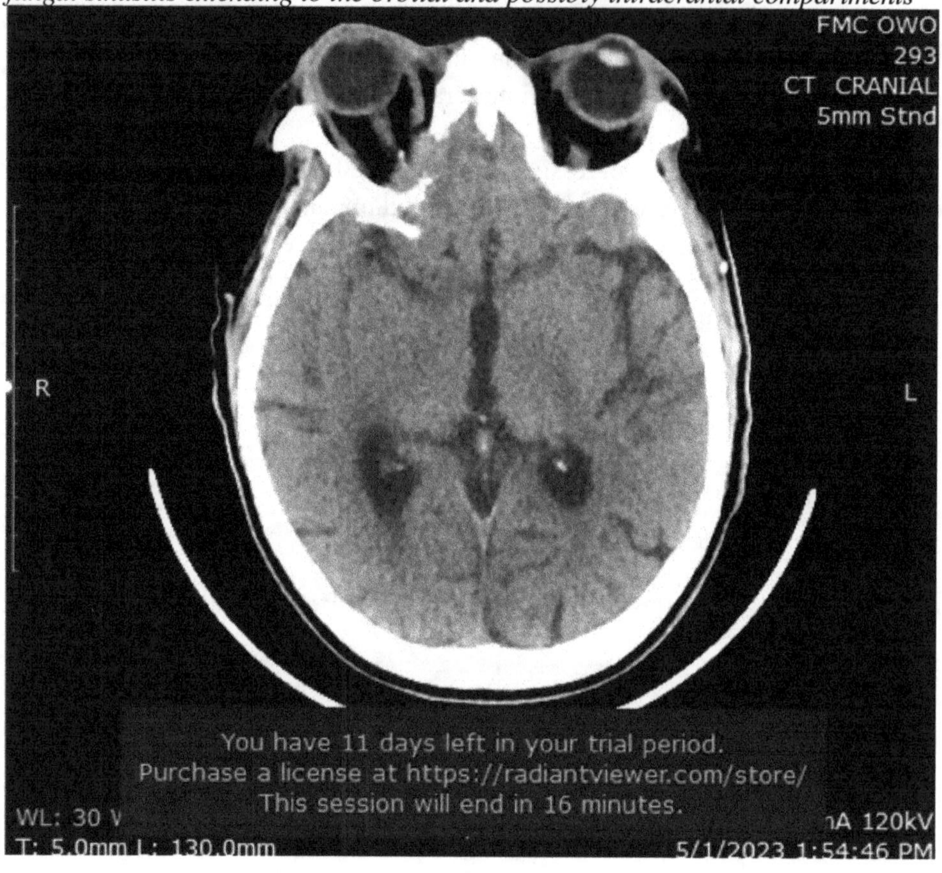

3.5 Case Summary of Extranodal NK/T-Cell Lymphoma With Unusual Sinonasal Tumor in an Elderly Female

A middle-aged to elderly woman, previously healthy, presented with a three-month history of progressive swelling over the nose and upper lip, associated with a rapidly enlarging left-sided nasal growth and blood-stained nasal discharge. There were no constitutional symptoms such as fever, night sweats, weight loss, or neurologic signs. Clinical examination revealed phymatoid nasal changes, bilaterally widened nasal cavities, and multiple firms, non-tender subcutaneous nodules (2–3 cm) on the upper and lower limbs (Figure 9a-b). No lymphadenopathy was observed.

Laboratory investigations showed elevated erythrocyte sedimentation rate (ESR) and absolute eosinophil count, with normal hematology, liver, and renal function. HIV and HBsAg tests were negative. Nasal endoscopy and smears for fungal and mycobacterial organisms were non-revealing. CT scan of the paranasal sinuses demonstrated complete obliteration of the left nasal cavity with mild haziness of the left maxillary sinus. Initial biopsy revealed non-specific findings numerous proliferating capillaries and perivascular lymphoplasmacytic infiltration which suggest granulomatous lesion (Figure 9c), but fungal and AFB cultures were negative. She was placed on antibiotics with a close OPD follow up.

A month later, she returned with a vascular, erythematous mass completely occluding the left nostril and edematous swelling of the right upper lip (Figure 9d). Repeat biopsy showed a dense infiltrate of atypical lymphoid cells with eosinophils, plasma cells, histiocytes, and skeletal muscle infiltration. Immunohistochemistry (IHC) was positive for T-cell markers CD3 and CD45RO, but negative for B-cell marker CD20. CD56 testing (NK-cell marker) was unavailable; however, clinical features and histopathology supported a diagnosis of extranodal nasal NK/T-cell lymphoma. She was referred to oncology for co-management and commenced on weekly intravenous methotrexate (50 mg for 12 weeks). In the 3rd month of her hospital admission, there was a significant regression of the nasal and facial was noticed. The summary of this case pinpoints diagnostic and rapid progression of NK/T-cell lymphomas in elderly patients. In future, AI-enabled wearables to monitor facial swelling, skin texture changes, or even local temperature, which will have a very detailed application in palliative healthcare management.

Figure 9. Clinical presentation of extranodal NK/T-Cell lymphoma in elderly female patients. (b) Edematous swelling of lower left limb. (b) Edema and swelling of the right upper limb showing lymphoproliferative. (c) Early nasal lesion presenting nasal dorsum mistaken for infection. (d) Advanced necrotic and fungating mass occluding the left nostril and distorting the nasal architecture

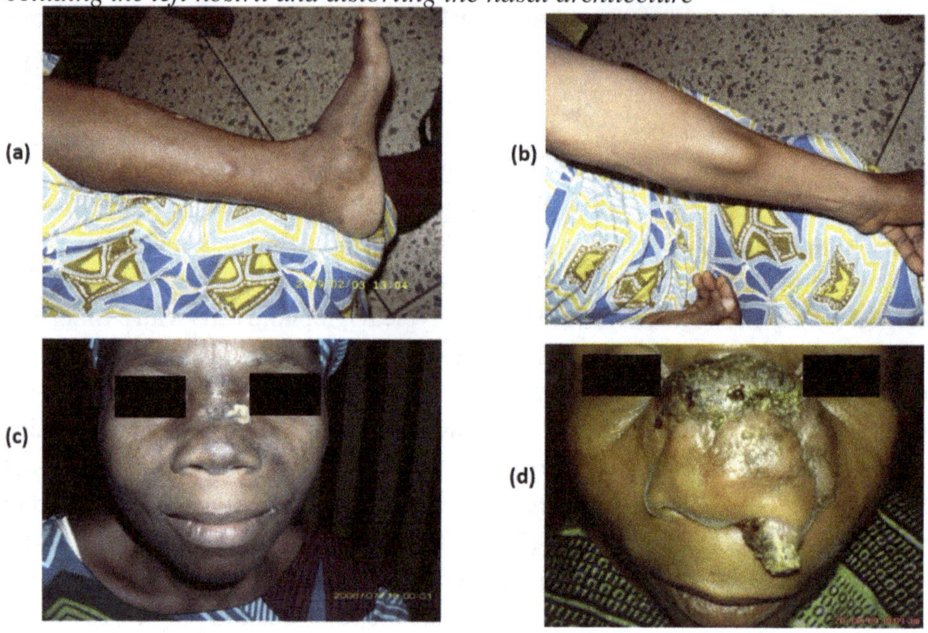

4.0 INTEGRATION OF AI INTO PALLIATIVE DECISION-MAKING

4.1 Integrated Monitoring and Predictive Interventions in Palliative Care

The integration of real-time monitoring and predicting incorporated into palliative cares defined a total turnaround for the healthcare delivery for elderly patients with complexity. Traditional palliative care depends on regularly clinical evaluations and reporting of related symptoms which might hampered timely intervention of medical personnel (Care, 2013). The AI-enabled wearable devices are developed to monitor physiological parameters like heart rate, respiratory, blood oxygen level and sleep patterns (Sethuraman et al. 2020). These devices give unhindered health data streaming, providing detailed view of condition of patients in real-time useful at home or hospice scenario.

The predictive analytics enhance the ability of AI to detect subtle trend or deviation in patient data which might prevent clinical deterioration (Thiele et al.,2025). The slight increment in heart rate or blood oxygen level may implies the onset of respiratory disorder or infection. The AI algorithm trained on large datasets can detect these subtle patterns and produce a predictive alert before the onset of symptoms. This early warning systems enabled the healthcare providers and caregiver workers to be able to respond timely by adjusting to desired medications or arrange emergency care. This intervention prevents complications, suffering and long-time hospitalization.

In general, elderly patients are often have multiple comorbidities, in such scenario, additional line of safety is established. The AI-enabled devices ensure that important health data are not missed when these routines are on-going (Guo et al., 2025). Likewise, special alerts are customized based on the individual patient's standard, making sure that the notification given are accurate, to avoid false alarms. For instance, special AI system can train to screen normal fluctuations in sleep pattern of patients and those that show pain and anxiety episode, thus giving a targeted intervention.

Getting the right actionable information is one the key advantage of palliative care to families and caregivers. They are not just ordinary observer but are actively participating in decision process of healthcare management (Murphree et al., 2021). These receive updates and guidance that help them to act decisively to changes in patient condition. As these technologies become more advanced and accessible, they are creating a new path for palliative care sharpen them into more personalized, and modern with emotion that aligns with core principle of comfort, dignity and quality service of life for elderly patients in their final stages of care.

Symptoms worsening has been attributed to delay self-reporting or missing of follow-up appointment, leading to missed opportunities. However, advent of AI-powered devices such as the Apple Watch Series 8 (Apple Inc.(n.d.)), Fitbit Sense Google LLC (n.d), Biovotion Everrion (Haveman et al., 2021). This allows continuous tracking of physiological indicators like heart rate, blood oxygen saturation (SpO_2), skin temperature and movement patterns. This device stream data in real time, giving healthcare teams continuous visibility into the wellbeing, even when they are at home or long-term care facilities.

Another important illustration is the application of Current Health, this is an AI-driven remote patient monitoring platform used in hospice setting in the United Kingdom (Current Health, n.d.). The system uses a device to monitor patient vital signs and fed into predictive model to detect any subtle psychological changes. In the documented pieces of evidence (Current Health, n.d.), a team of palliative care workers was able to detect sepsis in elderly cancer patient from abnormal increase in temperature and respiratory rate, these changes are captured by wearable. The sounded alarm will prompt the home-based antibiotic treatment to commence, this timely intervention prevent unnecessary hospitalization, with greater comfortability and relaxation at the comfort of home.

AI-enabled system is very vital to synthesize and interpret data stream. A very common application is PeraHealth's Rothman Index, which adopts data from hospital to generate predictive scores for patient deterioration, has been widely used in palliative healthcare management. (Open MedScience. (2024). This device embeds vital signs, laboratory results, nursing assessment, then output early warnings of clinical decline. In another scenario, a patient diagnosed with congestive heart failure wearing a BioSticker from BioIntelliSense showed reduction in physical activity, increase heart rate and body fatigue (BioIntelliSense, 2024). The system flagged this development and the clinicians adjust their diuretic treatment therapy to make sure the patients is in stable condition.

Apart from other physiological parameters measured, AI-enabled devices can incorporate data from patient report. Likewise, platforms like *CarePredict* embed location, motion, sleep quality and other conversations to detect behavioral changes. For example, when patience experience reduction in appetites and withdrawal symptoms, this can be syn of signal depressions or pain experienced by terminally ill patients. By synergistically linking all behavioral indicators with these biometric data, the predictive alert becomes more sensitive to give response that enhances symptom control.

The deployment of such Technology cares more about reducing the workload on caregivers. Families and care teams will receive a real-time notification when an intervention is needed which reduces frequent visit to hospitals. The technology aligns with the goals of palliative care, and this reduces suffering of patients and also provide a dignified, thus shifting a model from reactive to predictive model. This provides greater comfortability and stability for elderly patient nearing their final stages of life.

Figure 10. Application of AI in palliative care decision-making. This figure shows a conceptual framework of AI supporting palliative care via real-time monitoring, predictive dashboards and remote intervention

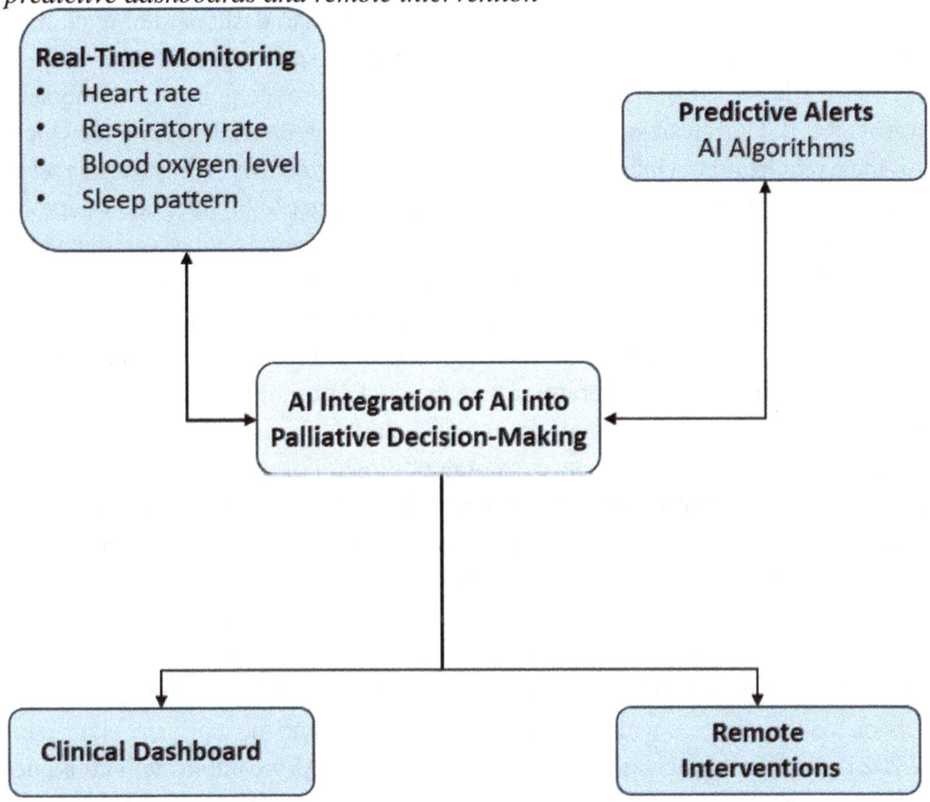

4.2 Clinical Dashboards for Physician Decision-Making in Palliative Care

In palliative care, timely, personalized and compassionate intervention are very crucial, clinical dashboards is a tool for supporting physical for taking real-time decision making. The dashboards display patient health data, such as progression, vital signs, adherence to prescription and psycho-social assessment enabling clinicians to access the condition of elderly patients and prioritize actions according (Oracle Cooperation, 2020). AI-enabled wearables have shifted the scope and functionality of these dashboards, which now offers holistic performance to the healthcare practitioners streaming a continuous physiological data that can give early warnings incase there is deterioration in health or side effects from medication (Mahajan et al., 2025).

An AI-enabled wearables device monitoring the heart rate variability, sleep patterns and physical activity, can send the real-time data into dashboard of attending physician, when the wearable detects abnormal pattern, such as reduced mobility or increased restlessness during sleep and these deviations are flagged in the dashboard (Li et al.,2023). The physician overseeing multiple patients can quickly predict which individual require urgent intervention, to enable him take decisive measure. In a pilot study carried in Netherlands. This study by Smeekes et al. (2024) integrate wearable data to central dashboard, it was revealed that emergency admission was reduced by 20% over the 6months, giving allowance to the physician to adjust treatment plan.

One of the importance of clinical dashboards was that it gives room for interdisciplinary collaboration. Since palliative cares often involve many professionals like doctors, nurses, physiotherapists and medical counselors working together. By providing a common interface, dashboard helps to align all these team together and be able understand patient current conditions. For example, if a wearable device monitors sign of respiratory disorders in elderly patient with also cancers, the dashboard will alert both the physician and as well as palliative care nurse and respiratory therapist which give rise to a well-coordinated and timely intervention.

Since these dashboards are predictive models, they are capable of forecasting patient decline path. This gives the physicians to commence conversations about the end-of-life planning on time, this will improve the quality of care and alignment in decision making process with patient and family taking the most priority (Dixon et al., 2024). As this AI technology advances, integrated AI-wearables will continue to change the method of palliative care, moving from predictive, to data-driven and to the patient-driven model.

4.3 Global Disparities in AI-Powered Wearables for Elderly Palliative Cares

The adoption of AI-enabled wearables in palliative care management has shown a significant shift for monitoring and comfort management in elderly patients., However, there exist global disparities in digital infrastructures, data accessibility and willingness of healthcare provider and healthcare services to further reduce previously existed inequalities gaps between the Global North and Global South (Rad, 2025; Li et al.,2025). In accordance to recent review carried out by Li et al. (2025), majority of adopted AI-enabled software are developed and validated using datasets from high-income countries (HICs), where there robust and effective digital facility with robust datasets suitable for such task. (Celi et al.,2022; Lopez et al.,2022). Invariably, low- and middle-income countries (LMICs) are often limited with such challenges such as non-availability of sophiscated digital infrastructure, no access to electronic health records combined with some cultural difference4s like the way patients are cared for at the end of life (Li et al.,2025). All these challenges all together lead to poorer performance of this AI-enabled models across global population.

According to the recent World Economic Forum (Onuh, 2025), which shows that AI-enabled would likely exclude up to 5billion people globally due to differences in the following like data representation, internet connectivity and affordability of this equipment to elderly patients from LMICs are already affected by the socio-economic disparities, because might find these unreliable and unsafe because the datasets used for its training are acquired from the developed countries. Furthermore, access to broadband internet, data integration, and insufficient training plan for clinicians can affect the adoption in poor regions of the world.

In conclusion, cultural and ethical believes in palliative care like different belief system about death, family involvement and autonomous decision making are the most time not incorporate in the design of these AI-enabled devices. Palliative care should incorporate empathy and personalization, to make this AI-enabled devices to generalize across various cultural background. It is very important that holistic policy intervention should be formulated, if not this digital gap will continue to deepened in healthcare management, and also reduced the level of trust among patients. When all these are achieved globally, it will enable the AI-driven palliative care available for elderly patient globally, rather than some selected minorities.

4.4 Economic Implications and Benefits of Wearables in Elderly Palliative Cares

The economic implications of integrating AI-enabled wearables into palliative care are multifaceted. For example, according to Li et al. (2025), AI-enabled technologies can reduce complicated healthcare operations, reduce administrative burden and lower cost of diagnosis and treatment. In palliative care, AI-wearables monitor psychological parameters to reduce hospital readmissions and home-based end-of-life management which reduce the expenses for healthcare in families. The strategy has demonstrated to save billions of dollars yearly via workflow automation and predictive analytics (Ronanki, 2024).

However, economic benefits are not uniformly distributed, it comes with certain initial investment like sensor development, cloud devices, cyber security and training for healthcare workers, which might pose little challenges for developing countries around the world. Li et al. (2025) highlighted that, AI-enabled screening tool in rural area of China cost about $430,000 for 2,000 patients, which is not easily at disposal of many community healthcare centers, which is also inline with assertion by World Economic Forum (Onuh, 2025) that global inequalities in technological management could exclude billions of people around the globe, making these devices of an access rather actual need.

With all the outlined challenges, the focus should be on an overall long-time benefit. These benefits include reduction of doctor's physical burnout, improve patient outcome and enhancement of healthcare efficiency and also promote inclusive economic growth via healthcare digital manufacturing. In order to maximize these outcomes, subsidy should be placed on AI-infrastructure in LMICs, making AI-algorithm to be an open source as possible and granting of funding for local inventors working in this field.

5.0 ETHICAL, PRACTICAL, AND IMPLEMENTATION CONSIDERATIONS

5.1 Data Privacy and Patient Consent

The integration of AI-powered wearables in palliative cares have shown immersed benefits to both patients and the healthcare staffs. Since all these devices are equipped to gather sensitive health data in continuous manner, which include heart rate, sleep patterns and so on, it therefore very necessary to make sure that the collected information are protected from unauthorized individual from accessing or even prevent misuse of this sensitive information. In order to ensure safety of this information, such data must comply with these regulations either United Stated law by Health Insurance Portability and accountability Act (HIPAA), (U.S. Department of Health & Human Services, 2013) or the European version of General Data Protection Regulation (GDPR) (European Union, 2016). These will ensure safety of patient information in digital healthcare management.

In deployment of these AI-enabled wearables, healthcare providers must get the consent from both patients and other legal representative of such entity. The consent obtained should expressly outlined the type of data collected, the intended usage of such data, potential risk of sharing the data with third parties like cloud-storage facilities and other AI-devices. In the scenario of palliative healthcare management, due to high sensitivity of elderly patient data, the consent letter must be clearly expressed to ensure that the elderly patients understand both risk and benefits of sharing their data.

Moreso, it is very crucial that healthcare sectors enforce a very effective and robust methods of preventing data breaches. This can be achieved through the usage of encrypted code, secured storage cloud or devices and strict access controls for healthcare professionals (Gangurde, 2023). In respect to AI-enabled wearables, it is crucial to maintain transparency in usage of data, and to clearly explain how this AI-algorithm make their decision, all these will make the patient to trust the judgement of this technology. By critically prioritizing data privacy, patient consent, healthcare providers can safely adopt these technologies into palliative cares which can respect the rights of these elderly patients.

Figure 11. Ethical and practical considerations of AI wearables in healthcare. The figure shows the significance of data privacy, patient consent and user-centered design for acceptability and usability among patients

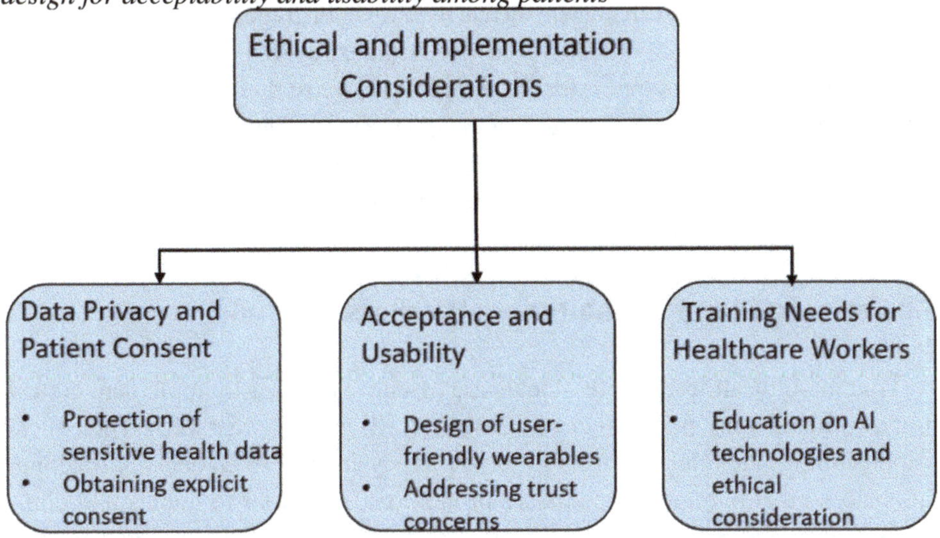

5.2 Acceptance and Usability among Elderly Patients

The integration of AI-enabled wearables into palliative care for elderly patients depend largely on acceptability and usability of these technologies. These wearables provide give good applicability such as real-time monitoring, predictive alerts for health deterioration and personalized care recommendations which depends on user engagement. As elderly patients are often face different challenges like inadequate digital literacy, physical impairments and cognitive decline that may prevent smooth adoption of these technologies (Bertolazzi et al., 2024). Therefore, engineering wearables with intuitive interfaces, voice-guided instructions, large displays and can greatly enhance the adaptability acceptance.

Trust is another important factor that influence the acceptability of AI-enabled wearable by elderly patient. As many elderly patients are really concerned about data privacy, equipment reliability and over relying on these AI technologies. To address these concerns, equipment producers must ensure transparency in data usage, provide integrated features into the product and maintain accuracy of equipment performance (Hanna et al., 2025). Previous study had shown that elder patients will adopt these technologies if they perceive direct benefits such great comfortability, reduction in hospitalization and staying in tact with caregivers (Schulz et al. 2020). Also, it is essential to involve these patients at early stage of design and pilot testing to meet the users' preferences and comfort levels (Zhao et al., 2022).

In summary, enhancing how the acceptability and usability of these devices are important in palliative care management that requires hybrid approach that incorporate both emotional and cognitive needs. Likewise, healthcare providers must incorporate training and continuous support for the caregivers to boost their confidence for long term adoption. When these devices are designed appropriately, the quality of life can be improved with a responsive and patient-centered useful for final stage of life. Figure 9 depicts ethical and practical considerations for implementing AI-enabled wearables in healthcare management.

5.3 Training Plan for Healthcare Workers

Training of healthcare professionals are essential in order to implement ethical framework and other practical consideration in AI-enabled wearables. The ethical responsibilities include patient safety, data privacy and informed decision-making, this places great burden on healthcare professionals in order to understand clinical, technical and ethical knowledge of these technologies. The training program is essential bridging gap, because many of the healthcare workers functioning in palliative cares might not be experienced in AI systems, data analytics and even wearable sensor technology.

In the practical sense of it, training program must cover the followings, like operations, interpretations, and integration systems. It also entails detecting emergency alerts, health records interpretation, differentiating between true emergency signals and false AI algorithmic errors (Bonnefoy et al., 2024). Moreover, training program should include a collaborative effort including patient-consent and autonomy in decision making process, especially when the recommendation of AI differs from patient and patient family values (Shaw et al.,2019). Knowing the limitations of these technologies is one the implementation strategies help know these technologies only serve as adjunct not to replace clinical judgement.

The training must be sustainable, potent and multidisciplinary involving clinicians, nurses, IT technicians and caregivers, to support this training is simulation labs and other interactive e-learning platforms which help to build the skills of these personnels (McLaney et al., 2022). Moreso, ethical training on patient confidentiality, informed consent and other algorithm bias avoidance should be incorporated to ensure responsive and equitable healthcare delivery. In summary, successful implementation of AI-enabled wearables into palliative care depends on availability of technology, competence of healthcare workers and readiness of healthcare workers to adopt these modern technologies.

6.0 RECOMMENDATIONS AND FUTURE DIRECTIONS

6.1 Clinical Guidelines for Implementation

The clinical implementation of AI-enabled wearables in palliative care requires specific, structured guidelines to ensure safety of patient, ethical compliance and clinical efficacy. First, eligibility criteria should be defined to defined to appropriate conditions based on cognitive function, digital literacy, comorbidities and end of life care. Let's examine patient with dementia or severe cognitive disorder might require assistance of AI-enabled wearables with caregiver assistance.

Secondly, the process of onboarding protocols should include standard procedures for initialization, patient education and equipment calibration. Clinical staffs need to ensure that wearables are programmed to monitor relevant parameters to palliative cares like respiratory rate, oxygen saturation, heart rate variability and sleep disorder. These devices should also be interoperable with previous Electronic Health Records (EHRs) to ensure real-time synchronization of data.

Thirdly, it is essential to set up threshold for clinical response, if AI algorithms can measure significant drop in oxygen saturation or restlessness, clinician review and response timeline should be specified clearly in the protocol, for instance response to high priority alerts should be within 30mins, this threshold must be customized to patient baseline.

Fourthly, length of data storage must be clearly stated in data management policies, under what conditions can these data be shared, who has access to this data is very important like caregiver workers, family and other palliative workers. Also, consent forms should explain clearly about data usage and how AI algorithm make decision, limitations and other rights of patient.

Finally, we need a review and feedback loop involving a regular clinical audits and caregiver surveys and algorithm performance evaluation should be done at regular intervals to allow improvements of wearable devices.

6.2 Research Gaps and Areas for Further Investigation

Despite growing interest in AI-enabled wearable for palliative care, several research gaps existed which hamper widespread acceptance of optimal implementation. One important research gap is the lack of large-scale longitudinal studies that explore long term impact of wearables and effectiveness of wearables on patient outcome in palliative management. Previous studies focused short-time pilot trials, limited understanding of device reliability, patient adherence over time. Additionally, there are insufficient research on performance of AI algorithms in diverse elderly populations with multi comorbidity and other cognitive impairment in different cultural and socioeconomic backgrounds.

Another area of research that have receive limited attention is the integration of psychological and emotional response of elderly patients for continuous health monitoring. Further investigation is needed to evaluate whether wearables can improve quality of life and autonomy and emotional wellbeing. There is limited evidence on integration of wearables data into previous healthcare systems, which include how clinicians interpret results of these AI algorithms. Future studies should consider more of ethical implementation of AI decision making especially for end-of-life care and developing a more transparent technique. Tackling these challenges will be vital in establishing a safe, personalized elderly patient AI-enabled technology for palliative care.

7.0 CONCLUSION

The growing population of elderly population, with increasing incidences of both chronic and multimorbidity require an urgent intervention of palliative care models. Traditional healthcare systems are often proactive, fragmented, and limited in their ability to respond to the dynamic needs to elderly patients. The integration of AI-enabled wearable technologies offers a dynamic shift toward continuous and patient-centered care. These technologies enable seamless connection and real-time analysis of vital physiological and behavioral data, enabling clinicians with right insight into diagnosis, symptom control and other decision making.

Wearable devices, supported by AI algorithms provide early warning of clinical deterioration and support timely remote intervention strategies to reduce unnecessary hospitalizations and to enhance comfort during end-of-life care management. By integrating knowledge of predictive analytics, using the clinical dashboards, these systems help healthcare team to integrate action plans with patients' goals and values. Moreso, ethical considerations like data privacy, consent statement, algorithm transparency and user acceptability are key guide to implementation.

Also, we have demonstrated few case studies and other related research. AI wearables provide a scalable solutions suitable to multi-facet healthcare domain. The continuous development and adoption enhanced by clinical guidelines, inter-disciplinary training and all-encompassing research to support delivery of palliative care. Finally, such integration provides elderly patients with wider experience in their final end of life stages with dignity and safety for quality of care.

REFERENCES

Abraham, W. T., Stevenson, L. W., Bourge, R. C., Lindenfeld, J. A., Bauman, J. G., & Adamson, P. B. (2016). Sustained efficacy of pulmonary artery pressure to guide adjustment of chronic heart failure therapy: Complete follow-up results from the CHAMPION randomised trial. *Lancet, 387*(10017), 453–461.

Adams, R., Henry, K. E., Sridharan, A., Soleimani, H., Zhan, A., Rawat, N., & Saria, S. (2022). Prospective, multi-site study of patient outcomes after implementation of the TREWS machine learning-based early warning system for sepsis. *Nature Medicine, 28*(7), 1455–1460.

Anagnostou, D. (2017). Palliative care improves quality of life and reduces symptom burden in adults with life-limiting illness. *Evidence-Based Nursing*.

Apple Inc. (n.d.). Track your vitals on Apple Watch. Apple Support. Retrieved June 6, 2025, from https://support.apple.com/guide/watch/vitals-apd15aa7ed96/watchos

. Arimany-Manso, J., Torralba, F., Lima, A. I., & Trill, M. D. (2025). A comprehensive approach to end-of-life care. Medical-legal, ethical, social, psychological and care aspects. *Medicina Clínica (English Edition).*

Assaad, R. H., Mohammadi, M., & Poudel, O. (2025). Developing an intelligent IoT-enabled wearable multimodal biosensing device and cloud-based digital dashboard for real-time and comprehensive health, physiological, emotional, and cognitive monitoring using multi-sensor fusion technologies. *Sensors and Actuators. A, Physical, 381*, 116074.

Atella, V., Piano Mortari, A., Kopinska, J., Belotti, F., Lapi, F., Cricelli, C., & Fontana, L. (2019). Trends in age-related disease burden and healthcare utilization. *Aging Cell, 18*(1), e12861.

Australian Institute of Health and Welfare. (2021). *Health and ageing*. In *Australia's health 2020: In brief* (pp. 66–69). AIHW. Retrieved June 4, 2025, from https://www.aihw.gov.au/getmedia/19dbc591-b1ef-4485-80ce-029ff66d6930/6_9-health-ageing.pdf.aspx

Awad, A., Trenfield, S. J., Pollard, T. D., Ong, J. J., Elbadawi, M., McCoubrey, L. E., & Basit, A. W. (2021). Connected healthcare: Improving patient care using digital health technologies. *Advanced Drug Delivery Reviews, 178*, 113958.

Bertolazzi, A., Quaglia, V., & Bongelli, R. (2024). Barriers and facilitators to health technology adoption by older adults with chronic diseases: An integrative systematic review. *BMC Public Health, 24*, 506. DOI: 10.1186/s12889-024-18036-5

BioIntelliSense. (2024). *A retrospective observational study of continuous wireless vital sign monitoring via a medical grade wearable device on hospitalized floor patients*. Journal of Clinical Medicine. Retrieved June 6, 2025, from https://www.biointellisense.com/wp-content/uploads/2024/12/BioIntelliSense_PRESS_JCM_Nov-2024.pdf

Bonfiglio, A. (2025). *The future of wearable bioelectronics in healthcare*. Nat Rev Electr Eng., DOI: 10.1038/s44287-025-00175-5

Bonnefoy, P. Y., Chaize, E., Mansuy, R., Mehdi, T. A. Z. I., & Heckel, S. (2024). *The Definitive Guide to Data Integration: Unlock the power of data integration to efficiently manage, transform, and analyze data*. Packt Publishing.

Care, H. (2013). *Clinical practice guidelines for quality palliative care*. Third National Consensus Project for Quality Palliative Care.

Celi, L. A., Cellini, J., Charpignon, M. L., Dee, E. C., Dernoncourt, F., Eber, R., & Yao, S. (2022). Sources of bias in artificial intelligence that perpetuate healthcare disparities—A global review. *PLOS Digital Health*, *1*(3), e0000022.

Chaikijurajai, T., Laffin, L. J., & Tang, W. H. W. (2020). Artificial intelligence and hypertension: Recent advances and future outlook. *American Journal of Hypertension*, *33*(11), 967–974.

Chan, P. Y., Ryan, N. P., Chen, D., McNeil, J., & Hopper, I. (2022). Novel wearable and contactless heart rate, respiratory rate, and oxygen saturation monitoring devices: A systematic review and meta-analysis. *Anaesthesia*, *77*(11), 1268–1280. DOI: 10.1111/anae.15834

Chen, S., Fan, S., Qiao, Z., Wu, Z., Lin, B., Li, Z., & Lim, C. T. (2025). Transforming healthcare: Intelligent wearable sensors empowered by smart materials and artificial intelligence. *Advanced Materials*, •••, 2500412.

Cicerchia, M., Ceci, M., Locatelli, C., Gianni, W., & Repetto, L. (2010). Geriatric syndromes in peri-operative elderly cancer patients. *Surgical Oncology*, *19*(3), 131–139.

Current Health. (n.d.). *Remote patient monitoring*. Retrieved June 6, 2025, from https://www.currenthealth.com/remote-patient-monitoring/

Dixon, D., Sattar, H., Moros, N., Kesireddy, S. R., Ahsan, H., Lakkimsetti, M., Fatima, M., Doshi, D., Sadhu, K., & Junaid Hassan, M. (2024). Unveiling the Influence of AI Predictive Analytics on Patient Outcomes: A Comprehensive Narrative Review. *Cureus*, *16*(5), e59954. DOI: 10.7759/cureus.59954

Dong, C., Ji, Y., Fu, Z., Qi, Y., Yi, T., Yang, Y., & Sun, H. (2025). Precision management in chronic disease: An AI empowered perspective on medicine-engineering crossover. *iScience*, *28*(3).

European Union. (2016). *General Data Protection Regulation (GDPR) 2016/679.* Official Journal of the European Union. https://eur-lex.europa.eu/legal-content/EN/TXT/?uri=CELEX%3A32016R0679

Funabashi, M., Wang, S., Lee, A. D., & Duarte, C K, F., Budgell, B., Stilwell, P., & Hogg-Johnson, S. (2022). Discomfort, pain and stiffness: What do these terms mean to patients? A cross-sectional survey with lexical and qualitative analyses. *BMC Musculoskeletal Disorders*, *23*(1), 283. DOI: 10.1186/s12891-022-05214-y

Gangurde, S. (2023). *Healthcare data security: Standards, measures & data breach protection.* CrelioHealth. https://blog.creliohealth.com/healthcare-data-security-standards-measures-and-data-breach-protection/. Accessed June 11, 2025.

Ghanem, M., Ghaith, A. K., & Bydon, M. (2024). Artificial intelligence and personalized medicine: transforming patient care. In *The New Era of Precision Medicine* (pp. 131–142). Academic Press.

Gianfredi, V., Nucci, D., Pennisi, F., Maggi, S., Veronese, N., & Soysal, P. (2025). Aging, longevity, and healthy aging: The public health approach. *Aging Clinical and Experimental Research*, *37*(1), 125.

Gobinath, A., Rajeswari, P., Anandan, M., & Kumar, N. S. (2025). AI in Imaging for Diagnosis. In *AI Insights on Nuclear Medicine* (pp. 51–76). IGI Global Scientific Publishing.

Google, L. L. C. (n.d.). Track your health metrics in the Fitbit app. Fitbit Help. Retrieved June 6, 2025, from https://support.google.com/fitbit/answer/14236917?hl=en

Guo, E., He, S., & Zheng, L. (2025). Health effects and mediating mechanisms of smart wearable devices on older people: Evidence from China. *Frontiers in Public Health*, *13*, 1578063.

. Habif, S., Constantin, A., Mueller, L., & Singh, H. (2020). 126-LB: Glycemic outcomes for people with type 1 and type 2 diabetes using Control-IQ Technology: real-world data from early adopters. *Diabetes, 69*(Supplement_1).

Hanna, M. G., Pantanowitz, L., Jackson, B., Palmer, O., Visweswaran, S., Pantanowitz, J., & Rashidi, H. H. (2025). Ethical and bias considerations in artificial intelligence/machine learning. *Modern Pathology*, *38*(3), 100686.

Haveman, M. E., van Melzen, R., Schuurmann, R. C., El Moumni, M., Hermens, H. J., Tabak, M., & de Vries, J. P. P. (2021). Continuous monitoring of vital signs with the Everion biosensor on the surgical ward: a clinical validation study. Expert review of medical devices, 18(sup1), 145-152.

Helmer, P., Glück, J., & Anastasiadis, A.. (2025). The use of wearable sensor technology to enhance supportive care in hospitalized palliative patients (Support trial): A prospective preliminary pilot study. *BMC Palliative Care*, *24*, 154. DOI: 10.1186/s12904-025-01794-3

Kamal, A., Currow, D., Bull, J., Ritchie, C., Kutner, J., & Abernethy, A. (2012). The Value of Data Collection to Palliative Care Program Sustainability and Growth (521). *Journal of Pain and Symptom Management*, *43*(2), 413–414.

Khan, H. T., Addo, K. M., & Findlay, H. (2024). Public health challenges and responses to the growing ageing populations. *Public Health Challenges*, *3*(3), e213.

Kuebler, K., Monroe, T., Ricciardi, R., Westlake, C., Sorenson, M., Pederson, J., & Bruera, E. (2024). Integration of palliative care in the management of multiple chronic conditions: An expert consensus paper with policy implications. *Nursing Outlook*, *72*(6), 102273.

Kumlin, M., Berg, G. V., Kvigne, K., & Hellesø, R. (2020). Elderly patients with complex health problems in the care trajectory: A qualitative case study. *BMC Health Services Research*, *20*, 1–10.

Lazzaroni, L., Bellotti, F., & Berta, R. (2024). An embedded end-to-end voice assistant. *Engineering Applications of Artificial Intelligence*, *136*, 108998.

Li, D. M., Parikh, S., & Costa, A. (2025). A critical look into artificial intelligence and healthcare disparities. *Frontiers in Artificial Intelligence*, *8*, 1545869.

Li, K., Cardoso, C., Moctezuma-Ramirez, A., Elgalad, A., & Perin, E. (2023). Heart Rate Variability Measurement through a Smart Wearable Device: Another Breakthrough for Personal Health Monitoring? *International Journal of Environmental Research and Public Health*, *20*(24), 7146. DOI: 10.3390/ijerph20247146

Li, Z., Zhang, Z., Ren, Y., Wang, Y., Fang, J., Yue, H., Ma, S., & Guan, F. (2021). Aging and age-related diseases: From mechanisms to therapeutic strategies. *Biogerontology*, *22*(2), 165–187. DOI: 10.1007/s10522-021-09910-5

Liu, Y., Zavareh, A. T., & Zoghi, B. (2024). Enhancing Well-Being and Alleviating Stress via Wearable-Driven Emotion Recognition and EQ Intentional Practice with Deep Reinforcement Learning. *IEEE Sensors Letters*.

López, D. M., Rico-Olarte, C., Blobel, B., & Hullin, C. (2022). Challenges and solutions for transforming health ecosystems in low-and middle-income countries through artificial intelligence. *Frontiers in Medicine*, *9*, 958097.

Mahajan, A., Heydari, K., & Powell, D. (2025). Wearable AI to enhance patient safety and clinical decision-making. *npj. Digital Medicine*, *8*(1), 176.

McLaney, E., Morassaei, S., Hughes, L., Davies, R., Campbell, M., & Di Prospero, L. (2022). A framework for interprofessional team collaboration in a hospital setting: Advancing team competencies and behaviours. *Healthcare Management Forum*, *35*(2), 112–117. DOI: 10.1177/08404704211063584

Murphree, D. H., Wilson, P. M., Asai, S. W., Quest, D. J., Lin, Y., Mukherjee, P., & Storlie, C. B. (2021). Improving the delivery of palliative care through predictive modeling and healthcare informatics. *Journal of the American Medical Informatics Association : JAMIA*, *28*(6), 1065–1073.

Nahavandi, D., Alizadehsani, R., Khosravi, A., & Acharya, U. R. (2022). Application of artificial intelligence in wearable devices: Opportunities and challenges. *Computer Methods and Programs in Biomedicine*, *213*, 106541.

Onuh, G. (2025, October 1). AI in healthcare risks could exclude 5 billion people: Here's what we can do about it. World Economic Forum. Retrieved November 10, 2025, from https://www.weforum.org/stories/2025/10/ai-in-healthcare-risks-could-exclude-5-billion-people-here-s-what-we-can-do-about-it/

Open MedScience. (2024, December 6). Healthcare reimagined: How virtual assistants are revolutionising patient care. Open MedScience. Retrieved June 6, 2025, from https://openmedscience.com/healthcare-reimagined-how-virtual-assistants-are-revolutionising-patient-care/

Petrie, J. R., Guzik, T. J., & Touyz, R. M. (2018). Diabetes, hypertension, and cardiovascular disease: Clinical insights and vascular mechanisms. *The Canadian Journal of Cardiology*, *34*(5), 575–584.

Pinsky, M. R., Bedoya, A., Bihorac, A., Celi, L., Churpek, M., Economou-Zavlanos, N. J., & Clermont, G. (2024). Use of artificial intelligence in critical care: Opportunities and obstacles. *Critical Care*, *28*(1), 113.

. Rad, J. "Health inequities: a persistent global challenge from past to future." *International Journal for Equity in Health* 24.1 (2025): 148.

Radhoe, S. P., Clephas, P. R., Mokri, H., & Brugts, J. J. (2023). The CardioMEMS Heart Failure System for chronic heart failure–a European perspective. *Expert Review of Medical Devices*, *20*(5), 349–356.

Ramachandran, A. K., Das, S., Joseph, A., Shenoy, G. G., Alex, A. T., & Mudgal, J. (2021). Neurodegenerative Pathways in Alzheimer's Disease: A Review. *Current Neuropharmacology, 19*(5), 679–692. DOI: 10.2174/1570159X18666200807130637

Ren, Z., Xu, Y., Sun, J., Han, Y., An, L., & Liu, J. (2023). Chronic diseases and multimorbidity patterns, their recent onset, and risk of new-onset Parkinson's disease and related functional degeneration in older adults: A prospective cohort study. *EClinicalMedicine*, •••, 65.

Roller-Wirnsberger, R., Thurner, B., Pucher, C., Lindner, S., & Wirnsberger, G. H. (2020). The clinical and therapeutic challenge of treating older patients in clinical practice. *British Journal of Clinical Pharmacology*, *86*(10), 1904–1911.

Ronanki, R. (2024). *Revolutionizing Health Care with AI: A New Era of Efficiency, Trust, and Care Excellence*. NEJM AI Sponsored.

Schulz, R., Beach, S. R., Czaja, S. J., Martire, L. M., & Monin, J. K. (2020). Family Caregiving for Older Adults. *Annual Review of Psychology*, *71*, 635–659. DOI: 10.1146/annurev-psych-010419-050754

Sethuraman, S. C., Kompally, P., Mohanty, S. P., & Choppali, U. (2020). MyWear: A smart wear for continuous body vital monitoring and emergency alert. *arXiv preprint arXiv:2010.08866.*

Shajari, S., Kuruvinashetti, K., Komeili, A., & Sundararaj, U. (2023). The emergence of AI-based wearable sensors for digital health technology: A review. *Sensors (Basel)*, *23*(23), 9498.

Shaw, J., Rudzicz, F., Jamieson, T., & Goldfarb, A. (2019). Artificial intelligence and the implementation challenge. *Journal of Medical Internet Research*, *21*(7), e13659.

Smeekes, O. S., De Boer, T. R., Van Der Mei, R. D., Buurman, B. M., & Willems, H. C. (2024). Receiving home care forms and the risk for emergency department visits in community-dwelling Dutch older adults, a retrospective cohort study using national data. *BMC Public Health*, *24*(1), 1792.

Sun, X., & Li, X. (2023). Editorial: Aging and chronic disease: public health challenge and education reform. *Frontiers in Public Health*, *11*, 1175898. DOI: 10.3389/fpubh.2023.1175898

Sutin, A. R., Stephan, Y., & Terracciano, A. (2018). Psychological Distress, Self-Beliefs, and Risk of Cognitive Impairment and Dementia. *Journal of Alzheimer's Disease*, *65*(3), 1041–1050. DOI: 10.3233/JAD-180119

Thiele, D., Rodseth, R., Friedland, R., Berger, F., Mathew, C., Maslo, C., & Nee, J. (2025). Machine Learning Models for the Early Real-Time Prediction of Deterioration in Intensive Care Units—A Novel Approach to the Early Identification of High-Risk Patients. *Journal of Clinical Medicine, 14*(2), 350.

United Nations. (2023). Second Committee approves 14 draft resolutions, including texts on agriculture development, biological diversity, combating sand and dust storms. UN Press. https://press.un.org/en/2023/gaef3587.doc.htm Retrieved June 13, 2025.

United Nations (UN). (2022). *Ageing* [Internet]. Retrieved June 4, 2025, from https://www.un.org/en/global-issues/ageing

U.S. Department of Health & Human Services. (2013). *Health Insurance Portability and Accountability Act of 1996 (HIPAA).* https://www.hhs.gov/hipaa/for-professionals/privacy/index.html

World Health Organization. (2024, October 1). *Ageing and health* [Fact sheet]. Retrieved June 3, 2025, from https://www.who.int/news-room/fact-sheets/detail/ageing-and-health

Zhao, W., Kelly, R. M., Rogerson, M. J., & Waycott, J. (2024, May). Older adults imagining future technologies in participatory design workshops: Supporting continuity in the pursuit of meaningful activities. In *Proceedings of the 2024 CHI Conference on Human Factors in Computing Systems* (pp. 1-18).

Zhou, L., Li, W., Wu, T., Fan, Z., Ismaili, L., Komolafe, T. E., & Zhang, S. (2024). Adaptive weighted stacking model with optimal weights selection for mortality risk prediction in sepsis patients. *Applied Intelligence, 54*(22), 11892–11913.

Zhou, L., Wu, R., Wang, S., Komolafe, T. E., Guo, J., Fan, Z., & Zhang, Z. (2025). An explicable machine learning approach for predicting 30-day septic mortality for ICU patients. *International Journal of Information and Communication Technology, 26*(9), 1–22.

Chapter 8

Home Health Care for Patients: Major Challenges and Strategic Solutions

Taha Hussein Musa
https://orcid.org/0000-0003-4452-1943
School of Medical and Health Sciences, Faculty of Pharmacy, Libyan International Medical University, Libya & Center of Medical Sociology, Darfur University College, Nyala, Sudan

Wafaa Ramadan Ahmed
https://orcid.org/0009-0005-5777-9988
School of Health and Medical Sciences, Libyan International Medical University, Libya & Faculty of Nursing, Assiut University, Egypt

Idriss Hussein Musa
School of Medicine, Darfur University College, Nyala, Sudan

Tosin Yinka Akintunde
https://orcid.org/0000-0002-9392-8726
Department of Sociology, Hohai University, China & Center for Medical Sociology, Darfur University College, Nyala, Sudan

Upama Ghimire
Nepal Health Research Council (NHRC), Ramshah Path, Kathmandu, Nepal

Prasoon Oli
Nepal Health Research Council (NHRC), Ramshah Path, Kathmandu, Nepal

Hassan Hussein Musa
Department of Medical Microbiology, Faculty of Medical Laboratory Sciences, University of Khartoum, Sudan

ABSTRACT

Home care has emerged as a cornerstone of contemporary health systems, driven by demographic aging, escalating chronic disease prevalence, and imperatives for

DOI: 10.4018/979-8-3373-4099-9.ch008

cost-effective, patient-centric models of care. This chapter critically interrogates the evolving landscape of home care delivery, foregrounding its most pressing challenges and strategic responses through the lenses of workforce deficits, technological discontinuities, regulatory disarticulation, and entrenched social inequities. Drawing on robust empirical evidence, it delineates pathways to fortify workforce capacity, harness digital health innovations, enhance care integration, and galvanize policy reform. It further explores transformative trends, including artificial intelligence, precision medicine, and pandemic preparedness, that increasingly intersect with domiciliary care. Bridging these systemic gaps holds the potential to reimagine home health care as an equitable, resilient, and high-quality alternative to institutional modalities.

INTRODUCTION

The global health landscape has changed significantly, with home healthcare now serving as a key component of modern health systems. Home healthcare, which provides skilled medical and non-medical care in patients' homes, has shifted from a secondary service to a strategic solution for persistent healthcare challenges(*Visiting Nurses Association of America (V.N.A.A.)*, n.d.) . This shift is driven by three main factors: rapid population aging, rising rates of chronic diseases, and growing demand for patient-centered care that supports autonomy and quality of life (Dellve et al., 2003). By 2050, the population aged 65 and older is projected to more than double, from 761 million in 2021 to 1.6 billion, indicating a major change in care needs (Koehlmoos et al., 2011; Zhang et al., 2020). Chronic conditions such as cardiovascular disease, diabetes, and respiratory illnesses now cause about 74% of global deaths, requiring long-term, complex care strategies(Thomas et al., 2023). These trends highlight the limitations of hospital-based models and the need for scalable, community-based alternatives.

Empirical evidence shows that home healthcare effectively addresses systemic gaps (El-Haddad et al., 2020; Juergens et al., 2010). High-quality home care programs improve patient satisfaction, treatment adherence, and functional outcomes, while significantly reducing unnecessary hospital use. A landmark meta-analysis by Jencks et al. (2009) found that structured post-discharge home visits reduced 30-day readmission rates by 25% among Medicare patients. This highlights home care's role as a vital bridge between acute and community-based care(Jencks et al., 2009). Interventions led by advanced practice nurses have shown particular promise, resulting in longer time to hospitalization, improved health outcomes for frail elderly patients, and significant cost savings. Home care also contributes to shorter hospital stays, fewer complications, and reduced anxiety and depression (Lei et al., 2023).

Additionally, it plays an active role in managing chronic heart failure (N. Zhang et al., 2024). Expanding home care in healthcare settings helps reduce costs, improve quality of care, and enhance patient well-being (Fajarini et al., 2025).

Nurse-led interventions have yielded promising outcomes, including delayed hospitalization and improved health metrics for frail elderly patients, alongside substantial cost savings for health systems (Curioni et al., 2023). Comparative analyses consistently show that home-based care offers significant economic advantages over institutional alternatives, particularly in chronic disease management and post-acute recovery(Thomas et al., 2023). The COVID-19 pandemic accelerated this recognition, with infection control imperatives and hospital bed shortages catalyzing rapid adoption of home-based care modalities and revealing both latent capacity and infrastructural deficits.

Despite these advantages, the home healthcare sector faces persistent systemic challenges that threaten its ability to scale effectively. Workforce shortages stemming from low pay, difficult conditions, and limited advancement drive high turnover and disrupt continuity of care. Over one-quarter of providers have had to refuse patients because of staffing deficits (Shahriari et al., 2024). Regulatory fragmentation reduces operational efficiency, as inconsistent licensing and scope-of-practice rules undermine effective workforce utilization. Technology adoption remains uneven, with many agencies ill-equipped for telehealth and remote monitoring(Shahriari et al., 2024). Significant disparities in access persist, especially in rural and marginalized communities where barriers such as inadequate insurance, language and cultural differences, and insufficient social determinant supports are pervasive (Beer et al., 2014; Masoumi et al., 2021). Even in well-resourced settings, disadvantaged groups remain vulnerable due to insurance and cultural barriers and lack of support for social determinants of health (Thomas et al., 2023). With global demand expected to reach 27 million individuals requiring chronic disease management by 2050 a likely underestimate given increased life expectancy and multimorbidity(Administration on Aging, 2006; Bedón-Molina et al., 2014) addressing these systemic challenges is imperative. This chapter outlines strategic, policy, and system-level recommendations for workforce development, regulatory harmonization, payment reform, and digital integration to ensure home healthcare's sustainability, equity, and resilience.

Figure 1. Modern Integrated Home-Based Care Ecosystem

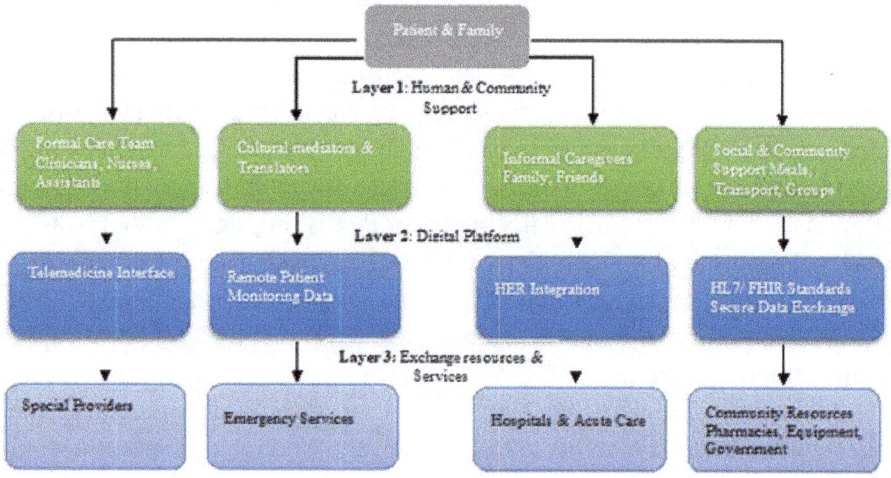

Adopted from: (Bedón-Molina et al., 2014).

The figure illustrates a modern, patient-centered home care system that replaces traditional step-by-step models with a more integrated approach. This model features three layers centered on the Patient & Family.

The first layer, Human & Community Support, includes clinicians, cultural mediators, family caregivers, and community services. It offers direct assistance and addresses social determinants of health. The second layer, the Digital Platform, supplies the technology for telemedicine, remote monitoring, EHR integration, and secure data exchange with HL7/FHIR standards. The third layer, External Resources & Services, covers specialist providers, emergency services, hospitals, and community resources that support care beyond the home.

This model enables seamless information flow. Human support works directly with patients, while the digital platform securely shares data with external services. It creates a responsive, coordinated care environment where technology enhances but does not replace human care. The approach stays holistic, prioritizing each patient's needs and preferences (Figure 1).

CURRENT LANDSCAPE OF HOME HEALTH CARE

Historical Development of Home-Based Care Models

In East Asia, Japan's home healthcare system has evolved into a model of integrated, institutionalized care, fundamentally shaped by key policy milestones since the 1980s. The 1981 inclusion of insulin self-administration under health insurance marked the beginning of strong institutional support for domiciliary care (Miura, 2015).

This effort expanded in 1986, when coverage was extended to bedridden elderly individuals under the revised Health and Medical Service Act for the Aged. By 1992, the Medical Service Law formally legitimized homes as sites for medical treatment, and in 1994, home care was incorporated fully into the national insurance framework. Although coverage initially targeted emergency cases, it soon broadened to encompass post-acute and chronic care. Further innovations included establishing 24-hour home care for bedridden elders in 1998, launching the Visiting Nurse Promotion Program in 2004, and supporting Home Care Support Clinics and Hospitals in 2006 and 2008, respectively. Despite these achievements, disparities in access persisted. The 2012 medical fee reform marked a pivotal shift allocating 150 billion yen to foster greater collaboration between physicians and nurses and establishing comprehensive community care, including 24-hour nurse visits, as a cornerstone of Japan's healthcare strategy (Miura, 2015).

FUTURE APPROACH TO HOME HEALTH CARE

The Comprehensive Community Care System expanded from 10 bases in 2011 to over 500 by 2013, connecting government, medical associations, and nursing services (Miura, 2015).

These bases are designed to provide integrated medical, nursing, and social support within a 30-minute radius. Providers are adopting digital health innovations, such as telemedicine and remote monitoring, to improve care for aging populations and those with chronic conditions(Leff & Burton, 2001). In the United States, home healthcare is a dynamic sector, driven by Medicare reimbursement reforms and the adoption of portable medical technologies (Landers, 2006). While home-based care has expanded globally, its effectiveness remains under discussion. The literature highlights improvements in patient outcomes, interdisciplinary care models, and the influence of policy and technology (Kao et al., 2009). In American primary care, 53% of family physicians continue to make home visits, though fewer younger practitioners do so (Cauthen, 1981). In the Pacific Islands, aging populations and chronic disease have increased healthcare burdens, prompting calls for national insurance reforms to improve access for homebound individuals (Fernandes et al., 2018).

CHALLENGES IN HOME HEALTH CARE DELIVERY

High Turnover Rates and Burnout

Challenges in home health care delivery despite its promise, home healthcare delivery is fraught with systemic challenges. High turnover rates and burnout among providers are exacerbated by poor working conditions, inadequate governance, and limited referral systems (Ajlouni et al., 2015; Samia et al., 2012). The World Health Organization projects a global shortfall of 10 million health workers by 2030, with the most severe deficits expected in low- and middle-income countries (Sibai et al., 2017). In the Arab League, underinvestment in nursing education and the migration of qualified professionals further compound the crisis (Babapour et al., 2022). The deficit of female nurses is caused by numerous factors, such as excessive work-related job stress (Babapour et al., 2022), cultural and family restrictions, and other social barriers these all present challenges for home care(Kaihlanen et al., 2023; Kayonga et al., 2025; Shahriari et al., 2024). Beyond personnel shortages, staff must deal with chronic labor deficits and reduced visitation, which forces them to rush tasks. Clients also experience isolation due to the social and physical seclusion of home care and the poverty-stricken working conditions in this field(Kallas et al., 2023). Their life expectancy and the resulting burden of NCDs among older populations amplify the impact of professional shortages, especially those lacking expertise in gerontology and geriatrics. These factors create a growing need for home care. For improvement, a reformed healthcare network, development of healthcare workers, and a new approach are required. There is also a need to close the gap through research, raising community awareness, and fostering connections among researchers, government organizations, and civil society(Sibai et al., 2017).

TECHNOLOGICAL AND INFRASTRUCTURE GAPS

Across the world, the emerging and rapid digital technologies revolutionising devices like digital health technologies (DHTs) like telemedicine and electronic health records (EHRs), mobile health (mHealth) applications, and remote monitoring systems, and artificial intelligence are rising in direction to augment all stages of the patient care continuum(Awad et al., 2021; Khan et al., 2025; Narayan et al., 2025). Apart can provide cutting-edge solutions for patients through the use of digital technology encompassing a variety of applications and services, which will play a promising complementary role in the care of the elderly population (Zhang et al., 2023). However, although the provision of quality care and disparities remain, it is a health care system. Therefore, system reforms for the emergence of digital health technologies will enable evidence-based solutions and also enable universal access to quality healthcare system (Rad, 2025). Those digital technologies moving away from the traditional approach of healthcare management towards digitizing devices have the potential outcome to improve and enhance healthcare delivery for individual patients (Gunasekeran et al., 2021). However, infrastructure and technology disparities is also becoming an emergent challenge towards decimate the efficiency of the provision of health care(Yao et al., 2022), and exacerbate healthcare disparities, and abate DHTs' ability to use maximum potential in home care, particularly among vulnerable populations are needed to guide future digital health research among vulnerable groups(Hamideh & Nebeker, 2020).

In the world, such global challenges in the form of limited internet and lack of knowledge about digital tools are barriers that need to be overcome to facilitate equitable access to digital health interventions in rural areas (Maita et al., 2024). For example, electronic health tools that have been said to significantly contribute to health care accessibility by offering patients new avenues of managing their own health information, interacting with health care physicians, and accessing remote care also minimises treatment time and cost to end treatment after initial screening (Avila et al., 2023) and patient satisfaction in such fields needs to be assessed towards health-care service effectiveness (Eldaly et al., 2022).

Although telehealth has huge potential for older individuals and aged care service delivery, privacy concerns can discourage its application and effective utilisation. Data from Saudi Arabia shows that the utilization of telehealth remains low in most regions, with facilitators and barriers influencing the uptake of telehealth among older persons. In addition, the use of digital technology advantages individuals in numerous ways, but some factors, like socioeconomic factors, play a determining role, as older persons from low-income families may not have equal access to digital resources and technology or Internet services required for telehealth (Alhussein et al., 2023; Alodhialah et al., 2024).

CULTURAL, LINGUISTIC, AND ENGAGEMENT BARRIERS

Homebound adults are increasing in the world, especially in the United States, and nearly 3.6 million of them require home-based care services that could lessen their suffering and delay their admission to a nursing home or hospital (Qiu et al., 2010). The chronic disease rates keep on showing increased prevalence among them, which leads to an effective and embraced development of care HBPC to meet the homebound individuals' needs(Cheng et al., 2020). However, the 'process of delivering home care services,' which emerged due to main challenges, includes Infrastructure and investment of sufficient time and resources and insurance for the development and enhancement of home care services, which are financial problems and challenges related to the process of home care services delivery (Shahriari et al., 2024). On the other hand, existing home-based care is found in fragmented services, which leads to coordination problems that reduce care effectiveness. Additionally, effective home health care requires cultural and linguistic competency. Language barrier worsens communication, reduces compliance with treatment, and worsens outcomes, especially in multicultural settings like the UAE (Al-Yateem et al., 2023).

In Saudi Arabia, the problems related to the culture and language differences of the health workforce have been documented, showing that there is a communication gap between patient and health care worker due to low cultural competency(Almutairi, 2015). Effective clinician-patient communication enhances trust, satisfaction, and health outcomes. Providers must adapt practices to language preferences to achieve accurate assessments and deliver patient-centered care. More than a training provision to clinicians is necessary to foster effective collaboration with these interpreters in interaction and activities of daily living(Al-Yateem et al., 2023). Optimal health outcomes depend on the involvement of patients and their families in treatment planning and decision-making processes. This could have contributed to improving health outcomes, improving satisfaction with the care experience, reducing costs, and even improving the clinician experience (Krist et al., 2017). Furthermore, patient engagement can influence the healthcare delivery system design (Krist et al., 2017).

In many Asian countries, families serve as the main caregivers for elderly relatives. Adult children manage daily activities. Daughters or daughters-in-law often handle medications and health appointments. These caregiving traditions shape views on privacy, decision-making, and the acceptance of outside help. Over 90% of older adults in rural China rely primarily on family. Formal home health services are often a last resort. They may signal family inadequacy(Hartanto et al., 2024; Jiang et al., 2024). In India, multigenerational households are common. Families usually seek professional home care only to supplement their efforts (Gustafsson et al., 2022). When cultural factors are ignored, service use is low. Trust in the provider falls. Adherence to care plans suffers. Effective home care models in Asia involve families as partners. Staff should communicate in ways that respect family roles and collective decisions.

Concepts such as patient activation, empowerment, participation, involvement, compliance, adherence, shared decision making, co-production of health, co-design, self-management, and self-care describe how patients become active participants in the management of health through their behaviors, attitudes, and processes. Active involvement is crucial in improving the quality and outcomes of care, especially in multiple chronic conditions

(Vick & Wolff, 2021). Encourage patient and family meaningful involvement, policymakers should develop and release detailed guidelines that enable healthcare providers to implement these practices as part of routine care. Proper use of patient and family involvement strategy can enhance patient safety, improve adherence to care plans, and enhance more patient-focused delivery of health care (Park & Giap, 2020) and also reduce patient harm and improve safety in practice as concerns one of the significant public health problems in developing and developed countries (Abdi et al., 2024).

REGULATORY AND REIMBURSEMENT COMPLEXITIES

Reimbursement policies for home healthcare vary globally, with each country having its own reimbursement policy that is unable to contain rising costs (Vanholder et al., 2012), with some countries relying heavily on direct out-of-pocket payments(e.g., Tunisia)(Abu-Zaineh et al., 2013; Gottret et al., 2008), the Iranian healthcare system (Hajizadeh & Nghiem, 2011), and Malawi (Mulaga et al., 2022), and others have partial state coverage (e.g., Kuwait). In African countries, there is similarity in the pricing and reimbursement policy of patent pharmaceuticals in Algeria, Morocco, and Tunisia (Dahmani et al., 2023). Studies found that reimbursement systems exert their influence by the choice of reimbursement system on many dimensions of patient care in the form of structure, process and outcome measures (Wagenschieber & Blunck, 2024). Asia and Europe represent heterogeneous models, with Japan and South Korea leading home-based care systems that are organized. There is a need to strengthen the integration of scattered long-term care services, and making community-based care for aging populations can attain high public satisfaction if properly designed. In middle-income countries, there is a lack of infrastructure for the provision of long-term care services. Therefore, middle-income countries should initiate preparations well ahead of the program of LTC implementation (Rhee et al., 2015).

One of the main obstacles is the lack of standard performance measures, as seen in Lebanon and Jordan, an Eastern Mediterranean country, where the inability of the national quality of a healthy referral system framework debilitates service evaluation(Aoun & Tajvar, 2024; El-Jardali & Fadlallah, 2017). Quality indicators (QIs) are increasingly utilised in overseeing standards of care, assessing the quality improvement tools, identifying gaps, and enabling benchmarking. In order to give quality care and allow trends over time to be studied in home healthcare(Dick et al., 2019). Overall, differences in financing, health regulation, and quality measurement suggest the need for more streamlined policies to foster accessible, good-quality home healthcare in both developed and developing countries.

SOCIAL AND ECONOMIC DISPARITIES

Socioeconomic status (SES) has a significant influence on health outcomes and home health care access, creating inequities between groups(Barnes et al., 2023; Marmot, 2005; Sindhukumari & Thomas, 2023). SES is lower with more medical care use in the home, emphasising its utilization for low-SES vulnerable older adults with restricted access to services (Hamasaki, 2025). Defamilization of long-term care integration of formal and informal care may potentially curtail health inequities, particularly among low-income populations (Floridi et al., 2021). This holds especially for the elderly in rural Japan, where health behavior and access to healthcare are determined by SES (Floridi et al., 2021; Kinjo et al., 2017). Expansion of home-visit care programs can promote affordability and availability of end-of-life care (Kinjo et al., 2017). Geographic and economic disadvantage exacerbate inequality. In rural Iraq and Algeria, limited infrastructure and scarcities of healthcare limit access for poorer populations (Eriksson et al., 2013). Women bear proportionately large responsibilities for caregiving worldwide. They facilitate waged work and unpaid care in Arab states, exacerbating gender inequalities(Charmes, 2022; Eriksson et al., 2013). Women facilitate home, agriculture, and care work in Nepal, constraining economic opportunities (Ghosh et al., 2023).

Home Health Care in Low- and Middle-Income Countries (LMICs)

Most research focuses on high-income countries, while home-based care in low- and middle-income countries faces unique challenges. In sub-Saharan Africa, formal home health systems are usually limited to urban areas. Unpaid family members, mainly women and girls, provide most care without sufficient training, protective equipment, or respite support(Sani et al., 2024). In rural Malawi and Uganda, community health workers (CHWs) are central but often overburdened, undercompensated, and lack strong links to formal health systems (Hassan et al., 2024; Pandya et al., 2022) . Out-of-pocket expenses further disadvantage the poorest families and worsen health inequalities. Exist in Tunisia and parts of the Middle East, where fragmented insurance systems often exclude homebound patients from coverage for nursing visits or medical equipment(Abu-Zaineh et al., 2013). Scalable, community-based models are needed to address these barriers. Effective strategies include training CHWs for expanded roles, implementing mobile supervision, and establishing public-private partnerships for equipment lending in resource-limited settings.

Strategies and Solutions for Effective Home Healthcare

Rising demand for home healthcare requires a comprehensive approach based on patient needs, workforce development, and technology. Effective home healthcare relies on person-centered care planning, clear caregiver communication, and satisfaction measurement to improve clinical and business outcomes (Evans et al., 2019). Building a strong workforce through rigorous hiring, training in clinical and cultural competence, and caregiver support systems is essential to prevent burnout (Burgdorf et al., 2022; Foster et al., 2019; Shoemake, 1994). Integrating technology such as telehealth, remote patient monitoring, and shared electronic health records enhances care coordination, accessibility, and patient satisfaction (Landers et al., 2016). These solutions should be supported by robust community partnerships that connect home health agencies with hospitals, long-term care, and social services to facilitate hospital-to-home transitions and reduce preventable readmissions(Evans et al., 2019; Mezzalira et al., 2024).

Effective sustainability involves providing policy settings, such as equitable payment systems ensuring fair compensation and culturally responsive care programs tailored for high-risk groups' backgrounds and needs(Mezzalira et al., 2024). Building on the importance of effective sustainability, workforce expansion through focused investment in training is particularly significant in meeting growing demand without sacrificing quality(Miller et al., 2022; Reckrey et al., 2017). Looking ahead, the intersection of new care models such as Hospital at Home programs and interdisciplinary collaboration will be particularly critical to chronic disease management and health equity achievement (Mezzalira et al., 2024). Moreover, the future of home healthcare relies on symbiotic integration of technological progress and person-centered delivery of care, backed by collaborative ecosystems and visionary policymaking (Foster et al., 2019; Steven Landers et al., 2016).

Strategic Solutions for High Turnover and Burnout

To address high turnover and burnout, strategic solutions include implementing competitive wage structures tied to certification levels (pay rates based on qualifications) and rural hardship allowances (extra compensation for work in difficult locations), as recent research confirms that financial incentives are a primary driver in stabilizing the nursing workforce(Allan & Vadean, 2023). Furthermore, reducing the administrative burden is critical; studies show home health nurses spend up to 30% of their time on documentation, but tools like voice-to-text HER (electronic health records) and scribe support (assistance with documentation) can reclaim this time for direct care(Alboksmaty et al., 2025). Finally, introducing mental health benefits and peer support circles (group discussions among peers for emotional support) can help mitigate isolation and emotional(Shalaby & Agyapong, 2020)(Kane et al., 2023).

Strategic Solutions to Technological and Infrastructure Gaps

Addressing technological and infrastructure gaps in healthcare requires a multi-faceted strategy. Overcoming data silos is critical and can be achived by promoting FHIR (Fast Healthcare Interoperability Resources) standards, which would enable seamless data exchange between home health agencies, hospitals, and primary care clinics. Bridging the digital divide also requires treating broadband as critical health infrastructure, with public funding for its expansion in underserved rural areas(Ne et al., 2023). In low-resource settings such as Low- and Middle-Income Countries (LMICs), implementing low-bandwidth telehealth solutions, including WhatsApp-based triage systems can help deliver essential services to populations with limited connectivity(Son et al., 2020)(Iyawa et al., 2016).

Strategic Solutions for Cultural, Linguistic, and Engagement Barriers

Healthcare institutions should mandate comprehensive cultural competence training for all clinical staff. In this context, cultural competence refers to ability of healthcare professionals to understand, respect, and interact effectively with people from diverse backgrounds. To ensure this, training should address patient cultural norms defined as beliefs and customs influencing behaviours, such as dietary restrictions, religious practices, and gender preferences. For instance, institutions should provide female-only caregivers for patients from conservative households. In addition, clear protocols for family inclusive decision-making meaning involving family members as active participants in healthcare decisions and the use of certified medical interpreters must be established. The use of ad-hoc interpreters, such as untrained family members or staff, should be prohibited due to increased risks of errors and confidentiality breaches(Juckett & Unger, 2014). Finally, the effectiveness of these initiatives should be measured through culturally stratified patient satisfaction surveys, which separate responses by cultural group, and by tracking specific clinical outcomes, such as reductions in adverse events and preventable hospital readmissions among racial, ethnic, and linguistic minority groups(Beach et al., 2006)(Price et al., 2005).

Strategic Solutions to Regulatory and Reimbursement Complexities

To promote high-quality, patient-centered care, policymakers and payers should support a transition to value-based payment models. These models reward positive health outcomes, such as reduced hospital readmissions and improved functional status, rather than the volume of services provided (Leao et al., 2023). It is also important to standardize scope-of-practice laws across states, enabling advanced practice providers, including nurses and physical therapists, to fully utilize their education and training in home-based settings. Removing these regulatory barriers increases access to care, especially in underserved areas, without compromising patient safety or quality (Frogner et al., 2023).

Strategic Solutions to Social and Economic Disparities

A two-pronged approach is recommended to address patients' social needs. First, systematic integration of screenings for social determinants of health (SDOH), such as housing instability and food insecurity, should be incorporated into standard home health assessments. Second, healthcare providers are encouraged to establish formal partnerships with community-based organizations to connect patients with essential wraparound services, including meal delivery and non-emergency medical transportation (Gottlieb et al., 2019; Yan et al., 2022) This integrated model of identifying social risks and facilitating interventions is vital for improving holistic patient outcomes.

FUTURE RESEARCH PRIORITIES IN HOME HEALTHCARE

As health care expands into the home, research in this area is adapting to new challenges and opportunities(Kim et al., 2002). Future studies should prioritize improving care quality, expanding access, and ensuring system sustainability (Ellenbecker et al., 2008; Juergens et al., 2010; Miller et al., 2022; Reckrey et al., 2017; Shahriari et al., 2024). Incorporating emerging technologies remains a key research focus (Foster et al., 2019; Steven Landers et al., 2016; Sibai et al., 2017; Yao et al., 2022). Artificial intelligence, the Internet of Things, robotics, and telehealth can improve care delivery, safeguard patient confidentiality, and provide alternatives to in-person visits (Gunasekeran et al., 2021; Rad, 2025). Workforce sustainability is also critical (Miller et al., 2022; Reckrey et al., 2017; Shahriari et al., 2024). Additional research should examine how long-term training, competitive compensation, and mental health benefits influence caregiver recruitment and retention (Burgdorf et al., 2022; Foster et al., 2019; Miller et al., 2022; Reckrey et al., 2017; Shoemake, 1994). Finally, addressing access gaps is essential, including identifying barriers for underserved populations and developing culturally responsive care models (Al-mutairi, 2015; Mezzalira et al., 2024).

Policy and payment model studies will be crucial to guiding the future of home healthcare. Studies will be required to contrast patient outcomes for multiple reimbursement models, that is, to assess if value-based payment models result in better patient outcomes than fee-for-service payment models at lower cost (Mukamel et al., 2022). Research standards should consider both direct health impacts and broader socioeconomic impacts, for example, how expanded coverage of home care can avert unnecessary institutionalization or enable family caregivers to remain on the payroll (Freedman et al., 2004; Goodridge et al., 2012). Integration of care models, especially those that are innovative and multidisciplinary, along with measures of success for hospital-to-home transitions, should also be prioritized (Labson, 2015).

In light of these advancing technologies and care models, there must also be research to address the newly arising ethical challenges of home healthcare. As technology evolves and care shifts to the home setting, research must address issues such as patient privacy, informed consent for AI-driven care, and equitable access to emerging technologies. Ethical principles will likely need revision to respond to these new realities without exploiting vulnerable populations. These interconnected priorities will drive increased quality, accessibility, and long-term sustainability of systems.

CONCLUSION

Home health care has become a central component of modern healthcare, addressing the needs of aging populations and the rise in long-term conditions. By reducing hospital readmissions, supporting patient autonomy, and providing cost-effective, personalized care, home-based models are transforming care delivery worldwide. However, significant challenges remain, including workforce shortages, limited technology, and persistent social inequalities, especially in low-resource settings where infrastructure and policy support are lacking. Despite these obstacles, new models are showing positive results globally. Workforce redesign, telehealth expansion, and artificial intelligence-based monitoring are improving outcomes, while adaptable models from the United States, India, and Scandinavia offer valuable guidance. Predictive analytics, home hospital initiatives, and personalized medicine are driving a major shift in practice, though these innovations also raise important concerns about data privacy and equitable access.

Building on these considerations around policy and innovative care models, the COVID-19 pandemic accelerated telehealth adoption and revealed weaknesses in existing care systems (Bouabida et al., 2022). As a result, there was increased use of Hospital-at-Home models, remote monitoring, and basic technologies to support isolated adults(Barrett et al., 2012; Getson & Nejat, 2021). Looking ahead, developments such as AI analytics, wearable sensors, assistive robots, and genomics are likely to play a role in personalized home care. These innovations, however, require strong ethical governance to prevent data misuse, bias, and the digital exclusion of vulnerable populations (Barrett et al., 2012).

Future home healthcare research must prioritize integrating emerging technologies, ensuring workforce sustainability, improving equitable access, developing ethical policies, and creating sustainable payment models to enhance care quality and accessibility.

Action for Advancing Home Healthcare

The full potential of home care is limited by fragmented services, staffing shortages, and inequitable access. To address these challenges, national health plans should prioritize home care, policymakers should invest in information technology and infrastructure, and long-term financing must be established to ensure equal access to high-quality home-based care. Health care providers should support team-based care, use technology to improve management, and deliver culturally competent care in partnership with families. Researchers should pilot scalable interventions, address rural inequities, and assess the implications of technology-enabled care. They need to evaluate the effects of home care interventions, develop solutions for high-risk areas, and consider the ethical impacts of technology in care delivery. Home healthcare redefines the value of medical services by shifting from high-tech hospital settings to dignified, home-based care. This approach places patient dignity at the center of technology-driven, relationship-focused health systems, fostering more humane and effective care worldwide.

REFERENCES

Abdi, Z., Ravaghi, H., Sarkhosh, S., Nafar, H., Khani, S., & Letaief, M. (2024). Patient and family engagement in patient safety in the Eastern Mediterranean Region: A scoping review. *BMC Health Services Research, 24*(1), 1–17. DOI: 10.1186/s12913-024-11198-3 PMID: 38918854

Abu-Zaineh, M., Ben Romdhane, H., Ventelou, B., Moatti, J.-P., & Chokri, A. (2013). Appraising financial protection in health: The case of Tunisia. *International Journal of Health Care Finance and Economics, 13*(1), 73–93. DOI: 10.1007/s10754-013-9123-8 PMID: 23381233

Administration on Aging. (2006). *A Profile of Older American.*

Ajlouni, M. T., Dawani, H., & Diab, S. M. (2015). Home Health Care (HHC) Managers Perceptions About Challenges and Obstacles that Hinder HHC Services in Jordan. *Global Journal of Health Science, 7*(4), 121–129. DOI: 10.5539/gjhs.v7n4p121 PMID: 25946949

Al-Yateem, N., Hijazi, H., Saifan, A. R., Ahmad, A., Masa'Deh, R., Alrimawi, I., Rahman, S. A., Subu, M. A., & Ahmed, F. R. (2023). Quality and safety issue: Language barriers in healthcare, a qualitative study of non-Arab healthcare practitioners caring for Arabic patients in the UAE. *BMJ Open, 13*(12), e076326. DOI: 10.1136/bmjopen-2023-076326 PMID: 38135338

Alboksmaty, A., Aldakhil, R., Hayhoe, B. W. J., Ashrafian, H., Darzi, A., & Neves, A.-L. (2025). The impact of using AI-powered voice-to-text technology for clinical documentation on quality of care in primary care and outpatient settings: A systematic review. *EBioMedicine, 118*. Advance online publication. DOI: 10.1016/j.ebiom.2025.105861 PMID: 40694861

Alhussein, M., Patel, B., & Liu, X. (2023). Closing the gap: Technology access and telehealth use among older adults in the U.S. Medicare beneficiaries. *Telematics and Informatics Reports, 12*, 100103. https://doi.org/https://doi.org/10.1016/j.teler.2023.100103

Allan, S., & Vadean, F. (2023). The Impact of Wages on Care Home Quality in England. *The Gerontologist, 63*(9), 1428–1436. DOI: 10.1093/geront/gnad032 PMID: 36964753

Almutairi, K. M. (2015). Culture and language differences as a barrier to provision of quality care by the health workforce in Saudi Arabia. *Saudi Medical Journal, 36*(4), 425–431. DOI: 10.15537/smj.2015.4.10133 PMID: 25828278

Alodhialah, A. M., Almutairi, A. A., & Almutairi, M. (2024). Telehealth Adoption Among Saudi Older Adults: A Qualitative Analysis of Utilization and Barriers. *Healthcare (Basel, Switzerland), 12*(23). Advance online publication. DOI: 10.3390/healthcare12232470 PMID: 39685092

Aoun, N., & Tajvar, M. (2024). Healthcare delivery in Lebanon: A critical scoping review of strengths, weaknesses, opportunities, and threats. *BMC Health Services Research, 24*(1). Advance online publication. DOI: 10.1186/s12913-024-11593-w PMID: 39334362

Avila, F. R., Carter, R. E., McLeod, C. J., Bruce, C. J., Guliyeva, G., Torres-Guzman, R. A., Maita, K. C., Ho, O. A., TerKonda, S. P., & Forte, A. J. (2023). The Role of Telemedicine in Prehospital Traumatic Hand Injury Evaluation. *Diagnostics (Basel, Switzerland), 13*(6). Advance online publication. DOI: 10.3390/diagnostics13061165 PMID: 36980474

Awad, A., Trenfield, S. J., Pollard, T. D., Ong, J. J., Elbadawi, M., McCoubrey, L. E., Goyanes, A., Gaisford, S., & Basit, A. W. (2021). Connected healthcare: Improving patient care using digital health technologies. *Advanced Drug Delivery Reviews, 178*, 113958. https://doi.org/https://doi.org/10.1016/j.addr.2021.113958 PMID: 34478781

Babapour, A. R., Gahassab-Mozaffari, N., & Fathnezhad-Kazemi, A. (2022). Nurses' job stress and its impact on quality of life and caring behaviors: A cross-sectional study. *BMC Nursing, 21*(1), 1–10. DOI: 10.1186/s12912-022-00852-y PMID: 35361204

Barnes, Lucy, & Hall, Peter A, & Taylor, Rosemary C R. (2023). The Structural Sources of Socioeconomic Inequalities in Health: A Cross-National Perspective. *Socius: Sociological Research for a Dynamic World, 9*, 23780231231174830. DOI: 10.1177/23780231231174832

Barrett, D., O'Connell, P., & Wyatt, J. (2012). Development and delivery of an SMS-based remote monitoring and support service: 'Simple Telehealth'. In *International Journal of Integrated Care* (Vol. 12, Issue Suppl1).

Beach, M. C., Gary, T. L., Price, E. G., Robinson, K., Gozu, A., Palacio, A., Smarth, C., Jenckes, M., Feuerstein, C., Bass, E. B., Powe, N. R., & Cooper, L. A. (2006). Improving health care quality for racial/ethnic minorities: A systematic review of the best evidence regarding provider and organization interventions. *BMC Public Health, 6*(1), 104. DOI: 10.1186/1471-2458-6-104 PMID: 16635262

Bedón-Molina, J., Lopez, M. J., & Derpich, I. S. (2014). A home-based smart health model. *Advances in Mechanical Engineering, 12*(6), 1687814020935282. DOI: 10.1177/1687814020935282

Beer, J. M., McBride, S. E., Mitzner, T. L., & Rogers, W. A. (2014). Understanding challenges in the front lines of home health care: A human-systems approach. *Applied Ergonomics*, *45*(6), 1687–1699. DOI: 10.1016/j.apergo.2014.05.019 PMID: 24958610

Bouabida, K., Lebouché, B., & Pomey, M.-P. (2022). Telehealth and COVID-19 Pandemic: An Overview of the Telehealth Use, Advantages, Challenges, and Opportunities during COVID-19 Pandemic. *Healthcare (Basel, Switzerland)*, *10*(11). Advance online publication. DOI: 10.3390/healthcare10112293 PMID: 36421617

Burgdorf, J. G., Arbaje, A. I., Chase, J.-A., & Wolff, J. L. (2022). Current practices of family caregiver training during home health care: A qualitative study. *Journal of the American Geriatrics Society*, *70*(1), 218–227. https://doi.org/https://doi.org/10.1111/jgs.17492 PMID: 34618918

Cauthen, D. B. (1981). The house call in current medical practice. *The Journal of Family Practice*, *13*(2), 209–213. PMID: 7252449

Charmes, J. (2022). Variety and change of patterns in the gender balance between unpaid care-work, paid work and free time across the world and over time: A measure of wellbeing? *Wellbeing, Space and Society*, *3*, 100081. https://doi.org/https://doi.org/10.1016/j.wss.2022.100081

Cheng, J. M., Batten, G. P., Cornwell, T., & Yao, N. (2020). A qualitative study of health-care experiences and challenges faced by ageing homebound adults. *Health Expectations*, *23*(4), 934–942. https://doi.org/https://doi.org/10.1111/hex.13072 PMID: 32476232

Curioni, C., Silva, A. C., Damião, J., Castro, A., Huang, M., Barroso, T., Araujo, D., & Guerra, R. (2023). The Cost-Effectiveness of Homecare Services for Adults and Older Adults: A Systematic Review. *International Journal of Environmental Research and Public Health*, *20*(4). Advance online publication. DOI: 10.3390/ijerph20043373 PMID: 36834068

Dahmani, H., Fradi, I., Achour, L., & Toumi, M. (2023). Pharmaceutical pricing and reimbursement policies in Algeria, Morocco, and Tunisia: Comparative analysis. *Journal of Market Access & Health Policy*, *11*(1), 2244304. DOI: 10.1080/20016689.2023.2244304 PMID: 37614557

Dellve, L., Lagerström, M., & Hagberg, M. (2003). Work-system risk factors for permanent work disability among home-care workers: A case-control study. *International Archives of Occupational and Environmental Health*, *76*(3), 216–224. DOI: 10.1007/s00420-002-0414-5 PMID: 12690496

Dick, A. W., Murray, M. T., Chastain, A. M., Madigan, E. A., Sorbero, M., Stone, P. W., & Shang, J. (2019). Measuring Quality in Home Healthcare. *Journal of the American Geriatrics Society*, *67*(9), 1859–1865. DOI: 10.1111/jgs.15963 PMID: 31063621

El-Haddad, C., Hegazi, I., & Hu, W. (2020). Understanding Patient Expectations of Health Care: A Qualitative Study. *Journal of Patient Experience*, *7*(6), 1724–1731. DOI: 10.1177/2374373520921692 PMID: 33457636

El-Jardali, F., & Fadlallah, R. (2017). A review of national policies and strategies to improve quality of health care and patient safety: A case study from Lebanon and Jordan. *BMC Health Services Research*, *17*(1), 1–13. DOI: 10.1186/s12913-017-2528-1 PMID: 28814341

Eldaly, A. S., Maniaci, M. J., Paulson, M. R., Avila, F. R., Torres-Guzman, R. A., Maita, K., Garcia, J. P., & Forte, A. J. (2022). Patient satisfaction with telemedicine in acute care setting: A systematic review. *Journal of Clinical and Translational Research*, *8*(6), 540–556. PMID: 36518201

Ellenbecker, C. H., Samia, L., Cushman, M. J., & Alster, K. (2008). Patient safety and quality in home health care. *Patient Safety and Quality: An Evidence-Based Handbook for Nurses*.

Eriksson, H., Sandberg, J., & Hellström, I. (2013). Experiences of long-term home care as an informal caregiver to a spouse: Gendered meanings in everyday life for female carers. *International Journal of Older People Nursing*, *8*(2), 159–165. DOI: 10.1111/j.1748-3743.2012.00340.x PMID: 22805660

Evans, R., Weech-Maldonado, R., Burke, D., Grammas, M., Jablonski, R., & Mehta, T. (2019). Developing a Strategic Group Typology for Home Health Care Agencies. *Home Health Care Management & Practice*, *32*(2), 87–94. DOI: 10.1177/1084822319882673

Fajarini, M., Setiawan, A., Sung, C.-M., Chen, R., Liu, D., Lee, C.-K., Niu, S.-F., & Chou, K.-R. (2025). Effects of advanced practice nurses on health-care costs, quality of care, and patient well-being: A meta-analysis of randomized controlled trials. *International Journal of Nursing Studies*, *162*, 104953. https://doi.org/https://doi.org/10.1016/j.ijnurstu.2024.104953 PMID: 39586168

Fernandes, R., Osarch, S., & Allen, N. E. (2018). Home Healthcare and Hospice: A Pacific Islands Perspective. *Home Healthcare Now*, *36*(4). https://journals.lww.com/homehealthcarenurseonline/fulltext/2018/07000/home_healthcare_and_hospice__a_pacific_islands.8.aspx PMID: 29979307

Floridi, G., Carrino, L., & Glaser, K. (2021). Socioeconomic Inequalities in Home-Care Use Across Regional Long-term Care Systems in Europe. *The Journals of Gerontology. Series B, Psychological Sciences and Social Sciences*, *76*(1), 121–132. DOI: 10.1093/geronb/gbaa139 PMID: 32996570

Foster, C. C., Agrawal, R. K., & Davis, M. M. (2019). Home Health Care For Children With Medical Complexity: Workforce Gaps, Policy, And Future Directions. *Health Affairs*, *38*(6), 987–993. DOI: 10.1377/hlthaff.2018.05531 PMID: 31158008

Freedman, V. A., Rogowski, J., Wickstrom, S. L., Adams, J., Marainen, J., & Escarce, J. J. (2004). Socioeconomic Disparities in the Use of Home Health Services in a Medicare Managed Care Population. *Health Services Research*, *39*(5), 1277–1298. https://doi.org/https://doi.org/10.1111/j.1475-6773.2004.00290.x PMID: 15333109

Frogner, B. K., Patterson, D. G., & Skillman, S. M. (2023). The Workforce Needed to Address Population Health. *The Milbank Quarterly*, *101*(S1), 841–865. DOI: 10.1111/1468-0009.12620 PMID: 37096630

Getson, C., & Nejat, G. (2021). Socially assistive robots helping older adults through the pandemic and life after covid-19. *Robotics (Basel, Switzerland)*, *10*(3). Advance online publication. DOI: 10.3390/robotics10030106

Ghosh, A., Singh, A., & Chigateri, S. (2023). A Trapeze Act : Women Balancing Paid Work and Unpaid Care Work in Nepal - National Report for Women's Economic Empowerment Policy and Programming. SSRN *Electronic Journal, October*. https://doi.org/DOI: 10.2139/ssrn.4660197

Goodridge, D., Hawranik, P., Duncan, V., & Turner, H. (2012). Socioeconomic disparities in home health care service access and utilization: A scoping review. *International Journal of Nursing Studies*, *49*(10), 1310–1319. https://doi.org/https://doi.org/10.1016/j.ijnurstu.2012.01.002 PMID: 22300550

Gottlieb, L. M., DeSalvo, K., & Adler, N. E. (2019). Healthcare Sector Activities to Identify and Intervene on Social Risk: An Introduction to the <em>American Journal of Preventive Medicine</em> Supplement. *American Journal of Preventive Medicine*, *57*(6), S1–S5. DOI: 10.1016/j.amepre.2019.07.009 PMID: 31753275

Gottret, P., Schieber, G., & Waters, H. R. (2008). *Good practices in health financing: lessons from reforms in low and middle-income countries*. World Bank Publications.

Gunasekeran, D. V., Tham, Y.-C., Ting, D. S. W., Tan, G. S. W., & Wong, T. Y. (2021). Digital health during COVID-19: Lessons from operationalising new models of care in ophthalmology. *The Lancet. Digital Health*, *3*(2), e124–e134. DOI: 10.1016/S2589-7500(20)30287-9 PMID: 33509383

Gustafsson, L.-K., Asztalos Morell, I., Johansson, C., & De, S. (2022). Informal caregiving from the perspectives of older people living alone in India. *International Journal of Older People Nursing*, *17*(6), e12468. DOI: 10.1111/opn.12468 PMID: 35466547

Hajizadeh, M., & Nghiem, H. S. (2011). Out-of-pocket expenditures for hospital care in Iran: Who is at risk of incurring catastrophic payments? *International Journal of Health Care Finance and Economics*, *11*(4), 267–285. DOI: 10.1007/s10754-011-9099-1 PMID: 21915727

Hamasaki, H. (2025). The Relationship Between Socioeconomic Status and Health Behaviors in Older Adults: A Narrative Review. *Healthcare (Switzerland)*, *13*(14), 1–22. DOI: 10.3390/healthcare13141669 PMID: 40724694

Hamideh, D., & Nebeker, C. (2020). The Digital Health Landscape in Addiction and Substance Use Research: Will Digital Health Exacerbate or Mitigate Health Inequities in Vulnerable Populations? *Current Addiction Reports*, *7*(3), 317–332. DOI: 10.1007/s40429-020-00325-9

Hartanto, A., Sim, L., Lee, D., Majeed, N. M., & Yong, J. C. (2024). Cultural contexts differentially shape parents' loneliness and wellbeing during the empty nest period. *Communications Psychology*, *2*(1), 105. DOI: 10.1038/s44271-024-00156-8 PMID: 39489810

Hassan, S. M., Okoli, E. C., Azike, C. A., Okoye, N. A., & Adindu, N. K. (2024). Assessing the Impact of Community Health Workforce on the Efficiency and Accessibility of Healthcare Delivery. *Archives of Current Research International*, *24*(10), 167–173. DOI: 10.9734/acri/2024/v24i10918

Iyawa, G. E., Herselman, M., & Botha, A. (2016). Digital Health Innovation Ecosystems: From Systematic Literature Review to Conceptual Framework. *Procedia Computer Science*, *100*, 244–252. https://doi.org/https://doi.org/10.1016/j.procs.2016.09.149

Jencks, S. F., Williams, M. V., & Coleman, E. A. (2009). Rehospitalizations among patients in the Medicare fee-for-service program. *The New England Journal of Medicine*, *360*(14), 1418–1428. DOI: 10.1056/NEJMsa0803563 PMID: 19339721

Jiang, N., Wu, B., & Li, Y. (2024). Caregiving in Asia: Priority areas for research, policy, and practice to support family caregivers. *Health Care Science*, *3*(6), 374–382. DOI: 10.1002/hcs2.124 PMID: 39735283

Juckett, G., & Unger, K. (2014). Appropriate use of medical interpreters. *American Family Physician*, *90*(7), 476–480. PMID: 25369625

Juergens, M. C., Seekatz, B., Moosdorf, R. G., Petrie, K. J., & Rief, W. (2010). Illness beliefs before cardiac surgery predict disability, quality of life, and depression 3 months later. *Journal of Psychosomatic Research*, *68*(6), 553–560. DOI: 10.1016/j.jpsychores.2009.10.004 PMID: 20488272

Kaihlanen, A.-M., Ruotsalainen, S., Väisänen, V., Corneliusson, L., Pesonen, T., & Sinervo, T. (2023). Job demand and job resource factors explaining stress and job satisfaction among home care nurses – a mixed-methods sequential explanatory study. *BMC Nursing*, *22*(1), 404. DOI: 10.1186/s12912-023-01568-3 PMID: 37891583

Kallas, J., Sterling, M. R., Ajayi, O., Mulroy, E., Kuo, E., Ming, J., Dell, N., & Avgar, A. C. (2023). Making a Bad Situation Worse: Examining the Challenges Facing Rural Home Care Workers. *Journal of Applied Gerontology : The Official Journal of the Southern Gerontological Society*, *42*(4), 768–775. DOI: 10.1177/07334648221134793 PMID: 36510645

Kane, L., Portman, R. M., Eberhardt, J., Walker, L., Proctor, E.-L., Poulter, H., & O'Neill, C. (2023). Peer supporters' mental health and emotional wellbeing needs: Key factors and opportunities for co-produced training. *Health Expectations*, *26*(6), 2387–2395. https://doi.org/https://doi.org/10.1111/hex.13836 PMID: 37565576

Kao, H., Conant, R., Soriano, T., & McCormick, W. (2009). The Past, Present, and Future of House Calls. *Clinics in Geriatric Medicine*, *25*(1), 19–34. DOI: 10.1016/j.cger.2008.10.005 PMID: 19217490

Kayonga, C. S., Ristolainen, H., & Lisko, I., Mäki- Petäjä-Leinonen, A., & Tiilikainen, E. (2025). Association Between Social Support and Quality of Life: Cross-Sectional Study Among Older Adults Receiving Home Care Services in Finland. *Home Health Care Management & Practice*. Advance online publication. DOI: 10.1177/10848223251385092

Khan, R., Khan, S., Almohaimeed, H. M., Almars, A. I., & Pari, B. (2025). Utilization, challenges, and training needs of digital health technologies: Perspectives from healthcare professionals. *International Journal of Medical Informatics*, *197*, 105833. https://doi.org/https://doi.org/10.1016/j.ijmedinf.2025.105833 PMID: 39954392

Kim, M.-J., Ahn, K.-H., & Jung, Y. (2002). Distribution of inorganic arsenic species in mine tailings of abandoned mines from Korea. *Chemosphere*, *49*(3), 307–312. https://doi.org/https://doi.org/10.1016/S0045-6535(02)00307-7 PMID: 12363309

Kinjo, K., Sairenji, T., Koga, H., Osugi, Y., Yoshida, S., Ichinose, H., Nagai, Y., Imura, H., South-Paul, J. E., Meyer, M., & Honda, Y. (2017). Cost of physician-led home visit care (Zaitaku care) compared with hospital care at the end of life in Japan. *BMC Health Services Research, 17*(1), 40. DOI: 10.1186/s12913-016-1961-x PMID: 28095906

Koehlmoos, T. P., Anwar, S., & Cravioto, A. (2011). Global health: chronic diseases and other emergent issues in global health. *Infectious Disease Clinics of North America, 25*(3), 623–638, ix. https://doi.org/DOI: 10.1016/j.idc.2011.05.008

Krist, A. H., Tong, S. T., Aycock, R. A., & Longo, D. R. (2017). Engaging Patients in Decision-Making and Behavior Change to Promote Prevention. *Studies in Health Technology and Informatics, 240*, 284–302. PMID: 28972524

Labson, M. C. (2015)... *Innovative and Successful Approaches To Improving Care Transitions From Hospital to Home., 33*(2), 88–95.

Landers, S., Madigan, E., Leff, B., Rosati, R. J., McCann, B. A., Hornbake, R., MacMillan, R., Jones, K., Bowles, K., Dowding, D., Lee, T., Moorhead, T., Rodriguez, S., & Breese, E. (2016). The Future of Home Health Care: A Strategic Framework for Optimizing Value. *Home Health Care Management & Practice, 28*(4), 262–278. DOI: 10.1177/1084822316666368 PMID: 27746670

Landers, S. H. (2006). Home care: A key to the future of family medicine? *Annals of Family Medicine, 4*(4), 366–368. DOI: 10.1370/afm.550 PMID: 16868241

Leao, D. L. L., Cremers, H.-P., van Veghel, D., Pavlova, M., & Groot, W. (2023). The Impact of Value-Based Payment Models for Networks of Care and Transmural Care: A Systematic Literature Review. *Applied Health Economics and Health Policy, 21*(3), 441 466. DOI: 10.1007/s40258-023-00790-z PMID: 36723777

Leff, B., & Burton, J. R. (2001). The future history of home care and physician house calls in the United States. *The Journals of Gerontology. Series A, Biological Sciences and Medical Sciences, 56*(10), M603–M608. DOI: 10.1093/gerona/56.10.m603 PMID: 11584032

Lei, Y.-Y., Ya, S. R. T., Zheng, Y.-R., & Cui, X.-S. (2023). Effectiveness of nurse-led multidisciplinary interventions in primary health care: A systematic review and meta-analysis. *International Journal of Nursing Practice, 29*(6), e13133. DOI: 10.1111/ijn.13133 PMID: 36658754

Maita, K. C., Maniaci, M. J., Haider, C. R., Avila, F. R., Torres-Guzman, R. A., Borna, S., Lunde, J. J., Coffey, J. D., Demaerschalk, B. M., & Forte, A. J. (2024). The Impact of Digital Health Solutions on Bridging the Health Care Gap in Rural Areas: A Scoping Review. *The Permanente Journal*, *28*(3), 130–143. DOI: 10.7812/TPP/23.134 PMID: 39135461

Marmot, M. (2005). Social determinants of health inequalities. *Lancet*, *365*(9464), 1099–1104. DOI: 10.1016/S0140-6736(05)71146-6 PMID: 15781105

Masoumi, N., Hosseinzadeh, M., VanSon, C., & Ghezeljeh, T. N. (2021). Home healthcare in Iran: A hybrid concept analysis. *Iranian Journal of Nursing and Midwifery Research*, *26*(3), 196–203. DOI: 10.4103/ijnmr.IJNMR_198_20 PMID: 34277369

Mezzalira, E., Canzan, F., Marini, G., Longhini, J., Leardini, C., Saiani, L., & Ambrosi, E. (2024). Introduction of novel complex integrated care models supported by digital health interventions in European primary settings: A scoping review. *Health Policy and Technology*, *13*(4), 100896. https://doi.org/https://doi.org/10.1016/j.hlpt.2024.100896

Miller, R. K., Morgan-Gouveia, M. D., & DeCherrie, L. V. (2022). Medical Training in Home Care Medicine: The Time is Now. *Journal of General Internal Medicine*, *37*(9), 2302–2305. DOI: 10.1007/s11606-022-07514-4 PMID: 35710677

Miura, H. (2015). Historical changes in home care service and its future challenges. *JMA Journal*, *58*(1–2), 1–5. PMID: 26557453

Mukamel, D. B., Ladd, H., Nuccio, E., Zinn, J. S., Sorkin, D. H., & Ettner, S. L. (2022). Home Health Care Quality, Its Costs and Implications for Home Health Value-Based Purchasing. *Medical Care Research and Review : MCRR*, *79*(1), 90–101. DOI: 10.1177/1077558720974528 PMID: 33233999

Mulaga, A. N., Kamndaya, M. S., & Masangwi, S. J. (2022). Decomposing socioeconomic inequality in catastrophic out-of-pocket health expenditures in Malawi. *PLOS Global Public Health*, *2*(2), e0000182. DOI: 10.1371/journal.pgph.0000182 PMID: 36962147

Narayan, S. M., Chung, M. K., Adedinsewo, D., Brant, L. C. C., Davis, L. L., Duncker, D., Hall, J. L., Han, J. K., Lam, C. S. P., Lewis, E., Loscalzo, J., Márquez, M. F., Rahimzadeh, V., Rodriguez, F., Sanders, P., Svennberg, E., Stein, K., Turakhia, M., Yancy, C., & Armoundas, A. A. (2025). Access to digital health technologies: Personalized framework and global perspectives. *Nature Reviews. Cardiology*. Advance online publication. DOI: 10.1038/s41569-025-01184-5 PMID: 40670723

Ne, L. S., Ne, L. S., & Ne, L. S. (2023). *The Honorable Jessica Rosenworcel Chairwoman Federal Communications Commission Washington, DC 20554 The Honorable Brendan Carr Commissioner Federal Communications Commission Washington, DC 20554 The Honorable Geoffrey Starks Commissioner Federal Communi. 14*, 1–6.

Pandya, S., Hamal, M., Abuya, T., Kintu, R., Mwanga, D., Warren, C. E., & Agarwal, S. (2022). Understanding Factors That Support Community Health Worker Motivation, Job Satisfaction, and Performance in Three Ugandan Districts: Opportunities for Strengthening Uganda's Community Health Worker Program. *International Journal of Health Policy and Management, 11*(12), 2886–2894. DOI: 10.34172/ijhpm.2022.6219 PMID: 35461208

Park, M., & Giap, T.-T.-T. (2020). Patient and family engagement as a potential approach for improving patient safety: A systematic review. *Journal of Advanced Nursing, 76*(1), 62–80. https://doi.org/https://doi.org/10.1111/jan.14227 PMID: 31588602

Price, E. G., Beach, M. C., Gary, T. L., Robinson, K. A., Gozu, A., Palacio, A., Smarth, C., Jenckes, M., Feuerstein, C., Bass, E. B., Powe, N. R., & Cooper, L. A. (2005). A systematic review of the methodological rigor of studies evaluating cultural competence training of health professionals. *Academic Medicine, 80*(6), 578–586. DOI: 10.1097/00001888-200506000-00013 PMID: 15917363

Qiu, W. Q., Dean, M., Liu, T., George, L., Gann, M., Cohen, J., & Bruce, M. L. (2010). Physical and Mental Health of Homebound Older Adults: An Overlooked Population. *Journal of the American Geriatrics Society, 58*(12), 2423–2428. https://doi.org/https://doi.org/10.1111/j.1532-5415.2010.03161.x PMID: 21070195

Rad, J. (2025). Health inequities: A persistent global challenge from past to future. *International Journal for Equity in Health, 24*(1). Advance online publication. DOI: 10.1186/s12939-025-02526-y PMID: 40410748

Reckrey, J. M., Ornstein, K. A., Wajnberg, A., Kopke, M. V., & DeCherrie, L. V. (2017). Teaching Home-Based Primary Care. *Home Healthcare Now, 35*(10). https://journals.lww.com/homehealthcarenurseonline/fulltext/2017/11000/teaching_home_based_primary_care.6.aspx PMID: 29095335

Rhee, J. C., Done, N., & Anderson, G. F. (2015). Considering long-term care insurance for middle-income countries: Comparing South Korea with Japan and Germany. *Health Policy (Amsterdam), 119*(10), 1319–1329. https://doi.org/https://doi.org/10.1016/j.healthpol.2015.06.001 PMID: 26117093

Samia, L. W., Ellenbecker, C. H., Friedman, D. H., & Dick, K. (2012). Home care nurses' experience of job stress and considerations for the work environment. *Home Health Care Services Quarterly*, *31*(3), 243–265. DOI: 10.1080/01621424.2012.703903 PMID: 22974083

Sani, D. K., Yunusa, U., Kombo, S. A., Ibrahim, A., Sani, H. M., Umar, S. S., & Ladan, M. A. (2024). Home-based care models for patients with terminal illnesses in low and middle-income countries: A systematic review of randomized and quasi-experimental studies. *Archives of Gerontology and Geriatrics*, *127*, 105580. DOI: 10.1016/j.archger.2024.105580 PMID: 39029345

Shahriari, M., Nia, D. H., Kalij, F., & Hashemi, M. S. (2024). Challenges of home care: A qualitative study. *BMC Nursing*, *23*(1), 215. DOI: 10.1186/s12912-024-01878-0 PMID: 38549100

Shalaby, R. A. H., & Agyapong, V. I. O. (2020). Peer Support in Mental Health: Literature Review. *JMIR Mental Health*, *7*(6), e15572. DOI: 10.2196/15572 PMID: 32357127

Shoemake, A. (1994). Solutions to the Home Healthcare Nursing Shortage. *Home Healthcare Now*, *12*(4). https://journals.lww.com/homehealthcarenurseonline/fulltext/1994/07000/solutions_to_the_home_healthcare_nursing_shortage.6.aspx PMID: 7960869

Sibai, A. M., Semaan, A., Tabbara, J., & Rizk, A. (2017). Ageing and health in the Arab region: Challenges, opportunities and the way forward. *Population Horizons*, *14*(2), 73–84. DOI: 10.1515/pophzn-2017-0007

Sindhukumari, S. U., & Varkey Thomas, K. (2023). Analyzing the Influence of Socioeconomic Status on Public Healthcare Access: An Interdisciplinary Framework. *EuroMid Journal of Business and Tech-Innovation (EJBTI)*, 33–48. https://doi.org/ DOI: 10.51325/ejbti.v2i2.176

Son, Y.-J., Lee, Y., & Lee, H.-J. (2020). Effectiveness of Mobile Phone-Based Interventions for Improving Health Outcomes in Patients with Chronic Heart Failure: A Systematic Review and Meta-Analysis. *International Journal of Environmental Research and Public Health*, *17*(5). Advance online publication. DOI: 10.3390/ijerph17051749 PMID: 32156074

Thomas, S. A., Browning, C. J., Charchar, F. J., Klein, B., Ory, M. G., Bowden-Jones, H., & Chamberlain, S. R. (2023). Transforming global approaches to chronic disease prevention and management across the lifespan: Integrating genomics, behavior change, and digital health solutions. *Frontiers in Public Health*, *11*, 1248254. DOI: 10.3389/fpubh.2023.1248254 PMID: 37905238

Vanholder, R., Davenport, A., Hannedouche, T., Kooman, J., Kribben, A., Lameire, N., Lonnemann, G., Magner, P., Mendelssohn, D., Saggi, S. J., Shaffer, R. N., Moe, S. M., Van Biesen, W., van der Sande, F., Mehrotra, R., & Nephrology, on behalf of the D. A. G. of the A. S. of. (2012). Reimbursement of Dialysis: A Comparison of Seven Countries. *Journal of the American Society of Nephrology, 23*(8). https://journals.lww.com/jasn/fulltext/2012/08000/reimbursement_of_dialysis__a_comparison_of_seven.7.aspx

Vick, J. B., & Wolff, J. L. (2021). A scoping review of person and family engagement in the context of multiple chronic conditions. *Health Services Research, 56 Suppl 1*(Suppl 1), 990–1005. https://doi.org/DOI: 10.1111/1475-6773.13857

Visiting Nurses Association of America (V.N.A.A.). (n.d.). https://www.vnaa.org/

Wagenschieber, E., & Blunck, D. (2024). Impact of reimbursement systems on patient care - a systematic review of systematic reviews. *Health Economics Review, 14*(1), 22. DOI: 10.1186/s13561-024-00487-6 PMID: 38492098

Yan, A. F., Chen, Z., Wang, Y., Campbell, J. A., Xue, Q.-L., Williams, M. Y., Weinhardt, L. S., & Egede, L. E. (2022). Effectiveness of Social Needs Screening and Interventions in Clinical Settings on Utilization, Cost, and Clinical Outcomes: A Systematic Review. *Health Equity*, *6*(1), 454–475. DOI: 10.1089/heq.2022.0010 PMID: 35801145

Yao, R., Zhang, W., Evans, R., Cao, G., Rui, T., & Shen, L. (2022). Inequities in Health Care Services Caused by the Adoption of Digital Health Technologies: Scoping Review. *Journal of Medical Internet Research*, *24*(3), e34144. DOI: 10.2196/34144 PMID: 35311682

Zhang, L., Zeng, Y., Wang, L., & Fang, Y. (2020). Urban-Rural Differences in Long-Term Care Service Status and Needs Among Home-Based Elderly People in China. *International Journal of Environmental Research and Public Health*, *17*(5). Advance online publication. DOI: 10.3390/ijerph17051701 PMID: 32150946

Zhang, N., Li, Q., Chen, S., Wu, Y., Xin, B., Wan, Q., Shi, P., He, Y., Yang, S., & Jiang, W. (2024). Effectiveness of nurse-led electronic health interventions on illness management in patients with chronic heart failure: A systematic review and meta-analysis. *International Journal of Nursing Studies*, *150*, 104630. DOI: 10.1016/j.ijnurstu.2023.104630 PMID: 38029453

Zhang, Y., Leuk, J. S. P., & Teo, W. P. (2023). Domains, Feasibility, Effectiveness, Cost, and Acceptability of Telehealth in Aging Care: Scoping Review of Systematic Reviews. *JMIR Aging*, *6*, 1–16. DOI: 10.2196/40460 PMID: 37071459

Chapter 9

Mindfulness-Based Interventions for Caregivers of Terminally Elderly Patients:

Reducing Burden, Enhancing Resilience, and Supporting Compassionate Care

Syed Zafar Sultan Rizvi
https://orcid.org/0009-0001-1927-9297
Mohammad Ali Jauhar University, India

Madiha Rehman
https://orcid.org/0009-0001-0620-4210
Blossom School, Aligarh, India

Arshy Kamal
https://orcid.org/0009-0008-3171-9380
Jawahar Lal Nehru Medical College, Aligarh, India

Ashba Javed
Blossom School, Aligarh, India

ABSTRACT

Caring for terminally ill elderly individuals imposes profound psychological, emotional, and physical stress on caregivers, often resulting in anxiety, depression, and anticipatory grief that diminish well-being and end-of-life care quality. Mindfulness-

DOI: 10.4018/979-8-3373-4099-9.ch009

Based Interventions (MBIs), rooted in Buddhist contemplative practice and supported by clinical research, offer an evidence-based means to reduce distress and enhance resilience and compassion. This chapter outlines the theoretical foundations and empirical evidence of MBIs in geriatric palliative care, presenting a practical "Mindfulness Care Pathway" featuring formal and brief practices adaptable for busy caregivers. Cultural adaptation, ethical concerns, and implementation strategies are discussed, alongside outcome measures such as caregiver burden and quality of life. Mindfulness emerges as a compassionate, scalable, and cost-effective approach to sustain caregiver wellness and deliver dignified end-of-life care.

1. INTRODUCTION

1.1 Global Challenges in Care-Giving for Terminally Ill Elderly

The globe is experiencing a swift demographic transition, characterized by a rapid rise in the share of senior populations. The World Health Organization (2020) projects that the global population aged 60 years and above will reach 2.1 billion by 2050. China alone is expected to have one of the world's largest ageing populations, with adults aged 60 years and above projected to comprise approximately 35% of the national population by 2050, equivalent to more than 400 million older adults (UN DESA, 2022). Countries in the Middle East, traditionally younger in demographic composition, are also undergoing accelerated ageing; the proportion of adults aged 60+ is expected to rise from 6% in 2020 to nearly 15% by 2050, with the steepest increases in Iran, Saudi Arabia, and Turkey (UN DESA, 2022). In Western nations, population ageing is even more pronounced: by 2050, adults aged 65 and over are estimated to constitute 26% of the population in Europe and 23% in North America (OECD, 2021). A substantial proportion of these older adults are likely to live with chronic and life-threatening conditions such as cancer, dementia, and multiple organ failure, requiring long-term caregiving and palliative support. This demographic shift exerts significant pressure on healthcare systems worldwide, particularly in low- and middle-income countries where geriatric and palliative care resources remain insufficient (Sleeman et al., 2019).

1.2 Burden on Family Caregivers & Healthcare Workers

Family caregivers frequently constitute the essential support for terminally ill older folks, delivering physical aid, emotional sustenance, and the orchestration of medical requirements. This function is linked to considerable psychological discomfort, financial hardship, and social isolation (Adelman et al., 2014). Healthcare professionals, especially nurses and palliative care personnel, may endure significant burnout, compassion fatigue, and moral anguish as a result of extended exposure to pain and mortality (Peters et al., 2013). Collectively, these costs undermine both caregiver welfare and the quality of care provided to patients.

1.3 Rationale for Mindfulness in This Context

The justification for mindfulness in this context is that, in recent years, mindfulness-based interventions (MBIs) have garnered recognition as effective tools for bolstering resilience and alleviating stress among caregivers. Mindfulness, characterized as the ability to focus on the present moment with receptivity and impartiality (Kabat-Zinn, 2003), has been linked to less emotional reactivity, greater coping mechanisms, and increased well-being. Recent data indicates that mindfulness-based interventions (MBIs) can alleviate caregiver stress, enhance emotional regulation, and elevate the overall quality of life for both familial and professional caregivers in palliative settings (Miroslav, 2020). Consequently, including mindfulness into care-giving models may offer a sustainable approach to enhance the mental health and resilience of individuals caring for terminally ill elderly patients.

2. CAREGIVER STRESS, GRIEF AND ECONOMICAL BURDEN

2.1 Psychological, Emotional, and Physical Dimensions

Providing care for terminally sick elderly adults entails considerable psychological, emotional, and physical challenges. Caregivers face an increased risk of depression, anxiety, and chronic stress due to extended uncertainty and the anticipatory aspect of loss (Pinquart & Sörensen, 2003). Caregivers frequently encounter feelings of shame, powerlessness, and role tension, especially when reconciling care-giving duties with familial and professional obligations (Kent et al., 2016). The ongoing physical demands of care-giving, including aiding mobility, overseeing prescriptions, and delivering personal care, have been associated with weariness, sleep disruptions, and a heightened risk of cardiovascular disease (Schulz & Sherwood, 2008).

2.2 Anticipatory Grief and Exhaustion

Caregivers of terminally ill patients often experience anticipatory grieving, characterized by mourning before to the patient's death (Lindauer & Harvath, 2014). This procedure may facilitate emotional preparedness, although it simultaneously exacerbates psychological pain, increasing susceptibility to burnout.

Burnout is defined as emotional weariness, depersonalization, and a diminished sense of achievement (Maslach & Leiter, 2016). Anticipatory grieving and fatigue diminish caregiver well-being and may restrict their ability to offer compassionate and enduring assistance.

2.3 Economical Analysis

Caring for terminally ill patients with serious life-threatening conditions such as advanced cancer, end-stage organ failure, or multiple organ dysfunction creates substantial economic and psychosocial burdens for family caregivers. These caregivers often face high out-of-pocket medical expenses, reduced work hours, and significant productivity loss. Studies show that informal-care costs are frequently underestimated, despite evidence that caregiving for advanced cancer and end-stage conditions requires intensive time investment and contributes to long-term financial strain (Mattingly et al., 2022; Iype et al., 2014).Economic evaluations indicate that home-based and hospice palliative care for severe illnesses can be cost-effective, reducing emergency visits, hospital admissions, and overall healthcare expenditures while improving caregiver well-being (Maresova, 2024; Salikhanov et al., 2023). However, many analyses still omit caregiver time, emotional labour, and their own health deterioration, leading to incomplete assessments of the true economic burden (Guzzon et al., 2023).Improving accessibility to formal palliative services—particularly respite care, caregiver training, and home-based support is essential for families caring for patients with terminal cancer or multiple organ failure, ensuring equitable and sustainable care.

Table 1. Dimensions of Caregiver Stress and Burden

Dimension	Description	Associated Risks
Psychological	Depression, anxiety, chronic stress from prolonged uncertainty	Mood disorders, impaired decision-making
Emotional	Guilt, helplessness, anticipatory grief, role strain	Emotional exhaustion, family conflict, compassion fatigue
Physical	Sleep disruption, fatigue, physical strain, cardiovascular vulnerability	Chronic illness, musculoskeletal pain, lowered immunity
Burnout	Emotional exhaustion, depersonalization, reduced accomplishment	Compassion fatigue, decreased quality of care, attrition
Impact on Care	Stress spilling over into care-giving quality, communication breakdown	Patient neglect, reduced satisfaction, unsafe care practices

3. NEUROBIOLOGICAL AND PSYCHO PHYSIOLOGICAL MECHANISMS UNDERPINNING STRESS AND MINDFULNESS IN CAREGIVERS OF TERMINALLY ILL PATIENTS

Care-giving for individuals with terminal illnesses—such as advanced cancer, end-stage renal disease, congestive heart failure, or progressive neurodegenerative conditions—induces chronic stress that activates multiple neurobiological pathways associated with psychological and physical morbidity. Persistent caregiving strain dysregulates the hypothalamic–pituitary–adrenal (HPA) axis, resulting in flattened diurnal cortisol slopes, elevated evening cortisol, and impaired cortisol reactivity—patterns consistently observed in caregivers of terminal cancer patients and associated with depression, fatigue, and immune suppression (Gao et al., 2020; Kim et al., 2021). Chronic sympathetic activation further contributes to heightened autonomic imbalance, marked by reduced heart rate variability (HRV), increased inflammatory markers (e.g., IL-6, CRP), and disrupted sleep–wake cycles, worsening emotional reactivity and decision-making fatigue (Zernicke et al., 2020). Mindfulness-based interventions (MBIs) modulate these stress pathways through well-characterized neural and physiological mechanisms. Neuroimaging studies demonstrate that mindfulness enhances prefrontal cortex (PFC) activation—supporting attentional control and cognitive reappraisal—while downregulating amygdala hyper-reactivity, thereby attenuating threat perception and emotional overload common among caregivers managing imminent loss (Taren et al., 2022). MBIs also strengthen connectivity within default mode (DMN) and salience networks, improving meta-awareness and reducing ruminative thinking, a known predictor of caregiver burnout (Liu et al., 2021). Physiologically, mindfulness practice restores autonomic balance by increasing HRV and parasympathetic tone, and early evidence in palliative caregiver trials suggests improved cortisol regulation and reductions in inflammatory markers following short MBI programs (Jones et al., 2022; Lengacher et al., 2019). Collectively, these mechanistic findings highlight that mindfulness not only reduces subjective distress but also exerts measurable neurobiological and psychophysiological effects that buffer caregivers against the cumulative toxicity of anticipatory grief, emotional labor, and prolonged exposure to suffering inherent in terminal care-giving. Furthered more, stress endured by caregivers directly affects the quality of patient care. Elevated caregiver stress correlates with heightened risks of medical errors, neglect, and diminished patient satisfaction in both familial and professional caring settings (Given et al., 2011). Furthermore, caregiver burden frequently results in impaired communication, less emotional availability, and weakened decision-making in end-of-life care (Reinhard et al., 2008). Consequently, caregiver well-being is not solely a concern of individual health but also a crucial factor influencing patient safety and quality results

4. THEORETICAL FOUNDATIONS OF MINDFULNESS

4.1 Historical Roots: From Buddhist Philosophy to Secular Adaptation

Mindfulness originates from Buddhist philosophy, specifically the Satipatthāna Sutta, which highlights awareness of the body, sensations, mind, and mental phenomena (Analayo, 2003). Historically, mindfulness was developed as a means to attain liberation from suffering. In the late 20th century, mindfulness techniques were incorporated into secular frameworks, particularly through Jon Kabat-Zinn's establishment of Mindfulness-Based Stress Reduction (MBSR) in the 1970s at the University of Massachusetts Medical School (Kabat-Zinn, 1990). This modification enabled the incorporation of mindfulness into healthcare, psychotherapy, and behavioral medicine.

4.2 Core Principles: Attention, Awareness, and Acceptance

Mindfulness is generally characterized as the practice of attentively engaging with present-moment events while maintaining openness, curiosity, and nonjudgmental acceptance (Bishop et al., 2004). Three fundamental concepts underpin the construct:

1. Attention — prolonged concentration on the current moment, minimizing rumination and distraction.
2. Awareness — metacognitive oversight of thoughts, emotions, and physiological experiences.
3. Acceptance – fostering a nonjudgmental and empathetic attitude towards one's experiences.

These principles promote self-regulation and resilience, rendering mindfulness especially pertinent for persons subjected to chronic stress, such as caretakers.

4.3 Mindfulness in Health Psychology and Palliative Care

In health psychology, mindfulness is defined as a strategy for mitigating stress and a resource for emotional regulation (Creswell, 2017). Mindfulness-based interventions (MBIs) in palliative care have been effective in improving quality of life, alleviating psychological distress, and fostering spiritual well-being for both patients and caregivers (Shennan et al., 2011). Mindfulness is fundamentally compatible with the comprehensive principles of palliative care, which prioritizes not only physical comfort but also psychological, social, and existential assistance.

5. EVIDENCE BASE FOR MINDFULNESS-BASED INTERVENTIONS (MBIS) IN CARE-GIVING

5.1 Overview

In the past twenty years, an expanding body of literature—including pilot randomized controlled trials (RCTs), pragmatic trials, systematic reviews, and meta-analyses—has assessed mindfulness-based interventions (MBIs) for informal family caregivers and healthcare professionals in palliative settings. Overall, data indicates modest enhancements in stress, depression, and caregiver burden, with certain research demonstrating increases in quality of life and emotional regulation capacity. Nonetheless, the heterogeneity of interventions, variability in outcome measurement, small sample sizes, and restricted long-term follow-up are significant limitations (Dharmawardene et al., 2015; Jaffray et al., 2016; Collins & Kishita, 2019).

5.2 Randomized Trials and Pilot Studies

Numerous rigorously executed randomized controlled trials (RCTs) and pilot RCTs especially focus on family caregivers of individuals with dementia, a common demographic in caregiver mindfulness-based intervention (MBI) research. Whitebird et al. (2013) conducted a randomized controlled trial comparing an 8-week Mindfulness-Based Stress Reduction (MBSR) program to an active comparator for family caregivers, revealing enhancements in mental health and diminished felt stress following the intervention. Brown et al. (2016) executed a pilot randomized controlled trial of an adapted Mindfulness-Based Stress Reduction (MBSR) program for dementia caregivers (N = 38) and discovered that MBSR resulted in rapid decreases in felt stress and mood disturbances; however, certain improvements were not maintained or did not differ from an active social-support comparator at follow-up. These randomized controlled trials (RCTs) demonstrate the feasibility and acceptability of Mindfulness-Based Stress Reduction (MBSR) for caregivers, while also highlighting the difficulty of identifying effects that surpass those attainable through well-organized social support or education (Whitebird et al., 2013; Brown et al., 2016).

Significant constraints in the existing evidence base encompass:

1. Limited sample sizes and pilot characteristics: Numerous trials are small, constraining statistical power and generalizability.
2. Diverse interventions: Differences in duration (single-session versus 8-week MBSR), mode of administration (in-person, group, mobile application), and "dose" complicate comparisons.

3. Active comparators: In comparison to active controls (social support, education), mindfulness-based interventions (MBIs) often exhibit diminished between-group differences, indicating the significance of nonspecific treatment characteristics (group support, attention).
4. Brief follow-up: Insufficient long-term outcome data; the sustainability of effects beyond 3–6 months remains uncertain.
5. Variability in outcome measurement: Diverse research employ distinct scales (stress, burden, depression), confounding meta-analytic aggregation.
6. Population bias: Numerous research concentrate on dementia caregivers in affluent nations; evidence for other care-giving populations (e.g., cancer, organ failure) and low-resource environments is limited.

These gaps provide avenues for additional investigation: Properly powered randomized controlled trials, standardized outcome measures (including both psychosocial and functional outcomes), consideration of cultural adaptation and delivery scalability, and comprehensive economic evaluations.

5.3 Systematic Reviews and Meta-Analyses

Numerous evaluations consolidate these experiments: A systematic review and meta-analysis of meditation therapies for informal caregivers and health professionals revealed small to moderate effects for stress, anxiety, and depression (Dharmawardene et al., 2015). Jaffray et al. (2016) examined informal palliative caregivers and determined that mindfulness-based interventions (MBIs) are possible and may be advantageous, especially for alleviating depression and caregiver burden; nevertheless, they acknowledged the limitations of small sample sizes and variability among research.

Recent meta-analyses focusing on caretakers of individuals with dementia indicate moderate effect sizes for depression and lower still significant effects for burden and stress; nevertheless, heterogeneity is common and the quality of studies varies (Collins & Kishita, 2019; Molero Jurado et al., 2020). Collectively, these syntheses reveal a coherent trend: Mindfulness-Based Interventions (MBIs) show potential for enhancing psychosocial outcomes for caregivers; however, the evidence base requires larger, more robust randomized controlled trials (RCTs) with standardized outcome measures and extended follow-up (Dharmawardene et al., 2015; Collins & Kishita, 2019; Molero Jurado et al., 2020).

5.4 Observed Outcomes

Commonly reported outcomes and effects across studies and meta-analyses include:

Perceived stress: decreases (small to moderate effect sizes).

Depression and anxiety: persistent reductions, frequently moderate for depression in meta-analytic summaries.

Caregiver burden: decreases observed, however effect sizes exhibit greater variability compared to mood symptoms.

Emotion regulation and experiential avoidance: enhanced in multiple randomized controlled trials, substantiating a molecular mechanism through which mindfulness-based interventions mitigate responsiveness to care-giving stressors.

Physiological markers: certain research assessed biomarkers (e.g., diurnal cortisol) yielding inconclusive results (Brown et al., 2016).

Quality of life/resilience: enhancements observed in certain trials and aggregated analyses; nevertheless, the evidence is less robust and more heterogeneous compared to mood/stress outcomes. Dharmawardene et al. (2015); Brown et al. (2016); Collins and Kishita (2019).

5.5 Gaps and Limitations

Significant constraints in the existing evidence base encompass:

1. Limited sample sizes and pilot characteristics: Numerous trials are small, constraining statistical power and generalizability.
2. Diverse interventions: Differences in duration (single-session versus 8-week MBSR), mode of administration (in-person, group, mobile application), and "dose" complicate comparisons.
3. Active comparators: In comparison to active controls (social support, education), mindfulness-based interventions (MBIs) often exhibit diminished between-group differences, indicating the significance of nonspecific treatment characteristics (group support, attention).
4. Brief follow-up: Insufficient long-term outcome data; the sustainability of effects beyond 3–6 months remains uncertain.
5. Variability in outcome measurement: Diverse research employ distinct scales (stress, burden, depression), confounding meta-analytic aggregation.
6. Population bias: Numerous research concentrate on dementia caregivers in affluent nations; evidence for other care-giving populations (e.g., cancer, organ failure) and low-resource environments is limited.

These gaps provide avenues for additional investigation: Properly powered randomized controlled trials, standardized outcome measures (including both psychosocial and functional outcomes), consideration of cultural adaptation and delivery scalability, and comprehensive economic evaluations.

5.6 Practical Interpretation for Palliative Care / Terminal Elderly Care-giving

Mindfulness-Based Interventions (MBIs), particularly structured programs such as Mindfulness-Based Stress Reduction (MBSR), are both practicable and acceptable to numerous caregivers and can be incorporated into palliative care support services. Anticipate consistent decreases in perceived stress and depressive symptoms, with moderate evidence indicating reductions in burden; however, mindfulness-based interventions (MBIs) should be provided in conjunction with, rather than as a replacement for, social support and practical assistance.

Due to heterogeneity, consider concise and accessible delivery modes (short group programs, combined online and phone support, app-based information) especially for caregivers with constrained time. Thorough local assessment is advised when modifying MBIs for different populations or resource-limited environments (Dharmawardene et al., 2015; Jaffray et al., 2016; Collins & Kishita, 2019).

6. MINDFULNESS PRACTICES FOR CAREGIVERS

6.1 Formal Practices

Formal mindfulness practices entail organized meditation activities necessitating committed time and space. Common strategies encompass: • Breathing meditation — concentrating on the breath's rhythm to foster present-moment awareness, hence diminishing rumination and autonomic arousal (Zeidan et al., 2010).Body scan meditation involves the systematic allocation of attention to various body regions to improve awareness of somatic sensations and alleviate muscle tension (Kabat-Zinn, 1990). Mindful walking — participating in slow, intentional walking while maintaining awareness of each step, beneficial for caregivers who struggle with extended periods of seated meditation (Teut et al., 2013). These activities assist caregivers in fostering relaxation, regulating emotions, and enhancing attentional control, therefore mitigating stress reactivity (Goyal et al., 2014).

6.2 Informal Practices

Informal practices incorporate mindfulness into everyday care-giving tasks, rendering them attainable even in time-restricted situations:

- Mindful eating involves attentively savoring the flavor, aroma, and texture of food at a deliberate pace, hence mitigating stress-induced eating behaviors (Allom et al., 2014).
- Mindful communication involves engaging in nonjudgmental listening and speaking with awareness during encounters with patients and their families, so fostering empathy and mitigating conflict (Beach et al., 2013).
- Routine activities - caregivers can cultivate attentive awareness during daily duties such as bathing the patient, delivering medication, or organizing the room, so transforming care-giving into a meditation practice.

These techniques bolster resilience by anchoring caregivers in the present while improving relational quality.

6.3 Loving-Kindness and Compassion Meditation

Compassion-focused techniques, like loving-kindness meditation (LKM), emphasize the development of affectionate and altruistic sentiments towards oneself, patients, and others (Hofmann et al., 2011). LKM fosters self-compassion and alleviates emotional weariness for caregivers who may encounter annoyance, resentment, or guilt. A thorough review indicated that compassion meditation correlates with heightened positive affect, enhanced empathy, and less depression symptoms (Galante et al., 2014).

Table 2. Sample Weekly Mindfulness Practice Schedule for Caregivers

Day	Formal Practice (10–20 min)	Informal Practice (throughout the day)	Compassion Practice (5–10 min)
Monday	Breathing meditation	Mindful eating	Loving-kindness meditation
Tuesday	Body scan	Mindful communication with patient	Compassion toward self
Wednesday	Mindful walking	Awareness during care-giving tasks	Sending compassion to patient
Thursday	Breathing meditation	Mindful awareness of fatigue signals	Loving-kindness for family
Friday	Body scan	Mindful listening in conversations	Compassion for healthcare workers

continued on following page

Table 2. Continued

Day	Formal Practice (10–20 min)	Informal Practice (throughout the day)	Compassion Practice (5–10 min)
Saturday	Mindful walking	Awareness while preparing meals	Loving-kindness for all beings
Sunday	Breathing meditation	Mindful reflection on the week	Compassion for self + patient

This adaptable plan can be modified based on caregiver availability, cultural preferences, and the intensity of care required. Significantly, even 5–10 minutes of daily mindfulness meditation can result in substantial decreases in stress and enhanced well-being (Creswell, 2017).

7. DEVELOPING A MINDFULNESS CARE PATHWAY

Mindfulness interventions for caretakers of terminally ill elderly patients must be systematic, practical, and culturally attuned. A care pathway offers a framework that incorporates mindfulness practices into caregiver routines while guaranteeing sustainability.

7.1 Step-by-Step Framework for Integrating Market-Based Instruments

1. Assessment Phase - Evaluate caregiver stress and burden utilizing validated instruments (e.g., Zarit Burden Interview, Perceived Stress Scale). Determine motivation, availability of time, and chosen mode of delivery (in-person, online, group, or self-directed).
2. Orientation and Psychoeducation Deliver introductory workshops elucidating the principles of mindfulness (awareness, acceptance, nonjudgment). Normalize caregiver stress and emphasize mindfulness as a means of fostering resilience rather than evasion.
3. Structured Mindfulness Training o Duration: 6–8 weeks, 1–2 sessions weekly (30–60 minutes each).Essential elements: breathing meditation, body scan, mindful walking, and compassion exercises. Customized modifications for low-energy caregivers (reduced session durations, auditory instructions, chair-based exercises).

   4.Incorporation into Routine Care-giving Promote informal methodologies during caring activities (e.g., attentive listening, conscientious medicine administration).

Utilize regular mindfulness journals for introspection and habit reinforcement.

5.Assistance and Reinforcement Weekly peer-support circles or online forums to discuss issues.

Support from healthcare professionals and regular follow-ups.

6.Assessment and Modification Reevaluate caregiver burden and stress at 8 to 12 weeks.

Adjust intensity and frequency according to caregiver requirements and preferences.

7.2 Individual versus Group Formats

- Individual Practice
  - -Adaptable, self-directed (applications, guided audio, or written directives).
  - -Appropriate for caretakers with erratic schedules or privacy apprehensions.
  - -Disadvantage: absence of peer support, potential compliance challenges.
- Group Practice
  - -Conducted by qualified specialists (psychologists, nurses, or meditation instructors).
  - -Offers social support, affirmation, and collaborative learning.
  - -Delivery can be conducted either in-person or electronically to address mobility and distance constraints.
  - -Disadvantage: necessitates scheduling, perhaps unsuitable for caretakers with significant time limitations.
  - -Research indicates that hybrid approaches, which combine brief individual practices with group reinforcement, produce optimal adherence and outcomes (Creswell, 2017).

7.3 Function of Healthcare Providers

Healthcare workers are essential in promoting the adoption of mindfulness among caregivers:

- Evaluation & Recommendation: Assessing caregivers for significant load and proposing mindfulness strategies.
- Facilitation: Directing brief exercises during hospital visits or tele-health consultations.

- Exemplifying Mindfulness: Providers who exhibit mindful communication bolster credibility and foster caregiver engagement.
- Integration with Palliative Care Teams: Affirms that mindfulness is regarded as an integral component of comprehensive care rather than an ancillary practice.

8. CASE VIGNETTES

Case vignettes provide realistic examples of how mindfulness-based therapies (MBIs) can be tailored to the actual experiences of caregivers. They emphasize several stressors—spousal caring, intergenerational obligations, and professional care-giving—and illustrate how mindfulness techniques can alleviate burden and enhance resilience.

Vignette 1: Spouse Attending to a Dementia Patient

Mrs. A, 68 years old, provides care for her husband who has been diagnosed with advanced Alzheimer's disease. She endures significant emotional distress owing to role confinement and anticipated grief. Her initial Zarit load Interview score signified a profound load.

- Mindfulness Strategy: She participated in an 8-week group Mindfulness-Based Stress Reduction program tailored for dementia caregivers. The practices encompassed breathing meditation, body scan, and loving-kindness meditation aimed at both her partner and herself.
- Outcome: Following the training, Mrs. A indicated enhanced emotional regulation, less irritation, and increased acceptance of her spouse's behavioral modifications. These results correspond with the findings of Whitebird et al. (2013), who reported a substantial reduction in burden among dementia caregivers following MBSR.

Vignette 2: Adult Offspring Managing Care-giving and Employment

Mr. B, a 42-year-old corporate professional, serves as the principal caregiver for his terminally ill mother while concurrently fulfilling work obligations and rearing two young children. He indicates experiencing role conflict and chronic weariness.

- Mindfulness Strategy: Owing to time limitations, he implemented app-based mindfulness practices, engaging in 10–15 minutes of daily guided meditation, complemented by mindful communication approaches during interactions with his mother.
- Outcome: He reported less stress, enhanced concentration at work, and increased attentiveness with his mother. Research indicates that digital Mindfulness-Based Interventions (MBIs) are useful for busy caregivers, namely in alleviating stress and improving well-being (Zhang et al., 2021).

Vignette 3: Nurse in Palliative Care Unit Experiencing Empathy Exhaustion

Ms. C, a 35-year-old palliative care nurse, is experiencing secondary traumatic stress and initial indications of burnout. She has emotional fatigue and perceives a disconnection from patients.

- Mindfulness Strategy: She engaged in a hospital-affiliated mindfulness training initiative for healthcare professionals, which included weekly group sessions featuring mindful walking, meditation, and reflective writing. Result: Ms. C indicated increased compassion fulfillment and less emotional weariness. These findings correspond with Irving et al. (2009), who demonstrated that MBSR diminishes the risk of burnout among healthcare professionals.

9. COMPARISON BETWEEN MBIS VS PSYCHOEDUCATION, CBT, PROBLEM-SOLVING THERAPY AND GROUP SUPPORT

Recent comparative research has evaluated the relative effectiveness of Mindfulness-Based Interventions (MBIs) against other evidence-based psychosocial approaches commonly offered to caregivers. Overall, findings suggest that MBIs perform comparably to structured psychotherapies for mood and stress outcomes, while offering unique benefits in emotional regulation and acceptance-based coping. For instance, MBIs and psychoeducation demonstrate similar reductions in caregiver stress; however, MBIs often produce superior improvements in mindfulness skills and emotional reactivity, which mediate long-term stress resilience (García-Campos et al., 2021). Comparative trials with Cognitive Behavioral Therapy (CBT) show that CBT may yield slightly stronger improvements in cognitive reframing and problem-solving, whereas MBIs provide greater gains in acceptance, nonreactivity, and self-compassion—mechanisms highly relevant for chronic caregiving stress (Burgdorf et al., 2019). Research comparing MBIs with Problem-Solving Therapy (PST) indicates that both interventions are effective, but MBIs may offer broader benefits for mood symptoms and overall well-being due to their emphasis on emotional regulation rather than task-oriented coping (Kalaf et al., 2020). Studies contrasting MBIs with group supportive interventions consistently report substantial improvements across both modalities; however, MBIs often show added benefits in reducing rumination and enhancing present-moment awareness, suggesting that mindfulness contributes unique mechanisms beyond general social support (Sun et al., 2022).

Collectively, these findings indicate that MBIs are a viable alternative or complement to psychoeducation, CBT, PST, and group therapy. MBIs may be especially beneficial for caregivers who experience chronic uncontrollable stressors—such as caring for individuals with terminal illnesses—where emotional acceptance, nonjudgmental awareness, and resilience-building capacities are crucial. These comparative results support integrating MBIs within multidisciplinary caregiver support programs to enhance psychological flexibility alongside traditional therapeutic approaches.

Table 3. Psychosocial Interventions for Caregivers of Terminally Ill Patients

Intervention	Relevance to Terminal Illness Caregiving	Key Benefits for Palliative-Care Caregivers	Limitations in Palliative Contexts
Mindfulness-Based Interventions (MBIs) (e.g., MBSR, MBCT)	Addresses chronic, uncontrollable stress typical of end-of-life caregiving; improves emotion regulation under sustained uncertainty.	• Reduces stress, depression, anxiety • Enhances acceptance and meaning-making • Supports anticipatory grief and resilience • Improves presence and compassion	• Requires consistent practice • Time demands may be challenging • Effects sometimes comparable to active controls
Psychoeducation (Disease- and Care-Specific)	Provides essential knowledge about cancer, organ failure, symptom progression, and caregiving demands.	• Increases preparedness • Improves decision-making confidence • Helpful during transitions such as home hospice	• Limited impact on emotional exhaustion • Does not address depression or grief • Benefits decline without reinforcement
Cognitive Behavioral Therapy (CBT)	Targets depression, anxiety, catastrophic thinking, and guilt common in terminal-illness caregiving.	• Reduces depressive symptoms and worry • Helps reframe hopelessness and guilt • Strengthens coping strategies	• Requires trained clinicians • Homework difficult for tired caregivers • Less focus on acceptance for irreversible decline
Problem-Solving Therapy (PST)	Useful for managing daily medical, logistical, and care-related challenges.	• Reduces burden through practical coping • Improves efficiency and control • Helps with daily medical decisions	• Does not address existential stress • Smaller mood effects vs CBT/ MBIs • Requires active participation
Supportive Group Therapy / Hospice Support Groups	Addresses loneliness, anticipatory grief, and emotional strain; aligns with hospice philosophy.	• Reduces isolation • Provides emotional validation • Encourages shared coping	• Benefits depend on group quality • Less structured; limited clinical symptom change • Lacks structured coping-skill training

10. CULTURAL AND SPIRITUAL ADAPTATIONS

Cultural and spiritual elements significantly impact care-giving methodologies and the receptiveness to mindfulness interventions. In India and several Asian nations, care-giving is frequently influenced by filial duties, familial hierarchy, and religious convictions. Mindfulness programs must honor these values while preserving their fundamental therapeutic concepts (Koenig, 2012; Sarfraz & Siddiqui, 2023).

10.1 Tailoring MBIs to Indian/Asian Cultural Contexts

1. Linguistics and Discourse

   -Employ vernacular languages (Hindi, Tamil, Bengali, etc.) in guided meditations to enhance understanding and participation (Sarfraz & Siddiqui, 2023).

   -Analogies and analogies must be culturally pertinent, such as references to local everyday practices, celebrations, or proverbs.

2. Collective Dynamics and Social Assistance

   -Family caregivers frequently favor group sessions that encompass several family members, fostering collective learning and shared accountability (Hudson et al., 2010).

   -Peer validation corresponds with the collectivist ethos characteristic to Indian culture.

10.2 Integration of Rituals and Religious Practices

-Mindfulness may be integrated with prayer, chanting, or puja practices, which are known to caregivers and enhance attentional focus and tranquility (Koenig, 2012).

-Brief contemplative activities can precede or succeed established rituals, smoothly incorporating mindfulness into regular spiritual habits.

10.3 Valuing Family Principles and Functions

-Programs must recognize gender roles, the participation of extended family, and intergenerational relationships.

-Flexibility in session scheduling is crucial to accommodate care-giving duties and religious practices.

`11. EXECUTION IN RESOURCE-LIMITED ENVIRONMENTS

Implementing mindfulness-based interventions (MBIs) in low-resource settings—prevalent in rural and semi-urban regions of India and other Asian nations—necessitates economical, accessible, and culturally relevant strategies. Resource limitations encompass a scarcity of qualified specialists, scheduling constraints on caretakers, and insufficient awareness of mental health interventions (Sarfraz & Siddiqui, 2023; Hudson et al., 2010).

11.1 Economical, Scalable Distribution Techniques

1. Digital Platforms
    - Smartphone applications or WhatsApp-based guided sessions offer audio and video mindfulness exercises.
    - Short courses lasting 5 to 15 minutes cater to caregivers with restricted time availability.

Evidence indicates that digital mindfulness-based interventions alleviate stress and enhance well-being, especially among caregivers with less prior experience to mindfulness (Zhang et al., 2021).

- Consistent phone calls or SMS reminders for mindfulness practice facilitate adherence reinforcement.

2. Telephonic Support

- Consistent phone calls or SMS reminders for mindfulness practice facilitate adherence reinforcement.
- Appropriate for regions with inadequate internet access or minimal smartphone usage.

3. Community and Group Sessions

- Local community centers, temples, or hospitals may conduct weekly group sessions facilitated by qualified professionals or volunteers.
- Group delivery utilizes peer support and collective motivation to enhance engagement (Hudson et al., 2010).

11.2 Educating Non-Experts

Task-shifting methods permit nurses, social workers, or trained volunteers to provide fundamental mindfulness instruction under supervision.

- Training encompasses:

  1. Comprehending fundamental mindfulness principles (attention, awareness, acceptance)
  2. Conducting brief guided meditations and promoting mindful communication
  3. Evaluating caregiver advancement and determining the necessity for specialist referral

- This methodology diminishes expenses and enhances scalability while preserving program integrity (Irving et al., 2009).

11.3 Comprehensive Execution Framework

1. Evaluation - Recognize caregiver stress and available resources (e.g., smartphone accessibility, reading levels).
2. Program Delivery — Integrate digital, telephonic, and community-oriented group methodologies.
3. Support and Reinforcement — Peer groups, telephonic follow-ups, and familial engagement.
4. Monitoring & Evaluation – Assess compliance, stress alleviation, and caregiver contentment utilizing standardized instruments (Zarit Burden Interview, Perceived Stress Scale).

This framework is adaptable for rural, semi-urban, and urban low-resource environments, guaranteeing accessibility and sustainability.

12. ETHICAL CONSIDERATIONS IN MINDFULNESS-BASED CARE-GIVING

Mindfulness therapies, albeit low-risk, necessitate meticulous ethical scrutiny to safeguard caregiver safety, autonomy, and well-being, and to avert their misuse as a replacement for professional medical treatment (Baer, 2015; Kabat-Zinn, 1990).

12.1 Guaranteeing Informed Consent and Psychological Security

- Caregivers must be provided with explicit information regarding the objectives, length, and substance of mindfulness therapies.
- Participants must recognize that involvement is voluntary and may be terminated at any moment without affecting clinical care.
- Psychological screening is advised to detect caregivers experiencing severe depression, PTSD, or acute anxiety, who may require professional help for mindfulness interventions (Crane et al., 2017).

12.2 Preventing the Misapplication of Mindfulness

- Mindfulness ought to augment, rather than supplant, medical, psychological, or social interventions.
- Ethical utilization entails acknowledging limitations: it is not a mechanism to "resolve" care-giving difficulties or alleviate systemic burdens.

Programs must avoid excessive focus on self-regulation that may unintentionally create guilt or pressure for caregivers (Van Dam et al., 2018).

12.3 Reconciling Caregiver Requirements with Patient Imperatives

- Mindfulness programs must take into account the well-being of both caregivers and patients.
- Scheduling sessions must not jeopardize patient care, and interventions should be adaptable to meet unforeseen caring requirements.
- Ethical frameworks prioritize non-maleficence, guaranteeing that mindfulness practices do not exacerbate stress or exhaustion for caregivers or patients (Shapiro et al., 2006).

13. MEASURING OUTCOMES

Precise measurement is crucial for evaluating the effects of mindfulness-based treatments (MBIs) on caregivers' psychological, emotional, and physical health. Multi-dimensional assessment facilitates the monitoring of stress reduction, burden alleviation, enhancements in quality of life, and alterations in compassion.

13.1 Tools: Zarit Burden Interview, Perceived Stress Scale, WHO-QOL

- **Zarit Burden Interview (ZBI):**
  - A 22-item questionnaire assessing felt strain in caretakers of elderly and terminally ill individuals.

    -Evaluates emotional, social, and financial burdens.

    -Extensively corroborated in Indian and Asian caregiver demographics (Zarit et al., 1980; Sarfraz & Siddiqui, 2023).

- Perceived Stress Scale (PSS):

A 10-item instrument evaluating the extent to which life situations are perceived as stressful.

Effective for assessing variations in stress levels prior to and following Mindfulness-Based Interventions (MBIs).

Exhibited dependability within caregiver demographics (Cohen et al., 1983).

- WHO Quality of Life-BREF (WHOQOL-BREF):-

  -A 26-item questionnaire assessing physical, psychological, social, and environmental domains.

  -Responsive to interventions that enhance overall life satisfaction and functional well-being (WHO, 1996).

13.2 Compassion Satisfaction and Secondary Traumatic Stress

- **Professional Quality of Life Scale (ProQOL):**
  - Assesses compassion satisfaction, burnout, and secondary traumatic stress.
  - Relevant for both professional and familial caregivers in palliative care (Stamm, 2010).

13.3 Monitoring Temporal Variations

- Pre- and post-intervention evaluations: Baseline, mid-point, and post-intervention metrics facilitate the assessment of progress.
- Subsequent evaluations: 3–6 months post-completion to examine the sustainability of benefits.
- Integrating quantitative metrics with qualitative feedback (such as interviews and diaries) yields comprehensive insights on caregiver experiences.

14. QUALITY IMPROVEMENT TOOLKIT

A Quality Improvement (QI) Toolkit guarantees the systematic delivery, effective monitoring, and adaptation of mindfulness-based interventions (MBIs) based on caregiver input. This toolbox is intended for caregivers, facilitators, and healthcare professionals in palliative and home care environments.

14.1. Checklists for Caregivers and Facilitators

Table 4. Caregiver Daily Practice Checklist

Day	Mindfulness Activity	Duration	Completed (/)	Notes/Reflections
Mon	Breathing meditation	10 min		
Tues	Body scan	10 min		
Wed	Mindful walking	15 min		
Thurs	Mindful eating	10 min		
Fri	Loving-kindness meditation	10 min		
Sat	Mindful communication	15 min		
Sun	Reflection & gratitude journaling	15 min		

- **Purpose:** Tracks daily mindfulness adherence and encourages reflection on practice outcomes (Creswell, 2017; Whitebird et al., 2013).

Table 5. Facilitator Session Checklist

Session	Component	Completed (/)	Notes
1	**Introduction & orientation**		
2	Breathing meditation		
3	Body scan		
4	Mindful walking		
5	Loving-kindness meditation		
6	Informal practices integration		
7	Group reflection & sharing		
8	Program review & follow-up plan		

- **Purpose:** Ensures all key components are delivered consistently and allows facilitators to **document engagement and challenges** (Irving et al., 2009).

14.2 Everyday Mindfulness Diary Template Instructions:

Instructions- Caregivers provide succinct comments on everyday mindfulness encounters.

Date Practice Category Duration Pre-Mood Post-Mood Obstacles Observations/ Insights.

- Assists in monitoring emotional regulation, stress alleviation, and compliance.
- Aids in qualitative assessment for facilitators and researchers (Sarfraz & Siddiqui, 2023).

14.3 Guidelines for Support Groups

- Frequency: Weekly or bimonthly meetings.
- Duration: 45 to 60 minutes.
- Elements:

    1. Registration and exchange of experience
    2. Concise directed mindfulness exercise.
    3. Examination of obstacles and methodologies for resolution.
    4. Evaluation of homework and preparation for the subsequent session.

- Facilitator Responsibilities: Uphold confidentiality, promote engagement, normalize difficulties, and observe stress indicators.
- Evaluation: Employ concise feedback forms to monitor satisfaction, perceived advantages, and recommendations for enhancement.

14.4 Incorporating Toolkit into Care Pathways

1. Preparation: Familiarize caregivers with the toolkit and elucidate the objectives of the checklists, diary, and group sessions.
2. Implementation: Promote daily practice, weekly evaluations, and monthly facilitator assessments.
3. Evaluation: Assess diary entries and checklist fulfillment; analyze trends in support groups.
4. Continuous Improvement: Modify frequency, content, or distribution method in response to caregiver feedback.

15. CONCLUSION

Caregivers of terminally ill older adults face profound and persistent stressors, including emotional exhaustion, anticipatory grief, physical strain, and the cumulative pressure of prolonged uncertainty. This chapter has examined these multidimensional burdens and demonstrated how Mindfulness-Based Interventions (MBIs) provide an evidence-supported pathway for reducing caregiver stress, mitigating burnout, and enhancing emotional resilience. Grounded in principles of present-moment awareness, acceptance, and compassionate attention, MBIs help caregivers develop healthier responses to overwhelming demands, thereby sustaining both their psychological well-being and caregiving capacity (Kabat-Zinn, 1990; Creswell, 2017).The overview of formal and informal mindfulness practices illustrates that structured techniques—such as body scans, breath meditation, and mindful movement—support physiological and emotional regulation. Informal practices such as mindful communication and mindful caregiving interactions further integrate these skills into daily routines, helping caregivers respond with clarity and compassion rather than reactive distress. Culturally and spiritually attuned adaptations, as discussed in the chapter, are essential for improving engagement and acceptability among caregivers across diverse sociocultural settings (Hudson et al., 2010; Sarfraz & Siddiqui, 2023). Additionally, strategies for low-resource contexts—including mobile-based mindfulness, telephonic guidance, and task-shifting to trained community workers—highlight how MBIs can be scaled ethically and effectively (Irving et al., 2009; Zhang et al., 2021).

Despite promising outcomes, important gaps remain. Long-term sustainability of MBI benefits is still insufficiently studied, especially beyond one year. Evidence on caregivers outside dementia—such as those caring for cancer patients or individuals with multiple organ failure—remains limited. Digital mindfulness interventions require more rigorous randomized trials to compare them with in-person delivery, particularly in low-resource environments. Furthermore, structural integration of MBIs into routine palliative care systems is underdeveloped, and culturally sensitive measures to evaluate spiritual and emotional congruence of interventions are still lacking

Policy Implications

1. Integrate MBIs as adjunctive components in national caregiver-support and palliative-care programs.
2. Train healthcare workers and community volunteers in foundational mindfulness facilitation to expand reach.
3. Prioritize funding for culturally tailored, scalable mindfulness research.

4. Support digital innovation—including apps, tele-health, and hybrid platforms—ensuring accessibility for underserved regions.
5. Use validated tools such as ZBI, PSS, WHOQOL, and ProQOL for continuous monitoring and evaluation of caregiver outcomes.

Future Directions

Hybrid Delivery Models: Combining digital and in-person formats to maximize accessibility while maintaining engagement.

- **Intergenerational Approaches:** Involving family networks to strengthen social support and reduce caregiver isolation.
- **Cross-Cultural Research:** Comparative studies across Asian, Middle Eastern, and Western populations to identify universal versus culture-specific mechanisms.
- **Integrated Therapies:** Exploring synergistic combinations of MBIs with cognitive-behavioral therapy, motivational interviewing, or pharmacological interventions to enhance impact.

Overall, the evidence presented in this chapter affirms that mindfulness-based interventions, when thoughtfully adapted and systematically implemented, hold significant potential to reduce stress, prevent burnout, and enhance overall well-being among caregivers of terminally ill older adults. As global ageing accelerates and caregiving demands intensify, MBIs offer an accessible, flexible, and compassionate approach to supporting those who shoulder the emotional and physical weight of end-of-life care.

REFERENCES

Adelman, R. D., Tmanova, L. L., Delgado, D., Dion, S., & Lachs, M. S. (2014). Caregiver burden: A clinical review. *Journal of the American Medical Association, 311*(10), 1052–1060. DOI: 10.1001/jama.2014.304

Allom, V., & Mullan, B. (2014). Individual differences in executive function predict distinct eating behaviours. *Appetite, 80*, 123–130. DOI: 10.1016/j.appet.2014.05.007

Analayo, B. (2003). *Satipatthāna: The direct path to realization.* Windhorse Publications. https://www.abhayagiri.org/media/discs/2015WinterRetreat/Sources/Analayo_Satipatthana-The-Direct-Path-to-Realization.pdf

Baer, R. A. (Ed.). (2015). *Mindfulness-Based Treatment Approaches: Clinician's Guide to Evidence Base and Applications* (2nd ed.). Academic Press.

Beach, M. C., Roter, D., Korthuis, P. T., Epstein, R. M., Sharp, V., Ratanawongsa, N., Cohn, J., Eggly, S., Sankar, A., Moore, R. D., & Saha, S. (2013). A multicenter study of physician mindfulness and health care quality. *Annals of Family Medicine, 11*(5), 421–428. DOI: 10.1370/afm.1507

Bishop, S. R., Lau, M., Shapiro, S., Carlson, L., Anderson, N. D., Carmody, J., Segal, Z. V., Abbey, S., Speca, M., Velting, D., & Devins, G. (2004). Mindfulness: A proposed operational definition. *Clinical Psychology : a Publication of the Division of Clinical Psychology of the American Psychological Association, 11*(3), 230–241. DOI: 10.1093/clipsy.bph077

Brown, K. W., Coogle, C. L., & Wegelin, J.. (2016). A pilot randomized controlled trial of mindfulness-based stress reduction for caregivers of family members with dementia. *Aging & Mental Health, 20*(11), 1157–1166. DOI: 10.1080/13607863.2015.1065790

Burgdorf, V., Szabo, Y. Z., & Abbott, M. J. (2019). A randomized comparison of mindfulness-based stress reduction and cognitive-behavioral therapy for family caregivers: Effects on stress and emotional regulation. *Journal of Contextual Behavioral Science, 13*, 27–35.

Cohen, S., Kamarck, T., & Mermelstein, R. (1983). A global measure of perceived stress. *Journal of Health and Social Behavior, 24*(4), 385–396. DOI: 10.2307/2136404

Collins, R. N., & Kishita, N. (2019). The effectiveness of mindfulness- and acceptance-based interventions for informal caregivers of people with dementia: A meta-analysis. *The Gerontologist, 59*(4), e363–e379. DOI: 10.1093/geront/gny024

Crane, R. S., Brewer, J., Feldman, C., Kabat-Zinn, J., Santorelli, S., Williams, J. M. G., & Kuyken, W. (2017). What defines mindfulness-based programs? The warp and the weft. *Psychological Medicine*, *47*(6), 990–999. DOI: 10.1017/S0033291716003317

Creswell, J. D. (2017). Mindfulness interventions. *Annual Review of Psychology*, *68*(1), 491–516. DOI: 10.1146/annurev-psych-042716-051139

Dharmawardene, M., Givens, J., Wachholtz, A., Makowski, S., & Tjia, J. (2015). A systematic review and meta-analysis of meditative interventions for informal caregivers and health professionals. *BMJ Supportive & Palliative Care*, *6*(2), 160–169. DOI: 10.1136/bmjspcare-2014-000819

Galante, J., Galante, I., Bekkers, M. J., & Gallacher, J. (2014). Effect of kindness-based meditation on health and well-being: A systematic review and meta-analysis. *Journal of Consulting and Clinical Psychology*, *82*(6), 1101–1114. DOI: 10.1037/a0037249

Gao, X., Sun, F., & Ko, E. (2020). Physiological stress responses in caregivers of patients with advanced cancer: Cortisol dysregulation and psychological burden. *Psycho-Oncology*, *29*(3), 486–494. DOI: 10.1002/pon.5273

García-Campos, N., Cebolla, A., & Soler, J. (2021). Mindfulness-based intervention versus psychoeducation for family caregivers: A controlled clinical trial. *Mindfulness*, *12*(4), 910–922.

Given, B., Sherwood, P. R., & Given, C. W. (2011). Support for caregivers of cancer patients: Transition after active treatment. *Cancer Epidemiology, Biomarkers & Prevention*, *20*(10), 2015–2021. DOI: 10.1158/1055-9965.EPI-11-0611

Goyal, M., Singh, S., Sibinga, E. M. S., Gould, N. F., Rowland-Seymour, A., Sharma, R., Berger, Z., Sleicher, D., Maron, D. D., Shihab, H. M., Ranasinghe, P. D., Linn, S., Saha, S., Bass, E. B., & Haythornthwaite, J. A. (2014). Meditation programs for psychological stress and well-being: A systematic review and meta-analysis. *JAMA Internal Medicine*, *174*(3), 357–368. DOI: 10.1001/jamainternmed.2013.13018

Guzzon, A.. (2023). Cost-effectiveness of supportive and palliative care interventions. *Systematic Reviews*.

Hofmann, S. G., Grossman, P., & Hinton, D. E. (2011). Loving-kindness and compassion meditation: Potential for psychological interventions. *Clinical Psychology Review*, *31*(7), 1126–1132. DOI: 10.1016/j.cpr.2011.07.003

Hudson, P. L., Remedios, C., & Thomas, K. (2010). A systematic review of psychosocial interventions for family carers of palliative care patients. *BMC Palliative Care*, *9*, 17. DOI: 10.1186/1472-684X-9-17

Irving, J. A., Dobkin, P. L., & Park, J. (2009). Cultivating mindfulness in health care professionals: A review of empirical studies of mindfulness-based stress reduction (MBSR). *Complementary Therapies in Clinical Practice, 15*(2), 61–66. DOI: 10.1016/j.ctcp.2009.01.002

Iype, T., Rani, P., & Kuriakose, R. (2014). The burden of caregiving for bedridden elderly patients in India. *International Journal of Community Medicine and Public Health, 1*(1), 12–17.

Jaffray, L., Bridgman, H., Stephens, M., & Skinner, T. (2016). Evaluating the effects of mindfulness-based interventions for informal palliative caregivers: A systematic literature review. *Palliative Medicine, 30*(2), 117–131. DOI: 10.1177/0269216315600331

Jones, B., Piet, J., Simonsen, J., & Zachariae, R. (2022). Mindfulness-based interventions and physiological stress markers in cancer caregivers: A randomized pilot trial. *Journal of Psychosocial Oncology, 40*(2), 237–255. DOI: 10.1080/07347332.2021.1872059

Jones, B., Piet, J., Simonsen, J., & Zachariae, R. (2022). Mindfulness-based interventions and physiological stress markers in cancer caregivers: A randomized pilot trial. *Journal of Psychosocial Oncology, 40*(2), 237–255. DOI: 10.1080/07347332.2021.1872059

Kabat-Zinn, J. (1990). *Full catastrophe living: Using the wisdom of your body and mind to face stress, pain, and illness.* Delta., DOI: 10.1037/e481272006-001

Kabat-Zinn, J. (1990). *Stress Reduction Clinic. Full catastrophe living : using the wisdom of your body and mind to face stress, pain, and illness. University of Massachusetts Medical Center/Worcester.* Delacorte Press.

Kabat-Zinn, J. (2003). Mindfulness-based interventions in context: Past, present, and future. *Clinical Psychology : a Publication of the Division of Clinical Psychology of the American Psychological Association, 10*(2), 144–156. DOI: 10.1093/clipsy.bpg016

Kalaf, E. P., de Souza, P., & Mari, J. J. (2020). Problem-solving therapy versus mindfulness intervention for caregivers of chronic patients: A randomized pilot study. *Clinical Psychology & Psychotherapy, 27*(2), 187–198.

Kent, E. E., Rowland, J. H., Northouse, L., Litzelman, K., Chou, W. Y. S., Shelburne, N., Timura, C., O'Mara, A., & Huss, K. (2016). Caring for caregivers and patients: Research and clinical priorities for informal cancer caregiving. *Cancer, 122*(13), 1987–1995. DOI: 10.1002/cncr.29939

Kim, Y., Carver, C. S., Shaffer, K. M., & Cannady, R. S. (2021). Cortisol patterns and psychological distress among spouses of patients with terminal cancer. *Health Psychology, 40*(8), 530–539. DOI: 10.1037/hea0001124

Koenig, H. G. (2012). Religion, spirituality, and health: The research and clinical implications. *ISRN Psychiatry, 2012*, 1–33. DOI: 10.5402/2012/278730

Lengacher, C. A., Reich, R., & Paterson, C.. (2019). Biobehavioral mechanisms of mindfulness-based interventions for cancer caregivers: A systematic review. *Supportive Care in Cancer, 27*(11), 4209–4222. DOI: 10.1007/s00520-019-04873-7

Lindauer, A., & Harvath, T. A. (2014). Pre-death grief in the context of dementia caregiving: A concept analysis. *Journal of Advanced Nursing, 70*(10), 2196–2207. DOI: 10.1111/jan.12411

Liu, X., Wang, S., Chang, K., & Chen, J. (2021). Mindfulness training modifies intrinsic brain networks associated with emotional regulation: A meta-analytic review of fMRI studies. *Neuroscience and Biobehavioral Reviews, 131*, 1211–1223. DOI: 10.1016/j.neubiorev.2021.11.019

Maresova, P. (2024). Cost-effectiveness of home-based palliative care. *Systematic Reviews.*

Maslach, C., & Leiter, M. P. (2016). Understanding the burnout experience: Recent research and its implications for psychiatry. *World Psychiatry; Official Journal of the World Psychiatric Association (WPA), 15*(2), 103–111. DOI: 10.1002/wps.20311

Mattingly, T. J., Silverman, E., & Lavenberg, J. (2022). Inclusion of informal caregiver costs in cost-of-illness studies: A systematic review. *Value in Health, 25*(3), 394–402.

Miroslav S. (2020). Mindfulness in Palliative Care - the Healing Effect of the Present Moment. Mindfulness/všímavost v paliativní péči - léčivý efekt přítomného okamžiku. *Klinicka onkologie: casopis Ceske a Slovenske onkologicke spolecnosti, 33*(Supplementum - 2), 138–140.

Molero Jurado, M. D. M., Pérez-Fuentes, M. C., Barragán Martín, A. B., Soriano Sánchez, J. G., Oropesa Ruiz, N. F., Sisto, M., & Gázquez Linares, J. J. (2020). Mindfulness in family caregivers of persons with dementia: Systematic review and meta-analysis. *Healthcare (Basel), 8*(3), 193. DOI: 10.3390/healthcare8030193

OECD. (2021). *OECD ageing population projections.* OECD Publishing.

Peters, L., Cant, R., Payne, S., O'Connor, M., McDermott, F., Hood, K., & Morphet, J. (2013). How death anxiety impacts nurses' caring for patients at the end of life: A review of literature. *The Open Nursing Journal*, *7*, 14–21. DOI: 10.2174/1874434601307010014

Pinquart, M., & Sörensen, S. (2003). Differences between caregivers and noncaregivers in psychological health and physical health: A meta-analysis. *Psychology and Aging*, *18*(2), 250–267. DOI: 10.1037/0882-7974.18.2.250

Reinhard, S. C., Given, B., Petlick, N. H., & Bemis, A. (2008). Supporting Family Caregivers in Providing Care. In Hughes, R. G. (Ed.), *Patient Safety and Quality: An Evidence-Based Handbook for Nurses*. Agency for Healthcare Research and Quality.

Salikhanov, I.. (2023). Economic evaluation of hospice and palliative care interventions. *Systematic Reviews*.

Sarfraz, A., & Siddiqui, S. (2023). Cultural adaptation of a mindfulness-based intervention for young adults: An application of heuristic framework. *Pakistan Journal of Social Research*, *5*(2), 40–53. DOI: 10.52567/pjsr.v5i02.1107

Schulz, R., & Sherwood, P. R. (2008). Physical and mental health effects of family caregiving. *The American Journal of Nursing*, *108*(9, Suppl), 23–27. DOI: 10.1097/01.NAJ.0000336406.45248.4c

Shapiro, S. L., Carlson, L. E., Astin, J. A., & Freedman, B. (2006). Mechanisms of mindfulness. *Journal of Clinical Psychology*, *62*(3), 373–386. DOI: 10.1002/jclp.20237

Shennan, C., Payne, S., & Fenlon, D. (2011). What is the evidence for the use of mindfulness-based interventions in cancer care? A review. *Psycho-Oncology*, *20*(7), 681–697. DOI: 10.1002/pon.1819

Sleeman, K. E., de Brito, M., Etkind, S., Nkhoma, K., Guo, P., Higginson, I. J., Gomes, B., & Harding, R. (2019). The escalating global burden of serious health-related suffering: Projections to 2060 by world regions, age groups, and health conditions. *The Lancet. Global Health*, *7*(7), e883–e892. DOI: 10.1016/S2214-109X(19)30172-X

Stamm, B. H. (2010). The concise ProQOL manual, *2nd edition*. Pocatello, ID: ProQOL.org.

Sun, H., Li, Q., & Zhang, W. (2022). Comparing mindfulness-based intervention with group supportive therapy for caregiver stress: A randomized controlled study. *Palliative & Supportive Care*, *20*(5), 620–629.

Taren, A. A., Creswell, J. D., & Gianaros, P. J. (2022). Neural mechanisms of mindfulness in stress reduction: Insights for caregivers of terminally ill patients. *Biological Psychiatry: Cognitive Neuroscience and Neuroimaging*, *7*(4), 396–405. DOI: 10.1016/j.bpsc.2021.04.006

Teut, M., Roesner, E. J., Ortiz, M., Reese, F., Binting, S., Roll, S., Fischer, H. F., Michalsen, A., Willich, S. N., & Brinkhaus, B. (2013). Mindful walking in psychologically distressed individuals: A randomized controlled trial. *Evidence-Based Complementary and Alternative Medicine : eCAM*, *489856*. Advance online publication. DOI: 10.1155/2013/489856

Van Dam, N. T., van Vugt, M. K., Vago, D. R., Schmalzl, L., Saron, C. D., Olendzki, A., Meissner, T., Lazar, S. W., Kerr, C. E., Gorchov, J., & Fox, K. C. R. (2018). Mind the hype: A critical evaluation and prescriptive agenda for research on mindfulness and meditation. *Perspectives on Psychological Science*, *13*(1), 36–61. DOI: 10.1177/1745691617709589

Whitebird, R. R., Kreitzer, M. J., Crain, A. L., Lewis, B. A., Hanson, L. R., & Enstad, C. J. (2013). Mindfulness-based stress reduction for family caregivers: A randomized controlled trial. *The Gerontologist*, *53*(4), 676–686. DOI: 10.1093/geront/gns126

World Health Organization. (1996). *WHOQOL-BREF: Introduction, administration, scoring, and generic version of the assessment*. WHO.

World Health Organization. (2020). *Decade of healthy ageing: Baseline report*. World Health Organization. https://www.who.int/publications/i/item/9789240017900

Zarit, S. H., Reever, K. E., & Bach-Peterson, J. (1980). Relatives of the impaired elderly: Correlates of feelings of burden. *The Gerontologist*, *20*(6), 649–655. DOI: 10.1093/geront/20.6.649

Zeidan, F., Johnson, S. K., Diamond, B. J., David, Z., & Goolkasian, P. (2010). Mindfulness meditation improves cognition: Evidence of brief mental training. *Consciousness and Cognition*, *19*(2), 597–605. DOI: 10.1016/j.concog.2010.03.014

Zernicke, K. A., Campbell, T. S., Speca, M., & Carlson, L. E. (2020). Autonomic and inflammatory correlates of caregiver stress and the potential role of mindfulness-based interventions. *Brain, Behavior, and Immunity*, *89*, 275–284. DOI: 10.1016/j.bbi.2020.06.005

Zhang, D., Lee, E. K. P., Mak, E. C. W., Ho, C. Y., & Wong, S. Y. S. (2021). Mindfulness-based interventions: An overall review. *British Medical Bulletin*, *138*(1), 41–57. DOI: 10.1093/bmb/ldab005

Chapter 10
Cultural and Religious Dimensions of Dying and the Respect for Diverse Beliefs and Rituals in End-of-Life Care:
Navigating Diversity in Dying Practices

Tosin Yinka Akintunde
https://orcid.org/0000-0002-9392-8726
Hohai University, China

Stanley Ologi Isangha
https://orcid.org/0000-0003-1177-0724
City University of Hong Kong, Hong Kong

Oluseye David Akintunde
https://orcid.org/0000-0001-9841-3206
Jilin University, China

Idriss Hussein Musa
Darfur University College, Sudan

Taha Hussein Musa
Libyan International Medical University, Libya

Wafaa R. Ahmed
https://orcid.org/0009-0005-5777-9988
Libyan International Medical University, Libya

ABSTRACT

End-of-life care in multicultural societies requires sensitivity to diverse cultural, religious, and trauma-informed perspectives. This work explores how beliefs rooted in Islam, Christianity, Buddhism, Confucianism, and African traditions shape dying experiences, family roles, and clinical decisions. It highlights tensions between

DOI: 10.4018/979-8-3373-4099-9.ch010

Western individualism and communal values, emphasizing the need for cultural safety, humility, and trust. Trauma histories further complicate care, especially among older adults with chronic illness. The analysis advocates for inclusive, personalized approaches that respect rituals, improve communication, and promote dignity in dying.

INTRODUCTION

The influence of culture and religious beliefs in end-of-life decision making and care remains complex and contentious among health professionals, particularly when it comes to dying and ensuring that quality health care is provided to older patients with chronic illnesses and their families in many multi-cultural and religiously diverse societies (Harwood et al., 2025). Recent developments indicate that dying is not solely private matter. With the increasing ageing Muslims population in Europe, North America and other multicultural societies, end-of-life decision making and care present significant challenges unless given substantial attention to cultural, religion and other contextual factors to ensure dying patients and their families receive satisfactory treatment (Bagheri, 2020; Kumari & Rajapaska, 2025). For instance, Islam teaches that death is inevitable but individuals are not permitted to end their own lives or request assisted death, even in the presence of pain, because life is a gift from God and any attempt to end it, is punishable by God. Muslims are expected to embrace pain as a test of their faith and spirituality. In contrast, some studies suggested that religion and cultural beliefs assist patients with serious and chronic health conditions, in coping with pain and suffering (Puchalski & Donnell, 2005) Consequently, reconciling diverse religious beliefs in end-of-life practices among dying patients and their families may be challenging for Western healthcare professionals whose objectives include ensuring quality care for patients at the end of life.

In Asia and Africa, there is a great need for end-of-life care as well. In many Asian countries such as Japan, Thailand, Singapore, Vietnam, Malaysia, Indonesia, the development of improved social amenities including improved healthcare systems has helped a lot of men and women live longer, controlled fertility rate and improved maternal and healthcare leading to increase in the number of aged adults or ageing populations that are vulnerable to several diseases(Sakamoto, 2025). The aged population and older adults in Asia are vulnerable to diseases as dementia, cardiovascular diseases, cancer, malignant neoplasms, chronic respiratory diseases, musculoskeletal diseases, and neurological and mental disorders that have continued to attract serious medical care (Feng, 2025; Goh, 2024; Prince, 2015). Asian societies are predominantly Buddhist and Confucius inclined and as end-of-life care progresses in many Asian countries as Hong Kong, Japan, South Korea, Singapore and Taiwan, end-of-life care discussion has been complicated and significantly influenced by cultural beliefs particularly the Confucius belief of filial piety where children are expected to care for their aged parents (Ho et al., 2022; Mori, 2025; Ohr, 2017). In Asian societies, the most preferred decision-maker and person with whom healthcare professionals are expected to discuss dying and end-of-life issues is a family member or children of the patients, contrary to the Western practice of individualism. Even when older Chinese patients decide on end-of-life care, it remains unclear under what conditions the patients would depend on health professionals rather than the family members. While studies suggested that Islam and Buddhism teach acceptance of death, the influence of psychological trauma on the end-of-life care choice of a dying patient experiencing pain and suffering is still unclear.

In Africa, there is also a significant need for end-of-life care considering the continent's aging population and efforts to reduce the spread of chronic diseases such as HIV&AIDS in South Africa (Sewpersad, 2024). End-of-life care is not new in Africa, though research on application and preferences has not yet to matured compared to Europe and Asia countries, despite the continent high share in the global burden of chronic diseases as HIV &AIDS (Donkor, 2024; Harding, 2003). Recent studies by the World Health Organization on global care treatment buttressed that Africa, to date, has remained one of the continents where implementation of end-of-life care has made less progress(Tripodoro et al., 2025)In African traditional societies where poverty and ignorance are rampant, discussing someone or another person's death, particularly that of a younger person, is considered a taboo or a death wish. The death of a person is usually perceived as a handiwork of a supernatural being, neighbor, or a vengeance for the sin committed. Even in African mega or big cities, the influence of religious belief in God and psychosocial supports from church members as Pentecostal Christians is huge and considered as antidote to HIV&AIDS among patients undergoing antiretroviral therapy(Azia, 2023; Chukwuneke, 2012; Ekore, 2016). However, limited studies have shown how religion and cultural beliefs influenced African older patients' perspectives on dying and preference for end-of-life decision and care.

Therefore, this study collates and compares diverse beliefs and ritual practices around death, as well as influence of these beliefs in Clinical Practice in End-of-Life care, in both developed countries of West and Europe and developing countries of Asia and Africa. It further examines the challenges and opportunities for end-of-life care.

DIVERSE BELIEFS AND RITUALS AROUND DEATH

Different cultural beliefs and ritual practices shaped how societies and individuals perceive dying and cope with the impending death of a family member or a loved one. In the medicine, the prevailing view is that death is either the cessation of breathing, the irreversible loss of brain function, or the death of the entire brain (Sarbey, 2016). There is a still general agreement that interpretations of "death" among healthcare professionals, patients, and family members influenced all patients, regardless of religious or cultural background. However, the concept of 'good death' is subjective and relatively different. While western patients' perspectives consider good death as often ranging from dying in one sleep, quietly, suddenly, and being pain-free, Western medical doctors consider the importance of adequate symptom control, family involvement, peacefulness, and lack of distress (Flaskerud, 2017). European or Westerns' beliefs around death are rooted in Christianity, which has shaped how Christian patients perceive death and how to cope with dying. Studies have shown that for European's, including the Nordic countries, although to a varying level, Christianity's belief in resurrection of the dead, religiosity, or someone's regular attendance in church, and abuse during childhood influenced belief or hope in life-after-death(Chen, 2025; Haraldsson, 2006). Dying patients' belief in life after death is significant in many ways, among which is that it helps to provide a psychological buffer against the fear of death and prepare their mind to accept death (Dezutter, 2008). In contrast, there are older dying patients who may not fear death and even prepare for their funeral ceremonies because they consider death a natural closure or a relief from life and something to long for, but still worry about dying because of their negative experiences in hospices or healthcare settings. These patients' beliefs about dying are influenced by the different thoughts and feelings they experience while they spend their last moments in has been described as a "boring and confined nursing home without a family and community," (Tjernberg, 2020).

Islam and Islamic faiths shaped individual's perspectives about death and dying. Islam teaches the belief that everyone will die, but any attempt to end one's life or that of another is a punishable offense by God. Islam, as a result, does not believe in brain death. According to Islam, death is the departure of the soul from the body, a belief that resonates with the conception of death as cessation of all functions of the body (Sarhill, 2001). Muslims generally believe that dying or death process, regardless of the illnesses, should be in agreement with Islamic faith and communities, such as receiving healthcare treatment at home with family members and reciting the Quran (Sheik, 1998; Suleman, 2023). Muslims believe that a dying patient should have the opportunity to recite verses from the Quran, hold prayer beads and access water from Makkah to guide the patient and family members on what to do and how to grieve or cope with the loss or bereavement of a dying patient. The dead or deceased is also expected to be washed and prepared for burial within 24hours. This belief has also shaped the narratives that surround the concept of a good death for Muslims. A dying Muslim patient would be said to have experienced a good death when the patient has experience of a good closure, dying with dignity, coming to peace, not dying alone, and having a religious engagement (Othman, 2025; Seise, 2021).

Similarly, many of African's beliefs do not cohere with the implementation of end-of-life care. Africans believe that death is not final but only a transition to another life for the dead. The Africans believe that life does not end when the body of a person ceases to function but rather that God gives the human body immortality, resurrection and the ability to become young after death According to this African belief about dying, a person is expected to live on earth for a specified period and after his or her death the person exist elsewhere in a supreme or supernatural form. The belief that the dead continue to live makes many Africans to engage in extravagant burial rituals to honor the person(Jock Agai, 2015). However, many Africans believe that it is a taboo to discuss their own death or that of their loved ones because death is an enemy of life. Therefore, it is difficult for Africans to write their own will or plan their funerals before their death or when they are still alive. Africans do not believe in discontinuity of life or taking a person's life even when the person is experiencing severe pain, as euthanasia an element of end-of-life care, because death is seen as an enemy and individuals must strive to preserve life rather than terminating it (Ekore, 2016b).

Africans' concept of good death is also different from the Europeans' perspectives and provides a coping strategy for dying patients and family members. In Africa's traditional societies, Africans believe the death of older adults is a 'good death' because it is a blessing followed by elaborate burial rites to enable the dead to join his or her ancestors to bring blessings to the family members and children who surround the dying patient on his bed. However, the death of a person without a child, who experienced a violent conflict or HIV infection, or infected person called 'walking dead' in South Africa, is considered a bad death. The death of older patients is believed to offer a possibility of passage into the world of the ancestors, but the latter does not attract much ceremonies and would be offered a possibility of reincarnation(Adinkrah, 2024). According to Traditional healers' experience of African Xhosa patients and their family members in South Africa, a good death is when dying patients are able to die without experiencing any form of suffering and surrounded by family members. The family gathering at the deathbed of dying patients provides enormous comfort for the dying patients to restore relationships, receive and give final wishes of family members, and give a verbal will (final spoken words). Africans' death rituals, therefore, provide a coping strategy for dying experience of older parents. In South Africa, ritual practices include washing or cleansing the home, sequestration of the family, and releasing the spirit and calling the spirit of the dead back home(Nichola et al., 2013).

In Asia, Buddhism and Confucius' teachings have shaped the concept of death, dying, and ritual practices. Buddhism teaches that death, suffering, and illness are parts of life, and individuals should accept and prepare for their death. According to Buddhism, death preparedness involves three stages, including engaging suffering, being open-minded about death and adhering to Buddhist practices, which help to maintain calmness, and peace when dying. Therefore, when individuals accept illnesses, suffering, and death as parts of life, they become open-minded and prepare for their death by engaging in religious practices such as practicing dharma, which enables them to sleep well and be happy before dying (Long, 2018; Upasen et al., 2022). Furthermore, the Buddhist belief in peaceful death has been dominant among Asian countries such as Thailand and Vietnam has often been used to describe a good death. A peaceful death is a peaceful state of mind in knowing that one's impending death is not a situation of suffering or being alone, but rather a time of being with family members who are not yet mourning one's death. The family members, friends and relatives are believed to help dying individuals achieve peaceful death by speaking words that help them avoid the fear of impending death, think of their merit and not to worry (Matchim et al., 2012). Confucius' teachings have also widely helped to shape Asian's perspectives about death, dying, and ritual practices. According to Confucius, man is not supposed to live in despair or speculate too much about his life and death but he's rather to embrace both as a matter of his fate and destiny. Man, therefore has certain responsibilities to prepare for both by cultivating virtue or living a good life, practicing filial piety (xiao) and fulfilling his role in society(Goh, 2024). The Confucius concept of filial piety is vital to the understanding how a dying patient accept and welcomes death and the family's duties in death rituals, as well as in Asia. Filial piety originally translated as Xiao, is depicted by a Chinese character that shows old at the top and son at the bottom, illustrating the hierarchical structure and the relationship of respect, care and support children provide to their parents (Li, 2021). Therefore, when it comes to death, the belief is that any Asian aged or adult who subscribed to and religiously followed Confucius' teachings should be able to accept and cope with death or dying experience without fear, worry or boredom.

Therefore, the tensions represented by these different perspectives regarding the meaning of death and dying ritual practices and after-life experiences not only contradict Western beliefs of individualism about healthcare but also affect preferences and discussions of end-of-life care among dying older patients in culturally and religiously diverse societies.

Table 1. Comparative Table: Belief Systems' Impact on End-of-Life Care (EOLC) Decisions

Belief System / Culture	Core Beliefs About Death	Concept of "Good Death"	Ritual Practices and Customs	Impact on EOLC Decisions	Coping and Bereavement Practices
Western / European (Christianity-based)	Death is the end of physical life but the beginning of eternal life; shaped by Christian belief in resurrection and salvation.	Peaceful, pain-free death; dying in sleep; family presence; emotional closure.	Prayer, last rites, funeral services, remembrance ceremonies.	Emphasis on medical symptom control, hospice care, and psychological comfort; acceptance of brain death; EOLC discussions are encouraged.	Faith in afterlife reduces death anxiety; family and clergy provide emotional support and comfort.
Islamic (Muslim)	Death occurs when the soul leaves the body; brain death is not accepted. Life and death belong to Allah.	Dying with dignity, at peace, surrounded by family, reciting Quran; death aligned with faith and religious rituals.	Reciting Quran, use of prayer beads, washing the body, burial within 24 hours.	Refusal of euthanasia or withdrawal of life support; preference for dying at home; emphasis on spiritual care and family presence.	Faith in divine will and afterlife strengthens acceptance; mourning guided by Islamic norms; community support vital.
African Traditional Beliefs	Death is not an end but a transition to ancestral world; soul continues to live in another realm.	Good death: old age, surrounded by family, elaborate burial; Bad death: violent, untimely, or childless death.	Cleansing rituals, family gathering, calling the spirit home, elaborate funerals.	Resistance to discussing or planning death (taboo); rejection of euthanasia; emphasis on life preservation and dignity.	Rituals reinforce social bonds and continuity; family unity helps the dying and bereaved cope spiritually and emotionally.
Buddhism (Asian countries like Thailand, Vietnam)	Death is a natural part of the life cycle; rebirth continues based on karma; acceptance of suffering as path to enlightenment.	Peaceful death with calm mind and spiritual readiness; dying without fear or attachment.	Meditation, reciting dharma, calm environment, family presence encouraging mindfulness.	Acceptance of palliative care; focus on inner peace over medical intervention; support spiritual preparation.	Calm acceptance, detachment from material concerns, family's compassionate support in achieving peaceful death.
Confucianism (China, East Asia)	Death is part of destiny; should not be feared; living a virtuous life ensures moral readiness for death.	Good death involves fulfilling filial duties, moral life, and family harmony.	Filial piety: family caring for elders, ritual mourning, maintaining ancestral ties.	Family plays major decision-making role; emphasis on respect and responsibility; less focus on individual autonomy.	Family-centered mourning; continuing bonds with ancestors; ritual respect and care after death bring emotional peace.

THEORETICAL FRAMEWORKS

Several models have emerged over the years with a focus to train and help healthcare professionals become culturally competent that can provide quality healthcare to patients that are culturally diverse. In 1988, the Giger and Davidhizar Transcultural Assessment model was developed in response to the need of nursing students attending undergraduate program to assess and provide care for patients that were culturally diverse. The educational model was simple and practical and focused on the influence of six cultural phenomena: communication, time, space, social organization, environmental control and biological variations on healthcare of patients of diverse cultural background (Giger & Davidhizar, 2002). However, Giger and Davidhizar Transcultural Assessment model lacks the systemic scope, continuous paradigms and ability to capture and address institutional factors and power dynamics that hinder healthcare delivery to patients of diverse cultures. Leninger's Transcultural Nursing Theory also emerged to promote the inclusion of culture into the nursing education and encouraged trained nurses to consider culture within the broader social contexts of their patients to provide effective healthcare (Leininger, 2002). The theory supported consideration of values of patients but can be limited in several ways such as inadequate focus on institutional inequalities which play vital role in healthcare in societies of diverse culture.

The study adopts Purnell Model of Cultural competence developed in 1995. The unique contributions of the model to the study of end-of-life decision making and care are laden in the assumptions that Cultural competence is a non-linear progression. According to Purnell, a culturally competent care provider is aware of his and her existence, sensations, thought and environment and does not allow those factors have effects on those he or she's is caring. Therefore, cultural competence is a conscious and non-linear process (Purnell, 2000). Purnell Model's focused on how the views of healthcare recipients, family and community are linked in a symbiotic relationship in which healthcare recipients (patients) who are trying to maintain their values and beliefs in constantly changing and advancing technologically diverse societies and the healthcare professionals to mutual share information that lead to quality healthcare (Purnell, 2000). The Model's 12 cultural domains and major concepts addressed family roles and organization, workforce, ethnic and racial origins and variations, spirituality and death rituals which make the theory relevant to the study of end-of-life decisions and care. The 12 domains contain series of questions to help healthcare provider to assess a group or person

RESPECTING BELIEFS IN CLINICAL PRACTICE IN END-OF-LIFE CARE

Clinical practice involves evidenced based activities that take place in clinics or outside between patients and health professionals including nurses and doctors as specified in the clinical practice guidelines in order to ensure an optimize patient care(Guerra-Farfan et al., 2023). Studies have identified that when it comes to standard clinical practice disease diagnosis, patient prognosis and diseases treatment are important aspects of evidence-based decision making for better health outcomes(Croft et al., 2015). Diagnosis provides healthcare nurses and doctors with the means to acquire, organize and interpret a range of information about clients particularly the diseases, symptoms, signs of diseases older patients at the end-of-life care. This helps to provide the foundation for clinicians to engage in a better and informed healthcare decision making, evidenced based recommendation and optimized health outcomes for patients.

Caring for older patients experiencing pain and suffering due to the chronic nature of their diseases can be overwhelming for healthcare professionals given the influence of different beliefs and values of patients and their families on health choices and health outcomes. A competent healthcare professional would follow ethical standards particularly the clinical practice guidelines that helped ensure optimized healthcare treatments that reduce the pain and suffering of patients in the intensive care units. The clinical practices of diagnosing, counseling, treating and showing care to patients can be enhanced through collaborative efforts of health professionals, patients and families (Qaseem, 2008). Clinical practice guidelines are global tools for improving quality of clinical practice around specific disease or clinical symptoms(Mertz & Strech, 2014). There are regular updates of clinical practice guidelines on online healthcare platforms to enhance trust and confidence of patients and their family in healthcare hospices and professionals to assist healthcare professionals on best and standard practices. Although, clinical practice guidelines have continued to improve over the years with advancements in modern technology tools, these clinical practice guidelines focused on specific diseases and their ethical issues(Vandvik et al., 2013). However, clinical practice guidelines that specifically focus on standard practice in end-of-life care and relationship between clients and healthcare professionals are still in their infant stage. South Korea is one of the countries healthcare professionals and researchers have taken a bold step to produce a clinical practice guideline of end-of-life care through the adaptation of 14 clinical practice guidelines both locally and internationally for clinicians, patients in dying process in hospices and ward and their families(Shin et al., 2020)

Consequently, end-of-life care in practice has often emerged as a contentious issue between healthcare professionals and the older dying patients agonizing in pain and suffering and their families. According to the Purnell Model for Cultural Competence, an effective end-of-life care in a multicultural society assumed that patients and healthcare workers mutual obligation to share information to obtain better outcomes(Purnell, 2000) (Purnell, 2000b). End-of-life conversations between doctors or nurses and patients and families are part of the daily medical protocol of end-of-life care. However, several studies have suggested that the sharing of information between patients, their families and health professionals has been limited, later than patients have requested and, in some cases, leading to delayed discussion of death, inadequate response to patients concerns over dying and disease progression and patient's discontinuation of disease-directed treatments(Knutzen et al., 2021). In some cases, patients and their family's preference for home both as a place of End-of-life care and place of death rather than hospitals in many European and North American countries has increased. Similar trends are also experienced in Asian and African countries where patients and their families would rather die at home than in the hospitals (Donkor, 2024; Pinto et al., 2024). In a nutshell, the indication is that patients and families are not clear about end-of-life conversation and the roles of clients, family and medical doctors which become complicated by the unconducive physical and organization environments of healthcare((Bergenholtz et al., 2019)).

Another tension between older patients at the end-of-life care, their families of patients and health professionals is the workforce and the increasing need for healthcare workforce to prioritize culture and religion of older patients. According to Purnell Model of Cultural Competence, healthcare organizations particularly workforce contributes to the competence of healthcare organizations and professionals to provide optimized care to patients of diverse cultural background. Purnell's diagram identified issues as acculturation, autonomy and language barriers affect the relationship between healthcare professional, patients and their families. The current study discovered that in many of the studies language barriers, difficulties in ascertaining patients' preference, late referrals and lack of workforce diversity led to mistrust and worse end-of-life outcomes among racial or ethnic minority older adults (Burke et al., 2023). In an urban tertiary hospital in the United States, a Mandaring Speaking 82 years old woman with advanced metastatic lung cancer had limited English proficiency but lives an adult daughter who could speak some English. The older patient admitted worsening dyspnea and pain. The hospital had no professional medical interpreter available for immediate meeting and the daughter volunteers to translate and was adopted to convey diagnostic and treatment information. During the meeting the doctors used clinical terms which were simplified, omitted, re-affirmed to align with what the daughter thought would protect her mother emotionally. She was distressed and worried about speaking directly to her mother about dying which limited them from asking clarifying questions. The aged women did not receive a clear, direct explanation of prognosis in her own language, understand dosing adjustments and report ongoing pain and anxiety. The family eventually could not make a fully informed decision. (Silva, 2016).

An older male migrant of African background, an Arabic speaker was admitted with a life-limiting illness in a Spanish public hospital. Discharge documents, instructional materials and telephone follow-up calls were all in Spanish and professional interpreters were not always available in the hospital. The Arab family members adopted an untrained neighbor as an ad-hoc interpreters in some cases. Consequently, a lot of medical changes and advance care information were misunderstood. The patient experienced unmanaged symptoms at home and the family reported confusion about prognosis and what to expect after discharge (Del Pino et al., 2020)

Researchers have addressed these cultural challenges by adopting two important basic concepts of cultural competency and cultural safety. Cultural competency seeks to incorporate teachings and knowledge, such as cross-cultural training of palliative healthcare among professionals, such as nurses (Orest Weber; Imane Semlali; Claudia Gamondi; Pascal Singy, 2021). However, cultural safety, which has replaced cultural competence, de-emphasized the sole importance of cultural competency among health professionals as the major pathway to achieve health equity in Western countries due to biases and stereotypical tendencies against patients of foreign backgrounds. Cultural safety, identified the 'focus for the delivery of healthcare through changes in thinking about power relationships and patients' rights. In a nutshell, cultural safety seeks to safeguard the culture of patients by removing multiple layers of oppressions in healthcare in order to improve access to healthcare among cultural minority groups and reducing disparity in healthcare outcomes in cultural and religious diverse societies as Australia and United Kingdom(Curtis, 2019; Rousseau, 2022)

Several strategies have emerged to ensure cultural safety when patients explore end-of-life care in healthcare settings, which are being investigated in the academic literature. Researchers and healthcare professionals agreed there is a strong connection between cultural humility and cultural safety when it comes to ensuring palliative and end-of-life care for patients in critical health conditions. Cultural humility has been described as "a mindset or practice whereby health providers self-evaluate their assumptions, biases, and values" which allows them to foster an understanding of the preferences of various patients(Singh et al., 2023). One of the strategies health professionals have been adopting is cultural humility which help them to engage in self-reflection enabling them to understand and appreciate their patients at all times. When doctors and nurses are genuinely interested, aware, and appreciate different perspectives of their patients to healthcare as well as the complex dynamic of social status and power that shape healthcare, they are able to create a safe atmosphere and engage in culturally safe healthcare treatments for patients(Zhang & Kong Metropolitan, 2024). There are other strategies, which include focusing on the organization and governance of health care settings, the hospital environment, service delivery, interpreters, clinical education, racism, culture and communication(Fowler & O'Loughlin, 2025). Three most critical strategies to ensure cultural safety are incorporated into ensuring health staffing of minority groups or workforce as interpreters or translators, and working together to spread the experience of cultural safety and strong governance in healthcare institutions.

TRAUMA-INFORMED SENSITIVITY: PAST-TRAUMA AND PATIENTS RESPONSES TO DYING AND MEDICAL INTERVENTION AND ENVIRONMENT

Trauma as a public health concern is not easy to define when investigating the meaning given by the Diagnostic and Statistical Manual of Mental Disorders 5th Edition, which define the concept as an "actual or threatened death, serious injury, or sexual violence" and the broad meaning of an "harmful event that causes lasting suffering" found in articles. It is however, reasonable for the sake of this study to argue that Trauma can be an event that translates into an actual experience and has adverse effects on the health of individuals(Gradus & Galea, 2023; Kimberg, 2019). The central questions to deal with in this section is how do past trauma shapes the way older patients respond to dying and what medical interventions are necessary to respond to their needs at the end-of-life care?

Studies suggested that 90% of older adults today might have experienced at least one traumatic event which includes military combat or violent conflict, unexpected death of someone close, serious illness or injury to self or someone close to them, spouse separation as adults and are also vulnerable to post-traumatic stress disorder. An example which can be related to civilians is the experience of the surviving male and female Vietnamese veterans who fought in the Vietnam War during the Cold War and were reported to have been involved in killing, inflicting severe injury or to have witnessed war atrocities, death of a child and spousal separation. The psychological trauma of these experiences has long-lasting impact that continues to affect these veterans and their healthcare(Korinek et al., 2017; Kuwert et al., 2013). Generally, older adults and individuals who have experienced trauma are at a higher risk of several chronic illnesses such as hypertension, coronary artery disease, diabetes as they grow older but the treatment of these illnesses can as well be impacted and adversely affected by the memory of their past trauma and trauma-related symptoms such as intrusion, avoidance, negative alterations in cognition and mood and hyperarousal which increase the level of their pain and decrease the level of their welfare at the end-of-life care (Ricks-Aherne, 2020). Nevertheless, post-traumatic stress disorder plays a vital role in the development or infection of these diseases among older adults even though a study conducted among older Vietnam veterans has suggested that older men are at a higher risk of hypertension which is a known risk factor for cardiovascular disease which is a major cause of death (Serier et al., 2025)

Studies have shown that trauma and post-traumatic stress disorder, which becomes prevalent at the end-of-life, greatly influence how dying patients respond to dying, and health professionals are required to be aware of existing trauma in order to understand their needs. Dying patients at the end of life generally depend on others, particularly family members for supports. However, trauma and post-traumatic stress disorder can disrupt family support networks by creating what has been called secondary traumatization, a condition in which spouse or family members of traumatized patients experience past symptoms and other forms of distress form being in a relationship with a traumatized individual. The dying patients without a family member also faced the risk of spending the remaining days of their life at healthcare institution settings without adequate care, and support leading to increased pain and depression at the end-of-life(Feldman, 2011). At the same time, dying patients as reported in the case of 'M'a 65-year-old ex-military male diagnosed with cancer, living in 'deep, persistent' poverty and with a prior experience of homelessness in Scotland suggested, may become withdrawn, indulge in drugs or alcohol and ambivalent toward staying in hospital or healthcare institutions and care and plan a way of escape which can increase their pain or suffering and worsen their health conditions until their death. This confirmed that dying patients dealing with chronic diseases, intense poverty and social deprivations and undisclosed history of undiagnosed trauma are vulnerable to posttraumatic stress disorder and PTSD syndromes such as his paranoia, unpredictability, decision to elope from the hospices and at home and avoiding or reluctance to accept personal care from nurses which posed a significant threat to his palliative care, health condition and lead to his painful death(Quinn et al., 2024).

Dying patients with undiagnosed trauma and posttraumatic stress disorder often face the constant challenge of interpretation or making sense of life because of their peculiar and painful health condition as they approach their death. Some patients without adequate coping strategies may avoid recollection of their lived experiences because they remind them of their trauma memories, while those who attempt to recollect their lived experiences may experience what has been termed "re-traumatization" a resurgence of their past suffering and loss. This process can also be complicated by nightmares, feelings of horror, troubling breathing and severe pain which these patients may be experiencing while undergoing medical interventions in the intensive care unit=gious beliefs have helped to shape how muslim patients with critical health conditions, such as infection of breast cancer and posttraumatic stress disorder, respond to disease treatment, PTSD symptoms, and dying or death.

Devoted Muslim patients are said to depend on religious and spiritual sources to cope with posttraumatic stress disorder and find meaning in their live, which helped them to gain inner strength and become healthy. They acknowledge their dependence on God through recitation of the holy Quran and application of psycho-spiritual therapy, which was a source of help to cope with pains and feelings of hopelessness and find meaning in their life(Abu Khait & Lazenby, 2021)

TRAUMA-SENSITIVE CARE AND OLDER PATIENTS AT THE END-OF-LIFE CARE

Health professionals such as nurses, doctors, and organizations may encounter patients with undisclosed histories of trauma or recent traumatic experiences, and it is required that they develop a Trauma-sensitive care approach or be sensitive to the special needs of these patients. Dying patients with a history of trauma require admission and medical interventions in the intensive care units, which need to be communicated to the health, professionals such as doctors, nurses, and the family. It is clear that patients' experiences require communication with nurses or medical doctors because some patients may feel the need to talk to avoid being lonely and hopeless while others may not. According to studies, communication may be limited for those that accept to have conversations with healthcare professionals for certain reasons. Nurses, when they are equipped with the right tools, knowledge and skills to deal with end-of-life issues and understand the importance of having conversations that surrounds the disease and end-of-life care of dying patients, may be limited by limited time, work overloads and the emotional stress of creating a sense of big family for the patients and having such conversation may have on them. Only few assistant nurses accepted they could manage and they adopted strategies that could only comfort, distract and disregard patients concerns about dying and death(Alftberg et al., 2018; Meyerson et al., 2023)

Nevertheless, communication helps to guarantee a satisfactory end-of-life care and it is important for ageing patients, relatives or family members and health professionals to avoid miscommunication. The previous section has explained that culture and religion influenced diverse beliefs regarding death, dying and end-of-life care in diverse religious and culturally diverse societies. However, it is important to observe the absence of effective communication between health workers and patients and their relatives or family members can lead to different issues such as divers expectations, intentions and outcomes which all health stakeholders want to avoid(Sullivan et al., 2023). Health professionals therefore need to communicate truthfully the prognosis of the ageing patients, disease progression, dying process as well as the pain management without including any medical jargons when trying to understand the preferences and wishes of patients as well as their family members in order to prepare them for what to expect in the future(Anderson et al., 2019).

CHALLENGES AND OPPORTUNITIES IN END-OF-LIFE CARE

End-of-life care offers great opportunities for older patients battling with life-threatening diseases and posttraumatic stress disorder which must reflect the religious and cultural diversities in today's world. A constant and active communication process between health professionals (doctor, nurses, therapist), aged or ageing patients and their family or caregivers remains an integral part of a successful palliative and end-of-life care in today's world of multiculturalism. A triad communication network that ensures that both patients and their family or/and caregivers of health professionals are able to understand, accept and prepare for the future both after diagnosis of the life-shortening chronic illnesses and at the time of death is necessary. However, this opportunity has often been marred by miscommunication caused by a complex combination of cultural misunderstanding and institutional or systemic barriers in healthcare hospitals and hospices. Most patients and family felt that health professionals would have been more open and host about the status of their health and illnesses and how they might have evolved or lead to death so they know what to expect and prepare for the future (Kallis, 2025). It is therefore imperative for healthcare professionals to ensure they deal with linguistic and communicative barriers that cause miscommunication between them and older patients and their family members through the use of medical interpreters and translators that can ease communication distress.

Communication can be greatly influenced by the unique culture and religion of both the dying patients and their family members and healthcare professionals need to carefully pay attention to how they shape their beliefs about dying and preferences for end-of-life care. The previous section has examined how cultural and religious influences interplay in individual's perception of death as a natural process or transition or fatalism. Nevertheless, health professional must understand and appreciate the importance of maintaining cultural humility in order to ensure that the right communication takes place between them and patients with Asia and African backgrounds(Mori, 2023).

Cultural competence is not enough to support healthcare professionals in end-of-life care activities because of it stereotypical and bias capacities. Health professional must demonstrate considerable efforts at cultural openness and empathy through active listening and flexibility in their healthcare practices. Culture is dynamic and unique changes may take place in ways family members and dying patients perceive death and end-of-life care treatments. Emerging studies have suggested that there are growing changes in the filial attitudes and actual filial behaviours of young adult Chinese in the Guangdong-Hong Kong-Macao Greater Bay Area (GBA) toward dying parents due to growing literacy about death and changing enactment of filial roles. This underscores a different attitude toward reluctance to disclose bad news regarding aged dying parents among Chinese and some Chinese would prefer actual information about their dying parents(Ng et al., 2024). It is also important to mention here the impacts of family burden and the patient's comfort and state of consciousness on the role and preference of younger family carers or caregivers and dying patients for life sustaining treatments in Chinese communities (Zhu et al., 2023). Therefore, healthcare professionals are expected to listen and be flexible when interacting with older patients and family members, and family care-givers of diverse generations and backgrounds to understand their unique roles, needs and preferences for end-of-life care.

Trust in healthcare settings and profession particularly in multicultural and religious diverse societies is a critical factor because many older patients at their dying stage are very vulnerable and have special needs and would require the best healthcare treatment that does not jeopardize their cultural safety. The existing academic literature and current emphasis on advancing health-related trust research steps toward the right direction and empirical evidence that trust still remains the foundation of "relationships marked by vulnerability and need as they are in healthcare"(Taylor et al., 2023). Many older dying patients facing posttraumatic stress disorder are vulnerable and their belief that they should be surrounded by family members has been shaped by trust issues including the trust in family built over the years through strong connection, care and supports can better safeguard their needs and wishes at their end-of-life. In societies with a history of oppression and injustice in terms of position and resource distribution against a particular group of people or generation by the government and government institutions such as healthcare organization, trust can be a big concern for patients coming from such backgrounds. In the United States of America black communities, the lower levels of trust Black and African Americans have in the healthcare institutions has played an important role in disparities in the end-of-life care and the low preference and attitude of Black and African Americans for hospices facilities and treatments(Ewy, 2025). This is contrary to the experience of U.S Chinese immigrants in the United States of America. Many U.S Chinese older patients who placed less emphasis on discussion with their family members and favored and engaged in a one-on-one counselling with healthcare doctors regarding their end-of-life care did so because they have a strong trust in the United States healthcare facilities and doctors(Kim et al., 2025). Therefore, it may be difficult for healthcare institutions and professionals to deal with trust issues among dying patients unless the narratives of injustices against these societies and groups are heard and addressed by the necessary government bodies and individuals. In a nutshell, it is highly imperative for government, healthcare organizations and professionals to build on trust as a core value that guides end-of-life care in cultural and religious diverse societies by listening to the views of minority groups and considering the best mechanisms to meet their needs for end-of-life care.

CONCLUSION

In today's world of multiculturalism, embracing diversity and personalized healthcare treatment in the provision of end-of-life care for older patients faced with life-threatening diseases and trauma has become very important for healthcare professionals such as nurses, doctors, healthcare administrators, and institutions. The rapid advancement in healthcare system has increased the number of older men and women now vulnerable to critical health diseases, trauma and posttraumatic stress disorder which complicate their health conditions and dying experience.

Cultural and religious beliefs define older patients' belief about death and dying and how they respond to or cope with their dying experiences, doctor's diagnosis of their diseases, trauma and their posttraumatic stress disorders and symptoms which affect their health outcomes. Developing cultural safety, humility and trust are critical factors to reduce the tensions that diverse cultural and religious beliefs generate in end-of-life care of older patients facing critical health conditions in many cultural and religious societies in diverse perspectives. Improving communication of end-of-life care to dying patients, family members and family caregivers remains inevitable in respecting diverse beliefs and ritual practices to prevent diverse expectations and health outcomes.

Education is crucial for promoting end-of-life care in multicultural societies, and all efforts should focus on improving death literacy among the younger generations in Asian and African societies. Patients and their family members, particularly younger adult children, can also be offered truth-disclosure supports to help them cope with discussing end-of-life care with healthcare professionals. Health professionals also need education on culture, religion, and the influence of disease and treatments to develop cultural humility and empathy for patients and their family members.

REFERENCES

Adinkrah, M. (2024). "We Will All Go, But What We All Seek Is Good Death": Cultural Notions of Good Death And Related Mortuary Rituals Among the Akan of Ghana. *Omega.*

Agai, J. (2015). Reading the near-death experience from an African perspective. *Theological Studies.*

Azia, I. N. (2023). Understanding the role of religious beliefs in adherence to antiretroviral therapy among Pentecostal Christians living with HIV in sub-Saharan Africa: A scoping review. *BMC Public Health*, •••, 1–12.

Bagheri, A. (2020). End of Life Issues: An Islamic Perspective. In A. Ahmad, *Ethics and Intercultural Issues in End of Life Care* (pp. 93-103). Springer Nature Link.

Chen, Z. J. (2025). Childhood predictors of belief in life after death across 22 countries. *Scientific Reports*, •••, 1–12.

Chukwuneke, F. (2012). Culture and Biomedical Care in Africa: The influence of culture on biomedical care in a traditional African society, Nigeria, West Africa. *Nigerian Journal of Medicine.*

Curtis, E. (2019). Why cultural safety rather than cultural competency is required to achieve health equity: a literature review and recommended definition.

Dezutter, J. (2008). The Role Of Religion in Death Attitudes: Distinguishing Between Religious Belief and Style of Processing Religious Contents. *Death Studies.*

Donkor, A. (2024). Prevalence of Preferences for End-of-Life Place of Care and Death Among Patients With Cancer in Low- and Middle-Income Countries: A Systematic Review and Meta-Analysis. *JCO Global Oncology.*

Ekore, R. I. (2016). *African Cultural Concept of Death and the Idea of Advance Care Directives.*

Feng, S. (2025). Global burden, risk factors, and projections of early-onset dementia: Insights from the Global Burden of Disease Study 2021. *Ageing Research Reviews.*

Flaskerud, J. H. (2017). Individual and Dynamic: Western Views of a Good Death. *Issues in Mental Health Nursing.*

Giger, J. N., & Davidhizar, R. (2002). Culturally competent care: Emphasis on understanding the people of Afghanistan, Afghanistan Americans, and Islamic culture and religion. *International Nursing Review*, *49*(2), 79–86.

Goh, R. S. (2024). The burden of cardiovascular disease in Asia from 2025 to 2050: A forecast analysis for East Asia, South Asia, South-East Asia, Central Asia, and high-income Asia Pacific regions. *The Lancet Regional Health. Western Pacific*, •••, 101138.

Haraldsson, E. (2006).. . *Nordic Psychology*.

Harding, R. (2003). Current HIV/AIDS end-of-life care in sub-Saharan Africa: A survey of models, services, challenges and priorities. *BMC Public Health*.

Harwood, J., Afsan, C., & Chetna. (2025). Measuring and monitoring the quality of dying in the UN Decade of Healthy Ageing. *The Lancelet Healthy Longevity*, 100739.

Ho, Kwong, & al., S. e. (2022). Decision-making preferences on end-of-life care for older people: Exploration and comparison of Japan, the Hong Kong SAR and South Korea in East Asia. *Journal of Clinical Nursing*.

Ho, L. Y. (2022). Decision-making preferences on end-of-life care for older people: Exploration and comparison of Japan, the Hong Kong SAR and South Korea in East Asia. *Journal of Clinical Nursing*.

Kallis, G. (2025). Exploring the challenges experienced by patients and families using palliative and end-of-life care services: A qualitative focus group study. *Palliative & Supportive Care*.

Kimberg, L. (2019). Trauma and Trauma-Informed Care. *Trauma-Informed Healthcare Approaches: A Guide for Primary Care*, 25-56.

Kumari, & Rajapaska. (2025). Global equality, complicated systems and assisted death in palliative care. *International Journal of Palliative Nursing*.

Leininger, M. (2002). Culture care theory: A major contribution to advance transcultural nursing knowledge and practices. *Journal of Transcultural Nursing*, *13*(3), 189–192.

Li, W. W. (2021). A Cross-Cultural Study of Filial Piety and Palliative Care Knowledge: Moderating Effect of Culture and Universality of Filial Piety. *Frontiers in Psychology*, •••, 787724.

Li, W. W. (2021). Death Acceptance in Vietnamese Cancer Patients: A Phenomenological Study. *journal of Transcultural Nursing*.

Long, N. H. (2018). Death Acceptance in Vietnamese Cancer Patients: A Phenomenological Study. *Journal of Transcultural Nursing*.

Matchim, W. K., & Chaipetch, O., & Yaowarat. (2012). Thai Buddhist families' perspective of a peaceful death in ICUs. *Nursing in Critical Care.*

Mori, M. (2023). Communication in Cancer Care in Asia: A Narrative Review. *JCO Global Oncology.*

Mori, M. (2025). Definition and recommendations of advance care planning: A Delphi study in five Asian sectors. *Palliative Medicine.*

Nichola, G., Gwyther, L., Tiso, T., & Harding, R. (2013). Traditional Healers' Views of the Required Processes for a ''Good Death'' Among Xhosa Patients Pre- and Post-Death. *Journal of Pain Symptoms and Management.*

Ohr, S. (2017). Cultural and religious beliefs and values, and their impact on preferences for end-of-life care among four ethnic groups of community-dwelling older persons. *Journal of Clinical Nursing*, •••, 1681–1689.

Othman, E. H. (2025). Death and Dying Through the Lens of Jordanian Muslim Patients and Caregivers. *Omega*, •••, 228–242.

Prince, M. J. (2015). The burden of disease in older people and implications for health policy and practice. *Lancet*, •••, 549–562.

Puchalski, & Donnel. (2005). Religious and spiritual beliefs in end of life care: how major religions view death and dying. 114-121.

Purnell, L. (2000). A description of the Purnell model for cultural competence. *Journal of Transcultural Nursing*, *11*(1), 40–46.

Qaseem, A. (2008). *Evidence-Based Interventions to Improve the Palliative Care of Pain, Dyspnea, and Depression at the End of Life: A Clinical Practice Guideline from the American College of Physicians.* American College of Physicians.

Ricks-Aherne, E. S. (2020). Practice Considerations for Trauma-Informed Care at End of Life. *Journal of Social Work in End-of-Life & Palliative Care*, •••, 313–329.

Ringdal, G. I. (2002). Health-related quality of life (HRQOL) in family members of cancer victims: Results from a longitudinal intervention study in Norway and Sweden. *Palliative Medicine.*

Rousseau, C. (2022). Safe enough? Rethinking the concept of cultural safety in healthcare and training. *The British Journal of Psychiatry*, •••, 587–588.

Sakamoto, R. (2025). Aging in Southeast Asia and Japan: Challenges and opportunities. *Geriatrics & Gerontology International*, •••, 837–854.

Sarhill, N. (2001). The terminally ill Muslim: Death and dying from the Muslim perspective. *American Journal of Hospice and Palliative Medicine®*.

Schefold, J. C. (2025). The impact of religion on changes in end-of-life practices in European intensive care units: A comparative analysis over 16 years. *Intensive Care Medicine*.

Seise, C. (2021). Dying a Good Death: Indonesian Rituals and Negotiations About the End of Life. *International Journal of Islam in Asia*, 168-190.

Sewpersad, S. (2024). Ageing in South Africa: Trends and Determinants. *Geriatrics & Gerontology International*.

Shalev, D. (2020). End-of-Life Care in Individuals With Serious Mental Illness. *Psychosomatics*, •••, 428–435.

Sheik, A. (1998). Death and dying-a Muslim perspective. *Journal of the Royal Society of Medicine*.

Singer, P. A. (1999). Quality end-of-life care. Patients' perspectives. *Journal of the American Medical Association*.

Sörensen, S. M. (2002). How effective are interventions with caregivers? an updated meta-analysis. *The Gerontologist*.

Stewart, S. (1998). Effects of a home-based intervention among patients with congestive heart failure discharged from acute hospital care. *Archives of Internal Medicine*.

Suleman, M. (2023). The balancing of virtues—Muslim perspectives on palliative and end of life care: Empirical research analysing the perspectives of service users and providers. *Bioethics*, •••, 57–68.

Tjernberg, J. (2020). Older persons' thoughts about death and dying and their experiences of care in end-of-life: A qualitative study. *BMC Nursing*.

Torrey, E. F. (2025). Epilogue 2025: How to Fix the Mental Illness Treatment System.

Tripodoro, V. A. (2025). First-Ever Global Ranking of Palliative Care: 2025 World Map Under the New WHO Framework. *Journal of Pain and Symptom Management*.

Upasen, R. (2022). Death Acceptance Process in Thai Buddhist Patients With Life-Limiting Cancer: A Grounded Theory. *Global Qualitative Nursing Research*.

Wenger, N. S. (2001). Quality indicators for end-of-life care in vulnerable elders. *Annals of Internal Medicine*, •••, 677–685.

Wenrich, M. D. (2003). Dying patients' need for emotional support and personalized care from physicians: Perspectives of patients with terminal illness, families, and health care providers. *Journal of Pain and Symptom Management*, •••, 236–246.

W.H.O. (2025). *News Release*. Retrieved from W.H.O.

Wong, L. P. (2015). Associations between religiosity and death attitudes: Different between christians and buddhists? *Psychology of Religion and Spirituality*.

Zanin, A. (2023). End-of-life decisions and practices as viewed by health professionals in pediatric critical care: A European survey study.

Zhu, T. (2023). Preferences and Attitudes Towards Life-Sustaining Treatments of Older Chinese Patients and Their Family Caregivers. *Clinical Interventions in Aging*, •••, 467–475.

Compilation of References

Aaronson, N. K., Ahmedzai, S., Bergman, B., Bullinger, M., Cull, A., Duez, N. J., Filiberti, A., Flechtner, H., Fleishman, S. B., Haes, J. C. J. M. D., Kaasa, S., Klee, M., Osoba, D., Razavi, D., Rofe, P. B., Schraub, S., Sneeuw, K., Sullivan, M., & Takeda, F. (1993). The European Organization for Research and Treatment of Cancer QLQ-C30 : A Quality-of-Life Instrument for Use in International Clinical Trials in Oncology. *Journal of the National Cancer Institute*, *85*(5), 365–376. DOI: 10.1093/jnci/85.5.365 PMID: 8433390

Abdi, Z., Ravaghi, H., Sarkhosh, S., Nafar, H., Khani, S., & Letaief, M. (2024). Patient and family engagement in patient safety in the Eastern Mediterranean Region: A scoping review. *BMC Health Services Research*, *24*(1), 1–17. DOI: 10.1186/s12913-024-11198-3 PMID: 38918854

Abernethy, A. P., Currow, D. C., Frith, P., Fazekas, B. S., McHugh, A., & Bui, C. (2003). Randomised, double blind, placebo controlled trial of sustained release morphine for the management of refractory dyspnea. *BMJ (Clinical Research Ed.)*, *327*(7414), 523–528. DOI: 10.1136/bmj.327.7414.523

Abernethy, A. P., McDonald, C. F., Frith, P. A., Clark, K., Herndon, J. E., Marcello, J., Young, I. H., Bull, J., Wilcock, A., Booth, S., Wheeler, J. L., Tulsky, J. A., Crockett, A. J., & Currow, D. C. (2010). Effect of palliative oxygen versus room air in relief of breathlessness in patients with refractory dyspnea: A double-blind, randomised controlled trial. *Lancet*, *376*(9743), 784–793. DOI: 10.1016/S0140-6736(10)61115-4

Abraham, W. T., Stevenson, L. W., Bourge, R. C., Lindenfeld, J. A., Bauman, J. G., & Adamson, P. B. (2016). Sustained efficacy of pulmonary artery pressure to guide adjustment of chronic heart failure therapy: Complete follow-up results from the CHAMPION randomised trial. *Lancet*, *387*(10017), 453–461.

Abu-Odah, H. M., Alex Liu, Justina. (2020). Challenges on the provision of palliative care for patients with cancer in low- and middle-income countries: A systematic review of reviews. *BMC Palliative Care*, *19*(1), 55–55. DOI: 10.1186/s12904-020-00558-5

Abu-Odah, H., Molassiotis, A., & Liu, J. Y. W. (2022). Global palliative care research (2002-2020): Bibliometric review and mapping analysis. *BMJ Supportive & Palliative Care, 12*(4), 376–387. PMID: 34373283

Abu-Zaineh, M., Ben Romdhane, H., Ventelou, B., Moatti, J.-P., & Chokri, A. (2013). Appraising financial protection in health: The case of Tunisia. *International Journal of Health Care Finance and Economics, 13*(1), 73–93. DOI: 10.1007/s10754-013-9123-8 PMID: 23381233

Achterberg, W., Lautenbacher, S., Husebo, B., Erdal, A., & Herr, K. (2019). Pain in dementia. *Pain Reports (Baltimore, Md.), 5*(1), e803–e803. DOI: 10.1097/PR9.0000000000000803

Adamek, M. E., Gebremariam Kotecho, M., Chane, S., & Gebeyaw, G. (2022). Challenges and assets of older adults in Sub-Saharan Africa: Perspectives of gerontology scholars. *Journal of Aging & Social Policy, 34*(1), 108–126. PMID: 34160333

Adam, R., & Murchie, P. (2014). Why are we not controlling cancer pain adequately in the community? *The British Journal of General Practice, 64*(626), 438–439. DOI: 10.3399/bjgp14x681229 PMID: 25179046

Adams, R., Henry, K. E., Sridharan, A., Soleimani, H., Zhan, A., Rawat, N., & Saria, S. (2022). Prospective, multi-site study of patient outcomes after implementation of the TREWS machine learning-based early warning system for sepsis. *Nature Medicine, 28*(7), 1455–1460.

Adelman, R. D., Tmanova, L. L., Delgado, D., Dion, S., & Lachs, M. S. (2014). Caregiver Burden : A Clinical Review. *Journal of the American Medical Association, 311*(10), 1052. DOI: 10.1001/jama.2014.304 PMID: 24618967

Adinkrah, M. (2024). "We Will All Go, But What We All Seek Is Good Death": Cultural Notions of Good Death And Related Mortuary Rituals Among the Akan of Ghana. *Omega*.

Administration on Aging. (2006). *A Profile of Older American.*

Adonteng-Kissi, B. (2021). Chronic life-limiting illness and informal care in Ghana: experiences of older people and their family carers.

Afolabi, O. A., Nkhoma, K., Maddocks, M., & Harding, R. (2021). What constitutes a palliative care need in people with serious illnesses across Africa? A mixed-methods systematic review of the concept and evidence. *Palliative Medicine, 35*(6), 1052–1070. PMID: 33860715

Agai, J. (2015). Reading the near-death experience from an African perspective. *Theological Studies*.

Aghaei, M. H., Vanaki, Z., & Mohammadi, E. (2021). Inducing a sense of worthiness in patients: The basis of patient-centered palliative care for cancer patients in Iran. *BMC Palliative Care, 20*(1). Advance online publication. DOI: 10.1186/s12904-021-00732-3 PMID: 33653323

Agom, D. A., Onyeka, T. C., Iheanacho, P. N., & Ominyi, J. (2021). Barriers to the Provision and Utilization of Palliative Care in Africa: A Rapid Scoping Review. *Indian Journal of Palliative Care, 27*(1), 3–17. DOI: 10.4103/ijpc.Ijpc_355_20 PMID: 34035611

Aguiar, J. P., Gama Marques, J., Leufkens, H. G., & Alves da Costa, F. (2022). Healthcare professionals' Views on the management of medication complexities in the elderly with mental health disorders: A cross-sectional study. *Frontiers in Psychiatry, 13*, 885216. PMID: 35677869

Ajlouni, M. T., Dawani, H., & Diab, S. M. (2015). Home Health Care (HHC) Managers Perceptions About Challenges and Obstacles that Hinder HHC Services in Jordan. *Global Journal of Health Science, 7*(4), 121–129. DOI: 10.5539/gjhs.v7n4p121 PMID: 25946949

Al Aboud, A. M., & Manna, B. (2025). Wound Pressure Injury Management(Archived). In *StatPearls*. Treasure Island (FL) ineligible companies. Disclosure: Biagio Manna declares no relevant financial relationships with ineligible companies.: StatPearls Publishing

Al Maqbali, M., Al Sinani, M., Al Naamani, Z., Al Badi, K., & Tanash, M. I. (2021). Prevalence of Fatigue in Patients With Cancer: A Systematic Review and Meta-Analysis. *Journal of Pain and Symptom Management, 61*(1), 167–189.e114. DOI: 10.1016/j.jpainsymman.2020.07.037

Alanazi, H. H. F., Alqarni, A. M. S., Alamri, A. A. H., Al-Faridi, S. G., Altawyan, Y. S. S., Al-Harbi, Z. B. B. H., Al Nemer, A. A. R., & Alqahtani, S. F. M. (•••). Palliative Care of Geriatrics-nursing Care Plans: An Updated Review. *International Journal of Health Sciences, 2*(S1), 444–456.

Al-Ansari, A. M., Abd-El-Gawad, W. M., AboSerea, S. M., ElShereafy, E. E. S., Ali, F. A. S., & ElSayed, M. A. E. (2021). The pattern of change in opioid and adjuvant prescriptions for cancer pain before and after referral to a comprehensive program in the Palliative Care Center in Kuwait. *BMC Palliative Care, 20*(1), 25. DOI: 10.1186/s12904-021-00717-2 PMID: 33536013

Alattas, I. M. (2025). Opiophobia: A Barrier to Pain Management. *Magalat Game'at al-Malik Abdul Aziz. Al-U'lum al-Tibyat, 23*(3), 1–7. DOI: 10.4197/med.23-3.1

Alboksmaty, A., Aldakhil, R., Hayhoe, B. W. J., Ashrafian, H., Darzi, A., & Neves, A.-L. (2025). The impact of using AI-powered voice-to-text technology for clinical documentation on quality of care in primary care and outpatient settings: A systematic review. *EBioMedicine, 118*. Advance online publication. DOI: 10.1016/j.ebiom.2025.105861 PMID: 40694861

Albrecht, T. A., & Taylor, A. G. (2012). Physical activity in patients with advanced-stage cancer: A systematic review of the literature. *Clinical Journal of Oncology Nursing, 16*(3), 293–300. DOI: 10.1188/12.Cjon.293-300

Alcalde, J., & Zimmermann, C. (2022). Stigma about palliative care: origins and solutions. *ecancermedicalscience, 16*, 1377.

Aleksandrowicz, H., Owczarczyk-Saczonek, A., & Placek, W. (2021). Venous Leg Ulcers: Advanced Therapies and New Technologies. *Biomedicines, 9*(11). Advance online publication. DOI: 10.3390/biomedicines9111569 PMID: 34829797

Alhussein, M., Patel, B., & Liu, X. (2023). Closing the gap: Technology access and telehealth use among older adults in the U.S. Medicare beneficiaries. *Telematics and Informatics Reports, 12*, 100103. https://doi.org/https://doi.org/10.1016/j.teler.2023.100103

Aljehani, M. S., Crenshaw, J. R., Rubano, J. J., Dellose, S. M., & Zeni, J. A. (2020). Falling risk in patients with end-stage knee osteoarthritis. *Clinical Rheumatology, 40*(1), 3–9. DOI: 10.1007/s10067-020-05165-6

Allan, S., & Vadean, F. (2023). The Impact of Wages on Care Home Quality in England. *The Gerontologist, 63*(9), 1428–1436. DOI: 10.1093/geront/gnad032 PMID: 36964753

Allom, V., & Mullan, B. (2014). Individual differences in executive function predict distinct eating behaviours. *Appetite, 80*, 123–130. DOI: 10.1016/j.appet.2014.05.007

Almutairi, K. M. (2015). Culture and language differences as a barrier to provision of quality care by the health workforce in Saudi Arabia. *Saudi Medical Journal, 36*(4), 425–431. DOI: 10.15537/smj.2015.4.10133 PMID: 25828278

Alodhialah, A. M., Almutairi, A. A., & Almutairi, M. (2024). Telehealth Adoption Among Saudi Older Adults: A Qualitative Analysis of Utilization and Barriers. *Healthcare (Basel, Switzerland), 12*(23). Advance online publication. DOI: 10.3390/healthcare12232470 PMID: 39685092

Alorfi, N. M. (2023). Pharmacological Methods of Pain Management: Narrative Review of Medication Used. *International Journal of General Medicine, 16*(16), 3247–3256. DOI: 10.2147/IJGM.S419239 PMID: 37546242

Al-Yateem, N., Hijazi, H., Saifan, A. R., Ahmad, A., Masa'Deh, R., Alrimawi, I., Rahman, S. A., Subu, M. A., & Ahmed, F. R. (2023). Quality and safety issue: Language barriers in healthcare, a qualitative study of non-Arab healthcare practitioners caring for Arabic patients in the UAE. *BMJ Open, 13*(12), e076326. DOI: 10.1136/bmjopen-2023-076326 PMID: 38135338

American Thoracic Society. (2012). An official American Thoracic Society statement: Update on the mechanisms, assessment, and management of dyspnea. [Note: This reference is formatted with the organizational author and the lead editor] [Parshall] [listed in the in-text citation, as per APA guidelines for edited works.]. *American Journal of Respiratory and Critical Care Medicine, 185*(4), 435–452. DOI: 10.1164/rccm.201111-2042ST

Amjad, H., Snyder, S. H., Wolff, J. L., Oh, E., & Samus, Q. M. (2019). Before Hospice: Symptom Burden, Dementia, and Social Participation in the Last Year of Life. *Journal of Palliative Medicine, 22*(9), 1106–1114. DOI: 10.1089/jpm.2018.0479 PMID: 31058566

Amoah, C. F. (2011). The central importance of spirituality in palliative care. *International Journal of Palliative Nursing, 17*(7), 353–358. DOI: 10.12968/ijpn.2011.17.7.353 PMID: 21841704

Anagnostou, D. (2017). Palliative care improves quality of life and reduces symptom burden in adults with life-limiting illness. *Evidence-Based Nursing*.

Analayo, B. (2003). *Satipatthāna: The direct path to realization*. Windhorse Publications. https://www.abhayagiri.org/media/discs/2015WinterRetreat/Sources/Analayo_Satipatthana-The-Direct-Path-to-Realization.pdf

Anandarajah, G., & Hight, E. (2001). Spirituality and medical practice: Using the HOPE questions as a practical tool for spiritual assessment. *American Family Physician, 63*(1), 81–89. PMID: 11195773

Anderson, R. E., & Grant, L. (2017). What is the value of palliative care provision in low-resource settings? *BMJ Global Health, 2*(1), e000139. PMID: 28588999

Anderson, T., Watson, M., & Davidson, R. (2008). The use of cognitive behavioural therapy techniques for anxiety and depression in hospice patients : A feasibility study. *Palliative Medicine, 22*(7), 814–821. DOI: 10.1177/0269216308095157 PMID: 18755828

Anekar, A. A., Cascella, M., & Hendrix, J. M. (2023). *WHO analgesic ladder*. National Library of Medicine; StatPearls Publishing. https://www.ncbi.nlm.nih.gov/books/NBK554435/

An, J., Ryu, H.-K., Lyu, S.-J., Yi, H.-J., & Lee, B.-H. (2021). Effects of Preoperative Telerehabilitation on Muscle Strength, Range of Motion, and Functional Outcomes in Candidates for Total Knee Arthroplasty: A Single-Blind Randomized Controlled Trial. *International Journal of Environmental Research and Public Health, 18*(11), 6071. DOI: 10.3390/ijerph18116071

Ansryan, L. Z., Aronow, H. U., Borenstein, J. E., Mena, V., Haus, F., Palmer, K., Chan, E., Swanson, J. W., Mass, S., & Rosen, B. (2018). Systems addressing frail elder care: Description of a successful model. *The Journal of Nursing Administration, 48*(1), 11–17. PMID: 29219905

Antonacci, R., Barrie, C., Baxter, S., Chaffey, S., Chary, S., Grassau, P., Hammond, C., Mirhosseini, M., Mirza, R. M., & Murzin, K. (2020). Gaps in hospice and palliative care research: A scoping review of the North American literature. *Journal of Aging Research, 2020*(1), 3921245. PMID: 33204532

Aoun, N., & Tajvar, M. (2024). Healthcare delivery in Lebanon: A critical scoping review of strengths, weaknesses, opportunities, and threats. *BMC Health Services Research, 24*(1). Advance online publication. DOI: 10.1186/s12913-024-11593-w PMID: 39334362

Apple Inc. (n.d.). Track your vitals on Apple Watch. Apple Support. Retrieved June 6, 2025, from https://support.apple.com/guide/watch/vitals-apd15aa7ed96/watchos

Argyropoulou, P., Patakas, D., Koukou, A., Vasiliadis, P., & Georgopoulos, D. (1993). Buspirone effect on breathlessness and exercise performance in patients with chronic obstructive pulmonary disease. *Respiration, 60*(4), 216–220. DOI: 10.1159/000196204

Aririguzoh, S. (2022). Communication competencies, culture and SDGs: Effective processes to cross-cultural communication. *Humanities & Social Sciences Communications, 9*(1), 1–11.

Armstrong, M., Flemming, K., Kupeli, N., Stone, P., Wilkinson, S., & Candy, B. (2019). Aromatherapy, massage and reflexology: A systematic review and thematic synthesis of the perspectives from people with palliative care needs. *Palliative Medicine, 33*(7), 757–769. DOI: 10.1177/0269216319846440

Assaad, R. H., Mohammadi, M., & Poudel, O. (2025). Developing an intelligent IoT-enabled wearable multimodal biosensing device and cloud-based digital dashboard for real-time and comprehensive health, physiological, emotional, and cognitive monitoring using multi-sensor fusion technologies. *Sensors and Actuators. A, Physical, 381*, 116074.

Atella, V., Piano Mortari, A., Kopinska, J., Belotti, F., Lapi, F., Cricelli, C., & Fontana, L. (2019). Trends in age-related disease burden and healthcare utilization. *Aging Cell, 18*(1), e12861.

Atomei, O.-L., Sânpălean, M., & Tarcea, M. (2024). Cultural Competence in Dietetic Practice. *Dietetics, 3*(4), 555–567.

Australian Institute of Health and Welfare. (2021). *Health and ageing*. In *Australia's health 2020: In brief* (pp. 66–69). AIHW. Retrieved June 4, 2025, from https://www.aihw.gov.au/getmedia/19dbc591-b1ef-4485-80ce-029ff66d6930/6_9-health-ageing.pdf.aspx

Avila, F. R., Carter, R. E., McLeod, C. J., Bruce, C. J., Guliyeva, G., Torres-Guzman, R. A., Maita, K. C., Ho, O. A., TerKonda, S. P., & Forte, A. J. (2023). The Role of Telemedicine in Prehospital Traumatic Hand Injury Evaluation. *Diagnostics (Basel, Switzerland), 13*(6). Advance online publication. DOI: 10.3390/diagnostics13061165 PMID: 36980474

Awad, A., Trenfield, S. J., Pollard, T. D., Ong, J. J., Elbadawi, M., McCoubrey, L. E., & Basit, A. W. (2021). Connected healthcare: Improving patient care using digital health technologies. *Advanced Drug Delivery Reviews, 178*, 113958.

Axelsson, B. (2022). The challenge: Equal availability to palliative care according to individual need regardless of age, diagnosis, geographical location, and care level. *International Journal of Environmental Research and Public Health, 19*(7), 4229. PMID: 35409908

Azia, I. N. (2023). Understanding the role of religious beliefs in adherence to antiretroviral therapy among Pentecostal Christians living with HIV in sub-Saharan Africa: A scoping review. *BMC Public Health, •••*, 1–12.

Azoulay, E., Chaize, M., & Kentish-Barnes, N. (2014). Involvement of ICU families in decisions : Fine-tuning the partnership. *Annals of Intensive Care, 4*(1), 37. DOI: 10.1186/s13613-014-0037-5 PMID: 25593753

Babapour, A. R., Gahassab-Mozaffari, N., & Fathnezhad-Kazemi, A. (2022). Nurses' job stress and its impact on quality of life and caring behaviors: A cross-sectional study. *BMC Nursing, 21*(1), 1–10. DOI: 10.1186/s12912-022-00852-y PMID: 35361204

Baer, R. A. (Ed.). (2015). *Mindfulness-Based Treatment Approaches: Clinician's Guide to Evidence Base and Applications* (2nd ed.). Academic Press.

Bae, S., & Kim, D. (2024). Improving home-like environments in long-term care units : An exploratory mixed-method study. *Scientific Reports, 14*(1), 13243. DOI: 10.1038/s41598-024-62328-0 PMID: 38853152

Baggetta, R., D'Arrigo, G., Torino, C., ElHafeez, S. A., Manfredini, F., Mallamaci, F., & Tripepi, G. (2018). Effect of a home based, low intensity, physical exercise program in older adults dialysis patients: A secondary analysis of the EXCITE trial. *BMC Geriatrics, 18*(1). Advance online publication. DOI: 10.1186/s12877-018-0938-5

Bagheri, A. (2020). End of Life Issues: An Islamic Perspective. In A. Ahmad, *Ethics and Intercultural Issues in End of Life Care* (pp. 93-103). Springer Nature Link.

Bakitas, M. A., Dionne-Odom, J. N., Ejem, D. B., Wells, R., Azuero, A., Stockdill, M. L., Keebler, K., Sockwell, E., Tims, S., Engler, S., Steinhauser, K., Kvale, E., Durant, R. W., Tucker, R. O., Burgio, K. L., Tallaj, J., Swetz, K. M., & Pamboukian, S. V. (2020). Effect of an Early Palliative Care Telehealth Intervention vs Usual Care on Patients With Heart Failure : The ENABLE CHF-PC Randomized Clinical Trial. *JAMA Internal Medicine, 180*(9), 1203–1213. DOI: 10.1001/jamainternmed.2020.2861 PMID: 32730613

Bandeali, S., des Ordons, A. R., & Sinnarajah, A. (2019). Comparing the physical, psychological, social, and spiritual needs of patients with non-cancer and cancer diagnoses in a tertiary palliative care setting. *Palliative & Supportive Care, 18*(5), 513–518. DOI: 10.1017/s1478951519001020

Banzett, R. B., & Lansing, R. W. (2021). Air hunger: A primal sensation and a primary element of dyspnea. *Comprehensive Physiology, 11*(2), 1449–1483. DOI: 10.1002/cphy.c200001

Baracho, V. D. S., Chaves, M. E. A., Huebner, R., Oliveira, M. X., Ferreira, P., & Lucas, T. C. (2021). Phototherapy (cluster multi-diode 630 nm and 940 nm) on the healing of pressure injury: A pilot study. *Journal of Vascular Nursing: Official Publication of the Society for Peripheral Vascular Nursing, 39*(3), 67–75. DOI: 10.1016/j.jvn.2021.06.002 PMID: 34507703

Barnes-Harris, M., Allcroft, S., & Johnson, M. J. (2019). Opioids for the palliation of refractory breathlessness in adults with advanced disease and terminal illness. *Cochrane Database of Systematic Reviews, 2019*(6), CD011008. Advance online publication. DOI: 10.1002/14651858.CD011008.pub3

Barnes, Lucy, & Hall, Peter A, & Taylor, Rosemary C R. (2023). The Structural Sources of Socioeconomic Inequalities in Health: A Cross-National Perspective. *Socius: Sociological Research for a Dynamic World*, *9*, 23780231231174830. DOI: 10.1177/23780231231174832

Barrett, D., O'Connell, P., & Wyatt, J. (2012). Development and delivery of an SMS-based remote monitoring and support service: 'Simple Telehealth'. In *International Journal of Integrated Care* (Vol. 12, Issue Suppl1).

Bastos, F., Garralda, E., Montero, A., Rhee, J. Y., Arias-Casais, N., Luyirika, E., Namisango, E., Pereira, J., Centeno, C., & Tripodoro, V. A. (2024). Comprehensive scoping review of palliative care development in Africa: Recent advances and persistent gaps. *Frontiers in Health Services*, *4*, 1425353. PMID: 39717493

Batchelor, N. H. (2010). Palliative or Hospice Care? Understanding the Similarities and Differences. *Rehabilitation Nursing*, *35*(2), 60–64. DOI: 10.1002/j.2048-7940.2010.tb00032.x

Bausewein, C., Booth, S., & Higginson, I. J. (2021). Measurement of dyspnea in the clinical rather than the research setting. *Current Opinion in Supportive and Palliative Care*, *2*(2), 95–99. DOI: 10.1097/SPC.0b013e3282fec4c5

Bayly, J., Edwards, B. M., Peat, N., Warwick, G., Hennig, I. M., Arora, A., & Maddocks, M. (2018). Developing an integrated rehabilitation model for thoracic cancer services: Views of patients, informal carers and clinicians. *Pilot and Feasibility Studies*, *4*, 160. DOI: 10.1186/s40814-018-0350-0

Beach, M. C., Gary, T. L., Price, E. G., Robinson, K., Gozu, A., Palacio, A., Smarth, C., Jenckes, M., Feuerstein, C., Bass, E. B., Powe, N. R., & Cooper, L. A. (2006). Improving health care quality for racial/ethnic minorities: A systematic review of the best evidence regarding provider and organization interventions. *BMC Public Health*, *6*(1), 104. DOI: 10.1186/1471-2458-6-104 PMID: 16635262

Beach, M. C., Roter, D., Korthuis, P. T., Epstein, R. M., Sharp, V., Ratanawongsa, N., Cohn, J., Eggly, S., Sankar, A., Moore, R. D., & Saha, S. (2013). A multicenter study of physician mindfulness and health care quality. *Annals of Family Medicine*, *11*(5), 421–428. DOI: 10.1370/afm.1507

Bedón-Molina, J., Lopez, M. J., & Derpich, I. S. (2014). A home-based smart health model. *Advances in Mechanical Engineering*, *12*(6), 1687814020935282. DOI: 10.1177/1687814020935282

Beer, J. M., McBride, S. E., Mitzner, T. L., & Rogers, W. A. (2014). Understanding challenges in the front lines of home health care: A human-systems approach. *Applied Ergonomics*, *45*(6), 1687–1699. DOI: 10.1016/j.apergo.2014.05.019 PMID: 24958610

Belgacem, B., Auclair, C., Fedor, M.-C., Brugnon, D., Blanquet, M., Tournilhac, O., & Gerbaud, L. (2013). A caregiver educational program improves quality of life and burden for cancer patients and their caregivers: A randomised clinical trial. *European Journal of Oncology Nursing*, *17*(6), 870–876. DOI: 10.1016/j.ejon.2013.04.006

Bellin, E. Y., Markis, W. T., Hellebrand, A. M., Busby, C. M., Wane, K. A., Jordan, C. R., & Kaufman, A. M. (2023). Improved nursing home end-stage renal disease patient participation in physical therapy with onsite, more frequent dialysis. *Hemodialysis International. International Symposium on Home Hemodialysis*, *27*(4), 465–474. DOI: 10.1111/hdi.13112

Bergerot, C. D., Soto-Perez-de-Celis, E., Thompson, C., Patel, R., Al-Mondhiry, J., Zhang, T., Dhawan, N., Burbage, D., McCollom, J., Tsang, M., Sedhom, R., & Rosa, W. E. (2025). Navigating Challenges in Palliative Care: A Survey on ASCO Guideline Adherence Among Health Care Providers in Low- and Middle-Income Countries. *JCO Global Oncology*, *11*. Advance online publication. DOI: 10.1200/go-24-00625 PMID: 40403199

Bertolazzi, A., Quaglia, V., & Bongelli, R. (2024). Barriers and facilitators to health technology adoption by older adults with chronic diseases: An integrative systematic review. *BMC Public Health*, *24*, 506. DOI: 10.1186/s12889-024-18036-5

Bhattacharyya, D. S., Hossain, M. H., Dutta, G. K., Snigdha, M. F., Nowrin, I., & Saif-Ur-Rahman, K. (2024). Service coverage and health workforce allocation strategies for geriatric and palliative care in low and middle-income countries: A systematic review. *Health Sciences Review (Oxford, England)*, *•••*, 100166.

Biney, A., Sarfo, J. O., Poku, C. A., Deegbe, D. A., & Atibila, F., Ti-enkawol Nachinab, G., Anaba, E., Dzansi, G., & Attafuah, P. Y. A. (2024). Challenges and coping strategies when caring for terminally ill persons with cancer: Perspectives of family caregivers. *BMC Palliative Care*, *23*(1), 175. PMID: 39020352

BioIntelliSense. (2024). *A retrospective observational study of continuous wireless vital sign monitoring via a medical grade wearable device on hospitalized floor patients*. Journal of Clinical Medicine. Retrieved June 6, 2025, from https://www.biointellisense.com/wp-content/uploads/2024/12/BioIntelliSense_PRESS_JCM_Nov-2024.pdf

Bishop, S. R., Lau, M., Shapiro, S., Carlson, L., Anderson, N. D., Carmody, J., Segal, Z. V., Abbey, S., Speca, M., Velting, D., & Devins, G. (2004). Mindfulness: A proposed operational definition. *Clinical Psychology : a Publication of the Division of Clinical Psychology of the American Psychological Association, 11*(3), 230–241. DOI: 10.1093/clipsy.bph077

Bökberg, C., Behm, L., & Ahlström, G. (2019). Quality of life of older persons in nursing homes after the implementation of a knowledge-based palliative care intervention. *International Journal of Older People Nursing, 14*(4), e12258. DOI: 10.1111/opn.12258 PMID: 31298499

Bondarchuk, O., Balakhtar, V., Pinchuk, N., Pustovalov, I., & Pavlenok, K. (2023). Adaptation of Coping Strategies to Reduce the Impact of Stress and Lonelines on the Psychological Well-Being of Adults - Digital Library NAES of Ukraine. *Iitta. gov.ua*. https://lib.iitta.gov.ua/id/eprint/738204/1/1852%2BLaw.pdf

Bonfiglio, A. (2025). *The future of wearable bioelectronics in healthcare*. Nat Rev Electr Eng., DOI: 10.1038/s44287-025-00175-5

Bonnefoy, P. Y., Chaize, E., Mansuy, R., Mehdi, T. A. Z. I., & Heckel, S. (2024). *The Definitive Guide to Data Integration: Unlock the power of data integration to efficiently manage, transform, and analyze data*. Packt Publishing.

Booth, S., Kelly, M. J., Cox, N. P., Adams, L., & Guz, A. (1996). Does oxygen help dyspnea in patients with cancer? *American Journal of Respiratory and Critical Care Medicine, 153*(5), 1515–1518. DOI: 10.1164/ajrccm.153.5.8630592

Booth, S., Moffat, C., Burkin, J., Galbraith, S., & Bausewein, C. (2018). Nonpharmacological interventions for breathlessness. *Current Opinion in Supportive and Palliative Care, 12*(3), 227–235. DOI: 10.1097/SPC.0000000000000362

Borasio, G. D. (2011). Translating the World Health Organization definition of palliative care into scientific practice. *Palliative & Supportive Care, 9*(1), 1–2. PMID: 21352612

Borgstrom, E., Schiff, R., Khan, S. A., Hindley, E., Thayabaran, D., Savage, E., Gough, N., & Holti, R. (2024). Practices, issues and possibilities at the interface between geriatrics and palliative care (InGaP): An exploratory study and knotworking. *Health Open Research, 6*(12), 12.

Borneman, T., Ferrell, B., & Puchalski, C. M. (2010). Evaluation of the FICA tool for spiritual assessment. *Journal of Pain and Symptom Management, 40*(2), 163–173. PMID: 20619602

Bouabida, K., Lebouché, B., & Pomey, M.-P. (2022). Telehealth and COVID-19 Pandemic: An Overview of the Telehealth Use, Advantages, Challenges, and Opportunities during COVID-19 Pandemic. *Healthcare (Basel, Switzerland), 10*(11). Advance online publication. DOI: 10.3390/healthcare10112293 PMID: 36421617

Bowden, L. G., Byrne, H. M., Maini, P. K., & Moulton, D. E. (2016). A morphoelastic model for dermal wound closure. *Biomechanics and Modeling in Mechanobiology, 15*(3), 663–681. DOI: 10.1007/s10237-015-0716-7 PMID: 26264498

Bradley, N., Dowrick, C., & Lloyd-Williams, M. (2022). Feasibility of Patient Reported Outcome Measures in Psychosocial Palliative Care : Observational Cohort Study of Hospice Day Care and Social Support Groups. *International Journal of Environmental Research and Public Health, 19*(20), 13258. DOI: 10.3390/ijerph192013258 PMID: 36293835

Brant, J. M., & Silbermann, M. (2021). Global perspectives on palliative care for cancer patients: Not all countries are the same. *Current Oncology Reports, 23*, 1–10. PMID: 33829323

Breitbart, W., Gibson, C., Poppito, S. R., & Berg, A. (2004). Psychotherapeutic Interventions at the End of Life : A Focus on Meaning and Spirituality. *Canadian Journal of Psychiatry, 49*(6), 366–372. DOI: 10.1177/070674370404900605 PMID: 15283531

Brighton, L. J., Miller, S., Farquhar, M., Booth, S., Yi, D., Gao, W., & Maddocks, M. (2019). Holistic services for people with advanced disease and chronic breathlessness: A systematic review and meta-analysis. *Thorax, 74*(3), 270–281. DOI: 10.1136/thoraxjnl-2018-211589

Brown, G. (2003). Long-term outcomes of full-thickness pressure ulcers: Healing and mortality. *Ostomy/Wound Management, 49*(10), 42–50. PMID: 14652420

Brown, J. V., Spicer, K. J., & French, E. (2021). Exploring the inclusion of cultural competence, cultural humility, and diversity concepts as learning objectives or outcomes in healthcare curricula. *Journal of Best Practices in Health Professions Diversity : Research, Education and Policy, 14*(1), 63–81.

Brown, K. W., Coogle, C. L., & Wegelin, J.. (2016). A pilot randomized controlled trial of mindfulness-based stress reduction for caregivers of family members with dementia. *Aging & Mental Health, 20*(11), 1157–1166. DOI: 10.1080/13607863.2015.1065790

Burgdorf, J. G., Arbaje, A. I., Chase, J.-A., & Wolff, J. L. (2022). Current practices of family caregiver training during home health care: A qualitative study. *Journal of the American Geriatrics Society*, *70*(1), 218–227. https://doi.org/https://doi.org/10.1111/jgs.17492 PMID: 34618918

Burgdorf, V., Szabo, Y. Z., & Abbott, M. J. (2019). A randomized comparison of mindfulness-based stress reduction and cognitive-behavioral therapy for family caregivers: Effects on stress and emotional regulation. *Journal of Contextual Behavioral Science*, *13*, 27–35.

Burge, A. T., Gadowski, A. M., Jones, A., Romero, L., Smallwood, N. E., Ekström, M., & Holland, A. E. (2024). Breathing techniques to reduce symptoms in people with serious respiratory illness: A systematic review. *European Respiratory Review : an Official Journal of the European Respiratory Society*, *33*(174), 240012. DOI: 10.1183/16000617.0012-2024

Burks, H. B., Des Bordes, J. K. A., Chadha, R., Holmes, H. M., & Rianon, N. J. (2021). Quality of Life Assessment in Older Adults with Dementia : A Systematic Review. *Dementia and Geriatric Cognitive Disorders*, *50*(2), 103–110. DOI: 10.1159/000515317 PMID: 34167127

Cain, C. L., Surbone, A., Elk, R., & Kagawa-Singer, M. (2018). Culture and Palliative Care : Preferences, Communication, Meaning, and Mutual Decision Making. *Journal of Pain and Symptom Management*, *55*(5), 1408–1419. DOI: 10.1016/j.jpainsymman.2018.01.007 PMID: 29366913

Cai, Y., & Lalani, N. (2022). Examining Barriers and Facilitators to Palliative Care Access in Rural Areas: A Scoping Review. *The American Journal of Hospice & Palliative Care*, *39*(1), 123–130. DOI: 10.1177/10499091211011145 PMID: 33906486

Caliskan, H., Sengul Aycicek, G., Ozsurekci, C., Dogrul, R. T., Balci, C., Sumer, F., Ozcan, M., Karabulut, E., Halil, M., Cankurtaran, M., & Yavuz, B. B. (2019). Turkish validation of a new scale from older people's perspectives : Older people's quality of life-brief (OPQOL-brief). *Archives of Gerontology and Geriatrics*, *83*, 91–95. DOI: 10.1016/j.archger.2019.04.002 PMID: 30991155

Campbell, C., & Parish, L. C. (2010). The decubitus ulcer: Facts and controversies. *Clinics in Dermatology*, *28*(5), 527–532. DOI: 10.1016/j.clindermatol.2010.03.010 PMID: 20797513

Campbell, M. L., Donesky, D., Sarkozy, A., & Reinke, L. F. (2021). Treatment of Dyspnea in Advanced Disease and at the End of Life. *Journal of Hospice &amp. Palliative Nursing*, *23*(5), 406–420. DOI: 10.1097/njh.0000000000000766

Campbell, M. L., & Templin, T. N. (2015). Intensity cut-points for the Respiratory Distress Observation Scale. *Palliative Medicine*, *29*(5), 436–442. DOI: 10.1177/0269216314564238

Campbell, M. L., Templin, T., & Walch, J. (2010). A Respiratory Distress Observation Scale for patients unable to self-report dyspnea. *Journal of Palliative Medicine*, *13*(3), 285–290. DOI: 10.1089/jpm.2009.0229

Candy, B., Jones, L., Larkin, P. J., Vickerstaff, V., Tookman, A., & Stone, P. (2015). Laxatives for the management of constipation in people receiving palliative care. *Cochrane Database of Systematic Reviews*, *2020*(1). Advance online publication. DOI: 10.1002/14651858.CD003448.pub4 PMID: 25967924

Care, H. (2013). *Clinical practice guidelines for quality palliative care*. Third National Consensus Project for Quality Palliative Care.

Castagna, A., Militano, V., Ruberto, C., Manzo, C., & Ruotolo, G. (2024). Comprehensive geriatric assessment and palliative care. *Aging Medicine (Milton, N.S.W.)*, *7*(5), 645–648. PMID: 39507225

Cauthen, D. B. (1981). The house call in current medical practice. *The Journal of Family Practice*, *13*(2), 209–213. PMID: 7252449

Cavalheri, V., Tahirah, F., Nonoyama, M., Jenkins, S., & Hill, K. (2014). Exercise training for people following lung resection for non-small cell lung cancer – A Cochrane systematic review. *Cancer Treatment Reviews*, *40*(4), 585–594. DOI: 10.1016/j.ctrv.2013.11.001

Celi, L. A., Cellini, J., Charpignon, M. L., Dee, E. C., Dernoncourt, F., Eber, R., & Yao, S. (2022). Sources of bias in artificial intelligence that perpetuate healthcare disparities—A global review. *PLOS Digital Health*, *1*(3), e0000022.

Cella, D. F. (1994). Quality of life : Concepts and definition. *Journal of Pain and Symptom Management*, *9*(3), 186–192. DOI: 10.1016/0885-3924(94)90129-5 PMID: 8014530

Centeno, C., & Arias-Casais, N. (2019). Global palliative care: From need to action. *The Lancet. Global Health*, *7*(7), e815–e816. PMID: 31129121

Cerullo, G., Figueiredo, T., Coelho, C., Campos, C. S., Videira-Silva, A., Carrilho, J., Midão, L., & Costa, E. (2024). Palliative care in the ageing European population: A cross-country comparison. *International Journal of Environmental Research and Public Health*, *21*(1), 113. PMID: 38276807

Chai, E., Meier, D., & Morris, J. (2014). *Geriatric palliative care*. OUP Us.

Chaikijurajai, T., Laffin, L. J., & Tang, W. H. W. (2020). Artificial intelligence and hypertension: Recent advances and future outlook. *American Journal of Hypertension, 33*(11), 967–974.

Chang, W.-Z. D., & Bourgeois, M. S. (2020). Effects of Visual Aids for End-of-Life Care on Decisional Capacity of People With Dementia. *American Journal of Speech-Language Pathology, 29*(1), 185–200. DOI: 10.1044/2019_ajslp-19-0028

Chan, P. Y., Ryan, N. P., Chen, D., McNeil, J., & Hopper, I. (2022). Novel wearable and contactless heart rate, respiratory rate, and oxygen saturation monitoring devices: A systematic review and meta-analysis. *Anaesthesia, 77*(11), 1268–1280. DOI: 10.1111/anae.15834

Chan, W.-L., Tai, Y.-L., Siu, W.-K. S., Hou, H. L.-Y., Yuen, K.-K., & Lee, V. H.-F. (2025). Use of mobile app “SUPPORT+” to enhance community palliative care in patients with advanced cancer : A prospective study. *Palliative Care and Social Practice, 19*, 26323524251351036. DOI: 10.1177/26323524251351036 PMID: 40606554

Chapman, A. E., Elias, R., Plotkin, E., Lowenstein, L. M., & Swartz, K. (2021). Models of care in geriatric oncology. *Journal of Clinical Oncology, 39*(19), 2195. PMID: 34043453

Chapman, E. J., Martino, E. D., Edwards, Z., Black, K., Maddocks, M., & Bennett, M. I. (2022). Practice review: Evidence-based and effective management of fatigue in patients with advanced cancer. *Palliative Medicine, 36*(1), 7–14. DOI: 10.1177/02692163211046754

Chapman, E. J., Pini, S., Edwards, Z., Elmokhallalati, Y., Murtagh, F. E. M., & Bennett, M. I. (2022). Conceptualising effective symptom management in palliative care: A novel model derived from qualitative data. *BMC Palliative Care, 21*(1), 17. DOI: 10.1186/s12904-022-00904-9 PMID: 35115005

Charmes, J. (2022). Variety and change of patterns in the gender balance between unpaid care-work, paid work and free time across the world and over time: A measure of wellbeing? *Wellbeing, Space and Society, 3*, 100081. https://doi.org/https://doi.org/10.1016/j.wss.2022.100081

Chen, C. Y., Chiang, I. H., Ou, K. L., Chiu, Y. L., Liu, H. H., Chang, C. K., & Tzeng, Y. S. (2020). Surgical treatment and strategy in patients with pressure sores: A single-surgeon experience. *Medicine, 99*(44), e23022. DOI: 10.1097/md.0000000000023022 PMID: 33126386

Cheng, C., & Christensen, M. (2024). Interventions Addressing Symptoms in Older Adults with Multimorbidity: An Umbrella Review. *Journal of Multidisciplinary Healthcare*, *17*, 3181–3192. DOI: 10.2147/jmdh.s452426 PMID: 39006878

Cheng, J. M., Batten, G. P., Cornwell, T., & Yao, N. (2020). A qualitative study of health-care experiences and challenges faced by ageing homebound adults. *Health Expectations*, *23*(4), 934–942. https://doi.org/https://doi.org/10.1111/hex.13072 PMID: 32476232

Chen, S., Fan, S., Qiao, Z., Wu, Z., Lin, B., Li, Z., & Lim, C. T. (2025). Transforming healthcare: Intelligent wearable sensors empowered by smart materials and artificial intelligence. *Advanced Materials*, ●●●, 2500412.

Chen, Y., Cai, T., Le, P., Zhang, L., Chen, Y., Wu, L., & Lu, Y. (2025). Family caregivers' perceptions and challenges in the care of pressure injuries in daily life: A qualitative study. *BMC Geriatrics*, *25*(1), 490. DOI: 10.1186/s12877-025-06114-1 PMID: 40610938

Chen, Y.-j., Li, X.-x., Ma, H.-k., Zhang, X., Wang, B.-w., Guo, T.-t., & Han, X.-m. (2020). Exercise Training for Improving Patient-Reported Outcomes in Patients With Advanced-Stage Cancer: A Systematic Review and Meta-Analysis. *Journal of Pain and Symptom Management*, *59*(3), 734–749.e710. DOI: 10.1016/j.jpainsymman.2019.09.010

Chen, Z. J. (2025). Childhood predictors of belief in life after death across 22 countries. *Scientific Reports*, ●●●, 1–12.

Chen, Z., Ding, Z., Chen, C., Sun, Y., Jiang, Y., Liu, F., & Wang, S. (2021). Effectiveness of comprehensive geriatric assessment intervention on quality of life, caregiver burden and length of hospital stay: A systematic review and meta-analysis of randomised controlled trials. *BMC Geriatrics*, *21*, 1–14. PMID: 34154560

Cheong, W. L., Mohan, D., Warren, N., & Reidpath, D. D. (2019). Palliative care research in the Asia Pacific region: A systematic review and bibliometric analysis of peer-reviewed publications. *Journal of Palliative Medicine*, *22*(5), 545–552. PMID: 30570416

Cheville, A. L., Kollasch, J., Vandenberg, J., Shen, T., Grothey, A., Gamble, G., & Basford, J. R. (2013). A home-based exercise program to improve function, fatigue, and sleep quality in patients with Stage IV lung and colorectal cancer: A randomized controlled trial. *Journal of Pain and Symptom Management*, *45*(5), 811–821. DOI: 10.1016/j.jpainsymman.2012.05.006

Chiang, I. H., Wang, C. H., & Tzeng, Y. S. (2018). Surgical treatment and strategy in patients with multiple pressure sores. *International Wound Journal, 15*(6), 900–908. DOI: 10.1111/iwj.12942 PMID: 29956467

Choudry, M., Gould, M., & Ganti, L. (2025). Treatment of agitation in dementia - a systematic review. *International Journal of Emergency Medicine, 18*(1), 101. DOI: 10.1186/s12245-025-00902-7

Chowdhury, R. A., Brennan, F. P., & Gardiner, M. D. (2020). Cancer Rehabilitation and Palliative Care-Exploring the Synergies. *Journal of Pain and Symptom Management, 60*(6), 1239–1252. DOI: 10.1016/j.jpainsymman.2020.07.030

Christensen, J. C., Paxton, R. J., Baym, C., Forster, J. E., Dayton, M. R., Hogan, C. A., & Stevens-Lapsley, J. E. (2020). Benefits of direct patient discharge to outpatient physical therapy after total knee arthroplasty. *Disability and Rehabilitation, 42*(5), 660–666. DOI: 10.1080/09638288.2018.1505968

Chukwuneke, F. (2012). Culture and Biomedical Care in Africa: The influence of culture on biomedical care in a traditional African society, Nigeria, West Africa. *Nigerian Journal of Medicine.*

Chu, W.-M., Tsai, H.-B., Chen, Y.-C., Hung, K. Y., Cheng, S.-Y., & Lin, C.-P. (2024). Palliative care for adult patients undergoing hemodialysis in Asia: Challenges and opportunities. *Journal of Hospice and Palliative Care, 27*(1), 1. PMID: 38449832

Cicerchia, M., Ceci, M., Locatelli, C., Gianni, W., & Repetto, L. (2010). Geriatric syndromes in peri-operative elderly cancer patients. *Surgical Oncology, 19*(3), 131–139.

Clegg, A., Young, J., Iliffe, S., Rikkert, M. O., & Rockwood, K. (2013). Frailty in elderly people. *Lancet, 381*(9868), 752–762. DOI: 10.1016/S0140-6736(12)62167-9 PMID: 23395245

Coger, V., Million, N., Rehbock, C., Sures, B., Nachev, M., Barcikowski, S., & Vogt, P. M. (2019). Tissue Concentrations of Zinc, Iron, Copper, and Magnesium During the Phases of Full Thickness Wound Healing in a Rodent Model. *Biological Trace Element Research, 191*(1), 167–176. DOI: 10.1007/s12011-018-1600-y PMID: 30552609

Cohen, S. R., Mount, B. M., Strobel, M. G., & Bui, F. (1995). The McGill Quality of Life Questionnaire : A measure of quality of life appropriate for people with advanced disease. A preliminary study of validity and acceptability. *Palliative Medicine, 9*(3), 207–219. DOI: 10.1177/026921639500900306 PMID: 7582177

Cohen, S., Kamarck, T., & Mermelstein, R. (1983). A global measure of perceived stress. *Journal of Health and Social Behavior, 24*(4), 385–396. DOI: 10.2307/2136404

Coleman, S., Nixon, J., Keen, J., Wilson, L., McGinnis, E., Dealey, C., & Nelson, E. A. (2014). A new pressure ulcer conceptual framework. *Journal of Advanced Nursing, 70*(10), 2222–2234. DOI: 10.1111/jan.12405 PMID: 24684197

Collins, R. N., & Kishita, N. (2019). The effectiveness of mindfulness- and acceptance-based interventions for informal caregivers of people with dementia: A meta-analysis. *The Gerontologist, 59*(4), e363–e379. DOI: 10.1093/geront/gny024

Conen, K., Guthrie, D. M., Stevens, T., Winemaker, S., & Seow, H. (2021). Symptom trajectories of non-cancer patients in the last six months of life: Identifying needs in a population-based home care cohort. *PLoS One, 16*(6), e0252814. DOI: 10.1371/journal.pone.0252814 PMID: 34129643

Corli, O., Santucci, C., Corsi, N., Radrezza, S., Galli, F., & Bosetti, C. (2019). The Burden of Opioid Adverse Events and the Influence on Cancer Patients' Symptomatology. *Journal of Pain and Symptom Management, 57*(5), 899–908.e6. DOI: 10.1016/j.jpainsymman.2019.02.009 PMID: 30776537

Cormie, P., Zopf, E. M., Zhang, X., & Schmitz, K. H. (2017). The Impact of Exercise on Cancer Mortality, Recurrence, and Treatment-Related Adverse Effects. *Epidemiologic Reviews, 39*(1), 71–92. DOI: 10.1093/epirev/mxx007

Corner, J., Plant, H., A'Hern, R., & Bailey, C. (1996). Non-pharmacological intervention for breathlessness in lung cancer. *Palliative Medicine, 10*(4), 299–305. DOI: 10.1177/026921639601000405

Cowdell, F., Jadotte, Y. T., Ersser, S. J., Danby, S., Walton, S., Lawton, S., Roberts, A., Gardiner, E., Ware, F., & Cork, M. (2014). Hygiene and emollient interventions for maintaining skin integrity in older people in hospital and residential care settings. *Cochrane Database of Systematic Reviews*. Advance online publication. DOI: 10.1002/14651858.CD011377 PMID: 32006460

Crane, R. S., Brewer, J., Feldman, C., Kabat-Zinn, J., Santorelli, S., Williams, J. M. G., & Kuyken, W. (2017). What defines mindfulness-based programs? The warp and the weft. *Psychological Medicine, 47*(6), 990–999. DOI: 10.1017/S0033291716003317

Crawley, L. M., Marshall, P. A., Lo, B., & Koenig, B. A., & for the End-of-Life Care Consensus Panel. (2002). Strategies for Culturally Effective End-of-Life Care. *Annals of Internal Medicine, 136*(9), 673–679. DOI: 10.7326/0003-4819-136-9-200205070-00010 PMID: 11992303

Creswell, J. D. (2017). Mindfulness interventions. *Annual Review of Psychology, 68*(1), 491–516. DOI: 10.1146/annurev-psych-042716-051139

Criss, M. G., Wingood, M., Staples, W. H., Southard, V., Miller, K. L., Norris, T. L., & Strunk, E. R. (2022). APTA Geriatrics' Guiding Principles for Best Practices in Geriatric Physical Therapy: An Executive Summary. *Journal of Geriatric Physical Therapy, 45*(2), 70–75. DOI: 10.1519/jpt.0000000000000342

Crombeen, A. M., & Lilly, E. J. (2020). Management of dyspnea in palliative care. *Current Oncology (Toronto, Ont.), 27*(3), 142–145. DOI: 10.3747/co.27.6413

Crowther, J., Horton, S., Wilson, K., & Lloyd-Williams, M. (2022). A UK qualitative study of living and dying with dementia in the last year of life. *Palliative Care and Social Practice, 16*, 26323524221096691–26323524221096691. DOI: 10.1177/26323524221096691

Curioni, C., Silva, A. C., Damião, J., Castro, A., Huang, M., Barroso, T., Araujo, D., & Guerra, R. (2023). The Cost-Effectiveness of Homecare Services for Adults and Older Adults: A Systematic Review. *International Journal of Environmental Research and Public Health, 20*(4). Advance online publication. DOI: 10.3390/ijerph20043373 PMID: 36834068

Current Health. (n.d.). *Remote patient monitoring*. Retrieved June 6, 2025, from https://www.currenthealth.com/remote-patient-monitoring/

Currow, D. C., Agar, M., & Abernethy, A. P. (2009). Tackling the challenge of breathlessness in advanced disease. *Progress in Palliative Care, 17*(4), 183–189.

Currow, D. C., Ekström, M., & Abernethy, A. P. (2020). Opioids for chronic refractory breathlessness: Patient predictors of beneficial response. *The European Respiratory Journal, 56*(4), 2002021. DOI: 10.1183/13993003.02021-2020

Curtis, E. (2019). Why cultural safety rather than cultural competency is required to achieve health equity: a literature review and recommended definition.

Dahmani, H., Fradi, I., Achour, L., & Toumi, M. (2023). Pharmaceutical pricing and reimbursement policies in Algeria, Morocco, and Tunisia: Comparative analysis. *Journal of Market Access & Health Policy, 11*(1), 2244304. DOI: 10.1080/20016689.2023.2244304 PMID: 37614557

Davidson, P. M., & Johnson, M. J. (2011). The use of palliative oxygen in advanced disease. *Progress in Palliative Care, 19*(2), 66–71.

Davies, B., & Bhutta, M. F. (2022). Geriatric medicine in the era of climate change. *Age and Ageing, 51*(1), afab199. PMID: 34651175

Dawson, A., Bowes, A., Kelly, F., Velzke, K., & Ward, R. (2015). Evidence of what works to support and sustain care at home for people with dementia: A literature review with a systematic approach. *BMC Geriatrics*, *15*, 59. DOI: 10.1186/s12877-015-0053-9

de Nooijer, K., Penders, Y. W., Pivodic, L., Van Den Noortgate, N. J., Pype, P., & Van den Block, L. (2020). Specialist palliative care services for older people in primary care: A systematic review using narrative synthesis. *Palliative Medicine*, *34*(1), 32–48. PMID: 31564214

Delgado-Guay, M. O., & Harding, A. (2021). Multidimensional Patient Assessment. *CRC Press EBooks*, 149–166. https://doi.org/DOI: 10.1201/9780429275524-20

Dellve, L., Lagerström, M., & Hagberg, M. (2003). Work-system risk factors for permanent work disability among home-care workers: A case-control study. *International Archives of Occupational and Environmental Health*, *76*(3), 216–224. DOI: 10.1007/s00420-002-0414-5 PMID: 12690496

desJardins-Park, H. E., Foster, D. S., & Longaker, M. T. (2018). Fibroblasts and Wound Healing: An Update. *Regenerative Medicine*, *13*(5), 491–495. DOI: 10.2217/rme-2018-0073 PMID: 30062921

Dezutter, J. (2008). The Role Of Religion in Death Attitudes: Distinguishing Between Religious Belief and Style of Processing Religious Contents. *Death Studies*.

Dharmarajan, T. (2021). Comprehensive geriatric assessment. In *Geriatric gastroenterology* (pp. 201–246). Springer.

Dharmawardene, M., Givens, J., Wachholtz, A., Makowski, S., & Tjia, J. (2015). A systematic review and meta-analysis of meditative interventions for informal caregivers and health professionals. *BMJ Supportive & Palliative Care*, *6*(2), 160–169. DOI: 10.1136/bmjspcare-2014-000819

Dick, A. W., Murray, M. T., Chastain, A. M., Madigan, E. A., Sorbero, M., Stone, P. W., & Shang, J. (2019). Measuring Quality in Home Healthcare. *Journal of the American Geriatrics Society*, *67*(9), 1859–1865. DOI: 10.1111/jgs.15963 PMID: 31063621

Diederichs, C., Berger, K., & Bartels, D. B. (2010). The Measurement of Multiple Chronic Diseases—A Systematic Review on Existing Multimorbidity Indices. *The Journals of Gerontology. Series A, Biological Sciences and Medical Sciences*, *66A*(3), 301–311. DOI: 10.1093/gerona/glq208

Dik, B. J., Daniels, D., & Alayan, A. J. (2024). Religion, spirituality, and the workplace: A review and critique. *Annual Review of Organizational Psychology and Organizational Behavior, 11*(1), 279–305.

Dingley, C., Ruckdeschel, A., Kotula, K., & Lekhak, N. (2021). Implementation and outcomes of complementary therapies in hospice care : An integrative review. *Palliative Care and Social Practice, 15*, 26323524211051753. DOI: 10.1177/26323524211051753 PMID: 34723183

Dixon, D., Sattar, H., Moros, N., Kesireddy, S. R., Ahsan, H., Lakkimsetti, M., Fatima, M., Doshi, D., Sadhu, K., & Junaid Hassan, M. (2024). Unveiling the Influence of AI Predictive Analytics on Patient Outcomes: A Comprehensive Narrative Review. *Cureus, 16*(5), e59954. DOI: 10.7759/cureus.59954

Dolibog, P., Dolibog, P., Franek, A., Brzezińska-Wcisło, L., Arasiewicz, H., Wróbel, B., & Błaszczak, E. (2018). Randomized, controlled clinical pilot study of venous leg ulcers treated with using two types of shockwave therapy. *International Journal of Medical Sciences, 15*(12), 1275–1285. DOI: 10.7150/ijms.26614 PMID: 30275753

Doñate-Martínez, A., Yang, J., Linklater, G., Bradley, C., Reppou, S., Panagiotis, P., Camacho, M., Fernandes, A., Gas, M. E., Giménez-Campos, M. S., Alhambra-Borrás, T., & Garcés-Ferrer, J. (2025). Care professionals' approach to early palliative care for non-malignant diseases shifted from relying on intuition to employing structured needs assessment. *International Journal of Integrated Care, 25*, 99–99. DOI: 10.5334/ijic.icic24047

Dong, C., Ji, Y., Fu, Z., Qi, Y., Yi, T., Yang, Y., & Sun, H. (2025). Precision management in chronic disease: An AI empowered perspective on medicine-engineering crossover. *iScience, 28*(3).

Donkor, A. (2024). Prevalence of Preferences for End-of-Life Place of Care and Death Among Patients With Cancer in Low- and Middle-Income Countries: A Systematic Review and Meta-Analysis. *JCO Global Oncology*.

Dreyfus, J., Gayle, J., Trueman, P., Delhougne, G., & Siddiqui, A. (2018). Assessment of Risk Factors Associated With Hospital-Acquired Pressure Injuries and Impact on Health Care Utilization and Cost Outcomes in US Hospitals. *American Journal of Medical Quality, 33*(4), 348–358. DOI: 10.1177/1062860617746741 PMID: 29262690

Dudgeon, D. (2019). Dyspnea, death rattle, and cough. In *Oxford Textbook of Palliative Medicine* (6th ed., pp. 340–355). Oxford University Press.

Dymarek, R., Kuberka, I., Walewicz, K., Taradaj, J., Rosińczuk, J., & Sopel, M. (2024). Is Shock Wave Application Effective on Various Chronic Wounds in the Geriatric Population? Preliminary Clinical Study. *Clinical Interventions in Aging, 19*, 665–679. DOI: 10.2147/cia.S448298 PMID: 38706636

Eckerblad, J., Theander, K., Ekdahl, A., Unosson, M., Wirehn, A.-B., Milberg, A., Krevers, B., & Jaarsma, T. (2015). Symptom burden in community-dwelling older people with multimorbidity: A cross-sectional study. *BMC Geriatrics, 15*(1). Advance online publication. DOI: 10.1186/1471-2318-15-1 PMID: 25559550

Eckerblad, J., Waldréus, N., Stark, Å. J., & Jacobsson, L. R. (2020). Symptom management strategies used by older community-dwelling people with multimorbidity and a high symptom burden - a qualitative study. *BMC Geriatrics, 20*(1). Advance online publication. DOI: 10.1186/s12877-020-01602-y PMID: 32539798

Ekore, R. I. (2016). *African Cultural Concept of Death and the Idea of Advance Care Directives.*

Ekström, M. P., Abernethy, A. P., & Currow, D. C. (2015). The management of chronic breathlessness in patients with advanced and terminal illness. *BMJ (Clinical Research Ed.), 349*, g7617. DOI: 10.1136/bmj.g7617

Eldaly, A. S., Maniaci, M. J., Paulson, M. R., Avila, F. R., Torres-Guzman, R. A., Maita, K., Garcia, J. P., & Forte, A. J. (2022). Patient satisfaction with telemedicine in acute care setting: A systematic review. *Journal of Clinical and Translational Research, 8*(6), 540–556. PMID: 36518201

El-Haddad, C., Hegazi, I., & Hu, W. (2020). Understanding Patient Expectations of Health Care: A Qualitative Study. *Journal of Patient Experience, 7*(6), 1724–1731. DOI: 10.1177/2374373520921692 PMID: 33457636

Elizabeth, J. T. (2015). *Oxford Textbook of Palliative Nursing* (R. F. Betty., Nessa, C., & Judith, A. P, Ed. 4th Edition ed.). Oxford University Press.

El-Jardali, F., & Fadlallah, R. (2017). A review of national policies and strategies to improve quality of health care and patient safety: A case study from Lebanon and Jordan. *BMC Health Services Research, 17*(1), 1–13. DOI: 10.1186/s12913-017-2528-1 PMID: 28814341

Ellenbecker, C. H., Samia, L., Cushman, M. J., & Alster, K. (2008). Patient safety and quality in home health care. *Patient Safety and Quality: An Evidence-Based Handbook for Nurses.*

Elsawy, A., & Elbehery, H., sweed, hala, & Sayed, A. (2024). Symptoms Burden In Elderly Male Patients Receiving Palliative Care .... *Egyptian Journal of Geriatrics and Gerontology*, *11*(1), 114–131. DOI: 10.21608/ejgg.2024.350629

Emanuel, E. J. (2000). Attitudes and Desires Related to Euthanasia and Physician-Assisted Suicide Among Terminally Ill Patients and Their Caregivers. *Journal of the American Medical Association*, *284*(19), 2460. DOI: 10.1001/jama.284.19.2460 PMID: 11074775

Engel, G. L. (1977). The Need for a New Medical Model : A Challenge for Biomedicine. *Science*, *196*(4286), 129–136. DOI: 10.1126/science.847460 PMID: 847460

Engel, M., Kars, M. C., Teunissen, S. C., & van der Heide, A. (2023). Effective communication in palliative care from the perspectives of patients and relatives: A systematic review. *Palliative & Supportive Care*, *21*(5), 890–913. PMID: 37646464

English, A. M. (2015). Physiotherapy in palliative care. In N. Cherny, M. Fallon, S. Kaasa, R. K. Portenoy, & D. C. Currow (Eds.), *Oxford Textbook of Palliative Medicine* (pp. 0): Oxford University Press.

Epstein, A. S., Liou, K. T., Romero, S. A. D., Baser, R. E., Wong, G., Xiao, H., & Mao, J. J. (2023). Acupuncture vs Massage for Pain in Patients Living With Advanced Cancer: The IMPACT Randomized Clinical Trial. *JAMA Network Open*, *6*(11), e2342482. DOI: 10.1001/jamanetworkopen.2023.42482

Eriksson, H., Sandberg, J., & Hellström, I. (2013). Experiences of long-term home care as an informal caregiver to a spouse: Gendered meanings in everyday life for female carers. *International Journal of Older People Nursing*, *8*(2), 159–165. DOI: 10.1111/j.1748-3743.2012.00340.x PMID: 22805660

Ester, M., Culos-Reed, S. N., Abdul-Razzak, A., Daun, J. T., Duchek, D., Francis, G., & Capozzi, L. C. (2021). Feasibility of a multimodal exercise, nutrition, and palliative care intervention in advanced lung cancer. *BMC Cancer*, *21*(1), 159. DOI: 10.1186/s12885-021-07872-y

European Union. (2016). *General Data Protection Regulation (GDPR) 2016/679.* Official Journal of the European Union. https://eur-lex.europa.eu/legal-content/EN/TXT/?uri=CELEX%3A32016R0679

Evans, R., Weech-Maldonado, R., Burke, D., Grammas, M., Jablonski, R., & Mehta, T. (2019). Developing a Strategic Group Typology for Home Health Care Agencies. *Home Health Care Management & Practice*, *32*(2), 87–94. DOI: 10.1177/1084822319882673

Fajarini, M., Setiawan, A., Sung, C.-M., Chen, R., Liu, D., Lee, C.-K., Niu, S.-F., & Chou, K.-R. (2025). Effects of advanced practice nurses on health-care costs, quality of care, and patient well-being: A meta-analysis of randomized controlled trials. *International Journal of Nursing Studies*, *162*, 104953. https://doi.org/https://doi.org/10.1016/j.ijnurstu.2024.104953 PMID: 39586168

Fang, M. L., Sixsmith, J., Sinclair, S., & Horst, G. (2016). A knowledge synthesis of culturally- and spiritually-sensitive end-of-life care : Findings from a scoping review. *BMC Geriatrics*, *16*, 107. DOI: 10.1186/s12877-016-0282-6 PMID: 27193395

Fasolino, T., Mayfield, M. E., Valentine, K., Rosa, W. E., & Koci, A. (2024). Palliative Care in Rural Communities. *AJN The American Journal of Nursing*, *124*(8), 50–55. DOI: 10.1097/01.Naj.0001027716.70431.35 PMID: 39051815

Fawole, O. A., Dy, S. M., Wilson, R. F., Lau, B. D., Martinez, K. A., Apostol, C. C., Vollenweider, D., Bass, E. B., & Aslakson, R. A. (2013). A Systematic Review of Communication Quality Improvement Interventions for Patients with Advanced and Serious Illness. *Journal of General Internal Medicine*, *28*(4), 570–577. DOI: 10.1007/s11606-012-2204-4 PMID: 23099799

Fayers, P., & Bottomley, A. (2002). Quality of life research within the EORTC—The EORTC QLQ-C30. *European Journal of Cancer*, *38*, 125–133. DOI: 10.1016/S0959-8049(01)00448-8 PMID: 11858978

Feinberg, I. Z., Owen-Smith, A., O'Connor, M. H., Ogrodnick, M. M., Rothenberg, R., & Eriksen, M. P. (2021). Strengthening culturally competent health communication. *Health Security*, *19*(S1), S–41–S–49. PMID: 33961489

Feinberg, L. F. (2014). Moving Toward Person- and Family-Centered Care. *The Public Policy and Aging Report*, *24*(3), 97–101. DOI: 10.1093/ppar/pru027

Feng, S. (2025). Global burden, risk factors, and projections of early-onset dementia: Insights from the Global Burden of Disease Study 2021. *Ageing Research Reviews*.

Fernandes, R., Osarch, S., & Allen, N. E. (2018). Home Healthcare and Hospice: A Pacific Islands Perspective. *Home Healthcare Now*, *36*(4). https://journals.lww.com/homehealthcarenurseonline/fulltext/2018/07000/home_healthcare_and_hospice__a_pacific_islands.8.aspx PMID: 29979307

Ferrans, C. E. (1990). Development of a quality of life index for patients with cancer. *Oncology Nursing Forum*, *17*(3, Suppl), 15–19. PMID: 2342979

Ferrans, C. E. (1996). Development of a conceptual model of quality of life. *Scholarly Inquiry for Nursing Practice*, *10*(3), 293–304. PMID: 9009823

Ferrans, C. E., & Powers, M. J. (1985). Quality of life index : Development and psychometric properties. *Advances in Nursing Science*, *8*(1), 15–24. DOI: 10.1097/00012272-198510000-00005 PMID: 3933411

Ferrell, B. R., & Paice, J. A. (2019). *Oxford textbook of palliative nursing*. Oxford University Press.

Fields, L., Shalev, D., Nathanson, M., & Shapiro, P. A. (2022). Palliative care training for geriatric psychiatry fellows: A national survey project. *The American Journal of Geriatric Psychiatry*, *30*(4), 504–510. PMID: 34535362

Fisher, A. R., Wells, G., & Harrison, M. B. (2004). Factors associated with pressure ulcers in adults in acute care hospitals. *Holistic Nursing Practice*, *18*(5), 242–253. DOI: 10.1097/00004650-200409000-00007 PMID: 15497604

Fitchett, G., Hisey Pierson, A. L., Hoffmeyer, C., Labuschagne, D., Lee, A., Levine, S., O'Mahony, S., Pugliese, K., & Waite, N. (2020). Development of the PC-7, a quantifiable assessment of spiritual concerns of patients receiving palliative care near the end of life. *Journal of Palliative Medicine*, *23*(2), 248–253. PMID: 31483184

Flaskerud, J. H. (2017). Individual and Dynamic: Western Views of a Good Death. *Issues in Mental Health Nursing*.

Fleischer, A., Campbell, C., & Polo, K. M. (2023). Cancer-Related Fatigue (2018-2022). *The American Journal of Occupational Therapy*, *77*(Suppl 1). Advance online publication. DOI: 10.5014/ajot.2023.77S10034

Floridi, G., Carrino, L., & Glaser, K. (2021). Socioeconomic Inequalities in Home-Care Use Across Regional Long-term Care Systems in Europe. *The Journals of Gerontology. Series B, Psychological Sciences and Social Sciences*, *76*(1), 121–132. DOI: 10.1093/geronb/gbaa139 PMID: 32996570

Fordjour, G. A., Yin, A., Ka-Ying Hui, V., & Lai, C. (2024). Comparative analysis of symptom burdens and influential factors among diverse terminally-ill patients. *Annals of Palliative Medicine*, *13*(3), 513–530. DOI: 10.21037/apm-23-565 PMID: 38769801

Foster, C. C., Agrawal, R. K., & Davis, M. M. (2019). Home Health Care For Children With Medical Complexity: Workforce Gaps, Policy, And Future Directions. *Health Affairs*, *38*(6), 987–993. DOI: 10.1377/hlthaff.2018.05531 PMID: 31158008

Fowlie, M., & Berkeley, J. (1987). Quality of Life—A Review of the Literature. *Family Practice*, *4*(3), 226–234. DOI: 10.1093/fampra/4.3.226 PMID: 3311862

Franek, A., Kostur, R., Polak, A., Taradaj, J., Szlachta, Z., Blaszczak, E., & Kucio, C. (2012). Using high-voltage electrical stimulation in the treatment of recalcitrant pressure ulcers: Results of a randomized, controlled clinical study. *Ostomy/Wound Management, 58*(3), 30–44. PMID: 22391955

Freedman, V. A., Rogowski, J., Wickstrom, S. L., Adams, J., Marainen, J., & Escarce, J. J. (2004). Socioeconomic Disparities in the Use of Home Health Services in a Medicare Managed Care Population. *Health Services Research, 39*(5), 1277–1298. https://doi.org/https://doi.org/10.1111/j.1475-6773.2004.00290.x PMID: 15333109

Frogner, B. K., Patterson, D. G., & Skillman, S. M. (2023). The Workforce Needed to Address Population Health. *The Milbank Quarterly, 101*(S1), 841–865. DOI: 10.1111/1468-0009.12620 PMID: 37096630

Frydenberg, K., & Brekke, M. (2012). Poor communication on patients' medication across health care levels leads to potentially harmful medication errors. *Scandinavian Journal of Primary Health Care, 30*(4), 234–240. PMID: 23050954

Frykberg, R. G., & Banks, J. (2015). Challenges in the Treatment of Chronic Wounds. *Advances in Wound Care (New Rochelle, N.Y.), 4*(9), 560–582. DOI: 10.1089/wound.2015.0635 PMID: 26339534

Funabashi, M., Wang, S., Lee, A. D., & Duarte, C K, F., Budgell, B., Stilwell, P., & Hogg-Johnson, S. (2022). Discomfort, pain and stiffness: What do these terms mean to patients? A cross-sectional survey with lexical and qualitative analyses. *BMC Musculoskeletal Disorders, 23*(1), 283. DOI: 10.1186/s12891-022-05214-y

Gaina, A.-M., Stefanescu, C., Szalontay, A.-S., Gaina, M.-A., Poroch, V., Mosoiu, D. V., Stefanescu, B.-V., Axinte, M., Tofan, C.-M., & Magurianu, L. A. (2024). A Systematic Review of Virtual Reality's Impact on Anxiety During Palliative Care. *Healthcare (Basel, Switzerland), 12*(24), 2517. DOI: 10.3390/healthcare12242517 PMID: 39765944

Galante, J., Galante, I., Bekkers, M. J., & Gallacher, J. (2014). Effect of kindness-based meditation on health and well-being: A systematic review and meta-analysis. *Journal of Consulting and Clinical Psychology, 82*(6), 1101–1114. DOI: 10.1037/a0037249

Galchutt, P. K. (2024). Spiritual assessment models for palliative care chaplains: A narrative review. *Journal of Health Care Chaplaincy, 30*(4), 329–345. PMID: 38900925

Galiano, R., Snyder, R., Mayer, P., Rogers, L. C., & Alvarez, O. (2019). Focused shockwave therapy in diabetic foot ulcers: Secondary endpoints of two multicentre randomised controlled trials. *Journal of Wound Care*, *28*(6), 383–395. DOI: 10.12968/jowc.2019.28.6.383 PMID: 31166864

Gamston, J. (2019). Pressure induced skin and soft tissue injury in the emergency department. *Emergency Medicine Journal: EMJ*, *36*(10), 631–634. DOI: 10.1136/emermed-2018-207807 PMID: 31311786

Gandarillas, M. Á., & Goswami, N. (2018). Merging current health care trends: Innovative perspective in aging care. *Clinical Interventions in Aging*, **•••**, 2083–2095. PMID: 30425463

Gangurde, S. (2023). *Healthcare data security: Standards, measures & data breach protection*. CrelioHealth. https://blog.creliohealth.com/healthcare-data-security-standards-measures-and-data-breach-protection/. Accessed June 11, 2025.

Gao, X., Sun, F., & Ko, E. (2020). Physiological stress responses in caregivers of patients with advanced cancer: Cortisol dysregulation and psychological burden. *Psycho-Oncology*, *29*(3), 486–494. DOI: 10.1002/pon.5273

García-Campos, N., Cebolla, A., & Soler, J. (2021). Mindfulness-based intervention versus psychoeducation for family caregivers: A controlled clinical trial. *Mindfulness*, *12*(4), 910–922.

Garcia, M. V., Agar, M. R., Soo, W.-K., To, T., & Phillips, J. L. (2021). Screening tools for identifying older adults with cancer who may benefit from a geriatric assessment: A systematic review. *JAMA Oncology*, *7*(4), 616–627. PMID: 33443547

Gardner, S. E., Frantz, R. A., & Doebbeling, B. N. (2001). The validity of the clinical signs and symptoms used to identify localized chronic wound infection. *Wound Repair and Regeneration*, *9*(3), 178–186. DOI: 10.1046/j.1524-475x.2001.00178.x PMID: 11472613

Gasparini, M., Moro, V., Amato, S., Vanacore, N., & Gambina, G. (2021). The evaluation of capacity in dementia: Ethical constraints and best practice. A systematic review. *Annali dell'Istituto Superiore di Sanita*, *57*(3), 212–225. DOI: 10.4415/ann_21_03_04

Getson, C., & Nejat, G. (2021). Socially assistive robots helping older adults through the pandemic and life after covid-19. *Robotics (Basel, Switzerland)*, *10*(3). Advance online publication. DOI: 10.3390/robotics10030106

Ghanem, M., Ghaith, A. K., & Bydon, M. (2024). Artificial intelligence and personalized medicine: transforming patient care. In *The New Era of Precision Medicine* (pp. 131–142). Academic Press.

Ghosh, A., Singh, A., & Chigateri, S. (2023). A Trapeze Act : Women Balancing Paid Work and Unpaid Care Work in Nepal - National Report for Women's Economic Empowerment Policy and Programming. SSRN *Electronic Journal, October*. https://doi.org/DOI: 10.2139/ssrn.4660197

Gianfredi, V., Nucci, D., Pennisi, F., Maggi, S., Veronese, N., & Soysal, P. (2025). Aging, longevity, and healthy aging: The public health approach. *Aging Clinical and Experimental Research*, *37*(1), 125.

Giger, J. N., & Davidhizar, R. (2002). Culturally competent care: Emphasis on understanding the people of Afghanistan, Afghanistan Americans, and Islamic culture and religion. *International Nursing Review*, *49*(2), 79–86.

Gijsberts, M.-J. H. E., Liefbroer, A. I., Otten, R., & Olsman, E. (2019). Spiritual Care in Palliative Care : A Systematic Review of the Recent European Literature. *Medical Sciences (Basel, Switzerland)*, *7*(2), 25. DOI: 10.3390/medsci7020025 PMID: 30736416

Gill, A., Chakraborty, A., & Selby, D. (2012). What is Symptom Burden: A Qualitative exploration of Patient Definitions. *Journal of Palliative Care*, *28*(2), 83–89. DOI: 10.1177/082585971202800204 PMID: 22860380

Girgis, B., & Duarte, J. A. (2018). High Voltage Monophasic Pulsed Current (HVMPC) for stage II-IV pressure ulcer healing. A systematic review and meta-analysis. *Journal of Tissue Viability*, *27*(4), 274–284. DOI: 10.1016/j.jtv.2018.08.003 PMID: 30177421

Given, B., Sherwood, P. R., & Given, C. W. (2011). Support for caregivers of cancer patients: Transition after active treatment. *Cancer Epidemiology, Biomarkers & Prevention*, *20*(10), 2015–2021. DOI: 10.1158/1055-9965.EPI-11-0611

Glass, G. E. (2021). Photobiomodulation: The Clinical Applications of Low-Level Light Therapy. *Aesthetic Surgery Journal*, *41*(6), 723–738. DOI: 10.1093/asj/sjab025 PMID: 33471046

Gobinath, A., Rajeswari, P., Anandan, M., & Kumar, N. S. (2025). AI in Imaging for Diagnosis. In *AI Insights on Nuclear Medicine* (pp. 51–76). IGI Global Scientific Publishing.

Goh, R. S. (2024). The burden of cardiovascular disease in Asia from 2025 to 2050: A forecast analysis for East Asia, South Asia, South-East Asia, Central Asia, and high-income Asia Pacific regions. *The Lancet Regional Health. Western Pacific*, •••, 101138.

Goh, S.-L., Persson, M. S. M., Stocks, J., Hou, Y., Welton, N. J., Lin, J., & Zhang, W. (2019). Relative Efficacy of Different Exercises for Pain, Function, Performance and Quality of Life in Knee and Hip Osteoarthritis: Systematic Review and Network Meta-Analysis. *Sports Medicine (Auckland, N.Z.)*, *49*(5), 743–761. DOI: 10.1007/s40279-019-01082-0

Goldsmith, J. V., & Wittenberg, E. (2024). The COMFORT model: Moving the initiative outside of the academy. *Health Communication*, *39*(14), 3514–3519. PMID: 38450611

Gomes, B., Calanzani, N., Curiale, V., McCrone, P. P., Higginson, I. J., & Brito, M. D. (2016). Effectiveness and cost-effectiveness of home palliative care services for adults with advanced illness and their caregivers. *São Paulo Medical Journal = Revista Paulista de Medicina*, *134*(1), 93–94. DOI: 10.1590/1516-3180.20161341T2 PMID: 26786605

Gomes-Ferraz, C. A., Rezende, G., Fagundes, A. A., & De Carlo, M. M. R. do P. (2022). Assessment of total pain in people in oncologic palliative care: Integrative literature review. *Palliative Care and Social Practice*, *16*, 263235242211252. DOI: 10.1177/26323524221125244 PMID: 36172038

Goodridge, D., Hawranik, P., Duncan, V., & Turner, H. (2012). Socioeconomic disparities in home health care service access and utilization: A scoping review. *International Journal of Nursing Studies*, *49*(10), 1310–1319. https://doi.org/https://doi.org/10.1016/j.ijnurstu.2012.01.002 PMID: 22300550

Google, L. L. C. (n.d.). Track your health metrics in the Fitbit app. Fitbit Help. Retrieved June 6, 2025, from https://support.google.com/fitbit/answer/14236917?hl=en

Gordon, B., Mason, B., & Smith, S. L. H. (2022). Leveraging Telehealth for Delivery of Palliative Care to Remote Communities : A Rapid Review. *Journal of Palliative Care*, *37*(2), 213–225. DOI: 10.1177/08258597211001184 PMID: 33730904

Gottlieb, L. M., DeSalvo, K., & Adler, N. E. (2019). Healthcare Sector Activities to Identify and Intervene on Social Risk: An Introduction to the <em>American Journal of Preventive Medicine</em> Supplement. *American Journal of Preventive Medicine*, *57*(6), S1–S5. DOI: 10.1016/j.amepre.2019.07.009 PMID: 31753275

Gottret, P., Schieber, G., & Waters, H. R. (2008). *Good practices in health financing: lessons from reforms in low and middle-income countries*. World Bank Publications.

Gould, L., Abadir, P., Brem, H., Carter, M., Conner-Kerr, T., Davidson, J., & Schmader, K. (2015). Chronic wound repair and healing in older adults: Current status and future research. *Wound Repair and Regeneration*, *23*(1), 1–13. DOI: 10.1111/wrr.12245 PMID: 25486905

Gould, L., Stuntz, M., Giovannelli, M., Ahmad, A., Aslam, R., Mullen-Fortino, M., & Gordillo, G. M. (2016). Wound Healing Society 2015 update on guidelines for pressure ulcers. *Wound Repair and Regeneration*, *24*(1), 145–162. DOI: 10.1111/wrr.12396 PMID: 26683529

Goyal, M., Singh, S., Sibinga, E. M. S., Gould, N. F., Rowland-Seymour, A., Sharma, R., Berger, Z., Sleicher, D., Maron, D. D., Shihab, H. M., Ranasinghe, P. D., Linn, S., Saha, S., Bass, E. B., & Haythornthwaite, J. A. (2014). Meditation programs for psychological stress and well-being: A systematic review and meta-analysis. *JAMA Internal Medicine*, *174*(3), 357–368. DOI: 10.1001/jamainternmed.2013.13018

Grant, L., Downing, J., Luyirika, E., Murphy, M., Namukwaya, L., Kiyange, F., Atieno, M., Kemigisha-Ssali, E., Hunt, J., Snell, K., Murray, S. A., & Leng, M. (2017). Integrating palliative care into national health systems in Africa: A multi-country intervention study. *Journal of Global Health*, *7*(1), 010419. DOI: 10.7189/jogh.07.010419 PMID: 28685037

Gravell, R. (2024). *Communication problems in elderly people: Practical approaches to management*. Taylor & Francis.

Graves, N., Birrell, F., & Whitby, M. (2005). Effect of pressure ulcers on length of hospital stay. *Infection Control and Hospital Epidemiology*, *26*(3), 293–297. DOI: 10.1086/502542 PMID: 15796283

Green, E. P., Lai, Y., Pearson, N., Rajasekharan, S., Rauws, M., Joerin, A., Kwobah, E., Musyimi, C., Jones, R. M., Bhat, C., Mulinge, A., & Puffer, E. S. (2020). Expanding Access to Perinatal Depression Treatment in Kenya Through Automated Psychological Support : Development and Usability Study. *JMIR Formative Research*, *4*(10), e17895. DOI: 10.2196/17895 PMID: 33016883

Grignoli, N., Di Bernardo, V., & Malacrida, R. (2018). New perspectives on substituted relational autonomy for shared decision-making in critical care. *Critical Care*, *22*(1), 260. DOI: 10.1186/s13054-018-2187-6 PMID: 30309384

Gülalp, B., Aldinç, H., Karagün, Ö., Çetinel, Y., & Benli, S. (2009). The complaint and outcome of geriatric patient in emergency department. *Turkish Journal of Emergency Medicine, 9*(2), 073–077.

Gunasekeran, D. V., Tham, Y.-C., Ting, D. S. W., Tan, G. S. W., & Wong, T. Y. (2021). Digital health during COVID-19: Lessons from operationalising new models of care in ophthalmology. *The Lancet. Digital Health, 3*(2), e124–e134. DOI: 10.1016/S2589-7500(20)30287-9 PMID: 33509383

Guo, E., He, S., & Zheng, L. (2025). Health effects and mediating mechanisms of smart wearable devices on older people: Evidence from China. *Frontiers in Public Health, 13*, 1578063.

Guppy, J. H., Widlund, H., Munro, R., & Price, J. (2024). Incivility in healthcare: The impact of poor communication. *BMJ Leader, 8*(1). PMID: 37419661

Gupta, A., Mahnken, J. D., Johnson, D. K., Thomas, T. S., Subramaniam, D., Polshak, T., & Sarnak, M. J. (2017). Prevalence and correlates of cognitive impairment in kidney transplant recipients. *BMC Nephrology, 18*(1). Advance online publication. DOI: 10.1186/s12882-017-0570-1

Gurwitz, J. H. (2023). The Paradoxical Decline of Geriatric Medicine as a Profession. *Journal of the American Medical Association, 330*(8), 693–694. DOI: 10.1001/jama.2023.11110 PMID: 37540519

Gustafsson, L.-K., Asztalos Morell, I., Johansson, C., & De, S. (2022). Informal caregiving from the perspectives of older people living alone in India. *International Journal of Older People Nursing, 17*(6), e12468. DOI: 10.1111/opn.12468 PMID: 35466547

Gutiérrez-Sánchez, D., Gómez-García, R., Cuesta-Vargas, A. I., & Pérez-Cruzado, D. (2020). The suffering measurement instruments in palliative care: A systematic review of psychometric properties. *International Journal of Nursing Studies, 110*, 103704. DOI: 10.1016/j.ijnurstu.2020.103704

Guzzon, A.. (2023). Cost-effectiveness of supportive and palliative care interventions. *Systematic Reviews*.

Hagarty, A. M., Bush, S. H., Talarico, R., Lapenskie, J., & Tanuseputro, P. (2020). Severe pain at the end of life: A population-level observational study. *BMC Palliative Care, 19*(1). Advance online publication. DOI: 10.1186/s12904-020-00569-2 PMID: 32354364

Hagelin, C. L., Melin-Johansson, C., Ek, K., Henoch, I., Österlind, J., & Browall, M. (2022). Teaching about death and dying—A national mixed-methods survey of palliative care education provision in Swedish undergraduate nursing programmes. *Scandinavian Journal of Caring Sciences*, *36*(2), 545–557. PMID: 34962307

Hajizadeh, M., & Nghiem, H. S. (2011). Out-of-pocket expenditures for hospital care in Iran: Who is at risk of incurring catastrophic payments? *International Journal of Health Care Finance and Economics*, *11*(4), 267–285. DOI: 10.1007/s10754-011-9099-1 PMID: 21915727

Hall, C. C., Cook, J., Maddocks, M., Skipworth, R. J. E., Fallon, M., & Laird, B. J. (2019). Combined exercise and nutritional rehabilitation in outpatients with incurable cancer: a systematic review. *Supportive care in cancer: official journal of the Multinational Association of Supportive Care in Cancer, 27*(7), 2371-2384. doi:DOI: 10.1007/s00520-019-04749-6

Hamasaki, H. (2025). The Relationship Between Socioeconomic Status and Health Behaviors in Older Adults: A Narrative Review. *Healthcare (Switzerland)*, *13*(14), 1–22. DOI: 10.3390/healthcare13141669 PMID: 40724694

Hamideh, D., & Nebeker, C. (2020). The Digital Health Landscape in Addiction and Substance Use Research: Will Digital Health Exacerbate or Mitigate Health Inequities in Vulnerable Populations? *Current Addiction Reports*, *7*(3), 317–332. DOI: 10.1007/s40429-020-00325-9

Hampton, M., Baydala, A., Bourassa, C., McKenna, B., & Saul, G., MckKay-McNabb, K., Goodwill, K., Clark, V., & Christiansen, J. (2011). Seven Years of Completing the Circle. *End-of-Life Care With Aboriginal Families.*, *43*(3), 119–125.

Han, G., & Ceilley, R. (2017). Chronic Wound Healing: A Review of Current Management and Treatments. *Advances in Therapy*, *34*(3), 599–610. DOI: 10.1007/s12325-017-0478-y PMID: 28108895

Hanna, J. R., McConnell, T., Harrison, C., Patynowska, K. A., Finucane, A. M., Hudson, B., Paradine, S., McCullagh, A., & Reid, J. (2022). 'There's something about admitting that you are lonely' – prevalence, impact and solutions to loneliness in terminal illness : An explanatory sequential multi-methods study. *Palliative Medicine*, *36*(10), 1483–1492. DOI: 10.1177/02692163221122269 PMID: 36081273

Hanna, M. G., Pantanowitz, L., Jackson, B., Palmer, O., Visweswaran, S., Pantanowitz, J., & Rashidi, H. H. (2025). Ethical and bias considerations in artificial intelligence/machine learning. *Modern Pathology*, *38*(3), 100686.

Hansen, M. B., Rojas-Concha, L., Petersen, M. A., Adsersen, M., & Groenvold, M. (2024). Differences in palliative care needs between cancer patients and non-cancer patients at the start of specialized palliative care: A nationwide register-based study. *Palliative Medicine*. Advance online publication. DOI: 10.1177/02692163241269705 PMID: 39194071

Haraldsson, E. (2006).. . *Nordic Psychology*.

Harding, R. (2003). Current HIV/AIDS end-of-life care in sub-Saharan Africa: A survey of models, services, challenges and priorities. *BMC Public Health*.

Hardman, R., Begg, S., & Spelten, E. (2021). Multimorbidity and its effect on perceived burden, capacity and the ability to self-manage in a low-income rural primary care population: A qualitative study. *PLoS One*, *16*(8), e0255802. DOI: 10.1371/journal.pone.0255802 PMID: 34370758

Harries, R. L., Bosanquet, D. C., & Harding, K. G. (2016). Wound bed preparation: TIME for an update. *Int Wound J, 13 Suppl 3*(Suppl 3), 8-14. doi:DOI: 10.1111/iwj.12662

Harris, K. A., Howell, D. S., & Spurgeon, D. W. (2018). Faith concepts in psychology: Three 30-year definitional content analyses. *Psychology of Religion and Spirituality*, *10*(1), 1.

Hartanto, A., Sim, L., Lee, D., Majeed, N. M., & Yong, J. C. (2024). Cultural contexts differentially shape parents' loneliness and wellbeing during the empty nest period. *Communications Psychology*, *2*(1), 105. DOI: 10.1038/s44271-024-00156-8 PMID: 39489810

Harwood, J., Afsan, C., & Chetna. (2025). Measuring and monitoring the quality of dying in the UN Decade of Healthy Ageing. *The Lancelet Healthy Longevity*, 100739.

Hassan, S. M., Okoli, E. C., Azike, C. A., Okoye, N. A., & Adindu, N. K. (2024). Assessing the Impact of Community Health Workforce on the Efficiency and Accessibility of Healthcare Delivery. *Archives of Current Research International*, *24*(10), 167–173. DOI: 10.9734/acri/2024/v24i10918

Haveman, M. E., van Melzen, R., Schuurmann, R. C., El Moumni, M., Hermens, H. J., Tabak, M., & de Vries, J. P. P. (2021). Continuous monitoring of vital signs with the Everion biosensor on the surgical ward: a clinical validation study. Expert review of medical devices, 18(sup1), 145-152.

Hedman, C., Fürst, P., Strang, P., Schelin, M. E. C., Lundström, S., & Martinsson, L. (2024). Pain prevalence and pain relief in end-of-life care – a national registry study. *BMC Palliative Care*, *23*(1), 171. DOI: 10.1186/s12904-024-01497-1 PMID: 39004730

Heerschap, C., Nicholas, A., & Whitehead, M. (2019). Wound management: Investigating the interprofessional decision-making process. *International Wound Journal*, *16*(1), 233–242. DOI: 10.1111/iwj.13017 PMID: 30393966

Heiskanen, V., & Hamblin, M. R. (2018). Photobiomodulation: Lasers vs. light emitting diodes? *Photochemical & Photobiological Sciences*, *17*(8), 1003–1017. DOI: 10.1039/c8pp90049c PMID: 30044464

Helmer, P., Glück, J., & Anastasiadis, A.. (2025). The use of wearable sensor technology to enhance supportive care in hospitalized palliative patients (Support trial): A prospective preliminary pilot study. *BMC Palliative Care*, *24*, 154. DOI: 10.1186/s12904-025-01794-3

Henderson, M., MacGregor, E., Sykes, N., & Hotopf, M. (2006). The use of benzodiazepines in palliative care. *Palliative Medicine*, *20*(4), 407–412. DOI: 10.1191/0269216306pm1151oa PMID: 16875110

Henry, C., & Hayes, A. (2009). Promoting high quality care for all at the end of life: Review of NHS National End of Life Care Programme 2004-2007 and implications for primary care. *London Journal of Primary Care*, *2*(2), 96–101. DOI: 10.1080/17571472.2009.11493261

Henry, M., Asuzu, C., Savard, S., Devault-Tousignant, C., Timmermans, S., Khosravi, K., Amin, A., Albert, J., Krochmalnek, T., & Odiyo, P. (2024). Psychosocial and palliative care in African national cancer control plans: A qualitative study. *Psycho-Oncology*, *33*(5), e6346. PMID: 38743345

Higginson, I. J. (2015). Palliative care delivery models. In N. Cherny, M. Fallon, S. Kaasa, R. K. Portenoy, & D. C. Currow (Eds.), *Oxford Textbook of Palliative Medicine* (pp. 0). Oxford University Press. https://doi.org/DOI: 10.1093/med/9780199656097.003.0012

Higginson, I. J., Bausewein, C., Reilly, C. C., Gao, W., Gysels, M., Dzingina, M., McCrone, P., Booth, S., & Jolley, C. J. (2014). An integrated palliative and respiratory care service for patients with advanced disease and refractory breathlessness: A randomised controlled trial. *The Lancet. Respiratory Medicine*, *2*(12), 979–987. DOI: 10.1016/S2213-2600(14)70226-7

Higginson, I. J., Reilly, C. C., Bausewein, C., Jolley, C. J., & Gysels, M. (2013). The quality of dying and death in a hospital setting for patients with advanced cancer. *Journal of Pain and Symptom Management, 45*(6), 1054–1064. DOI: 10.1016/j.jpainsymman.2012.06.010

Hirano, L. A., & Kang, G. (2023). Primary Palliative Care Education for Geriatricians: Lessons Learned. *Current Geriatrics Reports, 12*(3), 85–92.

Hofmann, S. G., Grossman, P., & Hinton, D. E. (2011). Loving-kindness and compassion meditation: Potential for psychological interventions. *Clinical Psychology Review, 31*(7), 1126–1132. DOI: 10.1016/j.cpr.2011.07.003

Hökkä, M., Melender, H.-L., Lehto, J. T., & Kaakinen, P. (2021). Palliative nursing competencies required for different levels of palliative care provision: A qualitative analysis of health care professionals' perspectives. *Journal of Palliative Medicine, 24*(10), 1516–1524. PMID: 33720785

Ho, Kwong, & al., S. c. (2022). Decision-making preferences on end-of-life care for older people: Exploration and comparison of Japan, the Hong Kong SAR and South Korea in East Asia. *Journal of Clinical Nursing.*

Holzer, K. J., Vaughn, M. G., Loux, T. M., Mancini, M. A., Fearn, N. E., & Wallace, C. L. (2022). Prevalence and correlates of antisocial personality disorder in older adults. *Aging & Mental Health, 26*(1), 169–178. PMID: 33107330

House, S. A., Schoo, C., & Ogilvie, W. A. (2025). Advance Directives. In *StatPearls* [Internet]. StatPearls Publishing., https://www.ncbi.nlm.nih.gov/books/NBK459133/

Hudson, P. L., Remedios, C., & Thomas, K. (2010). A systematic review of psychosocial interventions for family carers of palliative care patients. *BMC Palliative Care, 9*, 17. DOI: 10.1186/1472-684X-9-17

Hudson, P., Collins, A., Boughey, M., & Philip, J. (2021). Reframing palliative care to improve the quality of life of people diagnosed with a serious illness. *The Medical Journal of Australia, 215*(10), 443. PMID: 34676567

Hui, D., Abdelghani, E., Chen, J., Dibaj, S., Zhukovsky, D., Dev, R., Tanco, K., Haider, A., Azhar, A., Reddy, A., Epner, D., Arthur, J., Dalal, S., Heung, Y., Reddy, S., De La Cruz, M., Liu, D., & Bruera, E. (2020). Chronic Non-Malignant Pain in Patients with Cancer Seen at a Timely Outpatient Palliative Care Clinic. *Cancers (Basel), 12*(1), 214. DOI: 10.3390/cancers12010214 PMID: 31952220

Hui, D., & Bruera, E. (2020). Models of palliative care delivery for patients with cancer. *Journal of Clinical Oncology, 38*(9), 852–865. PMID: 32023157

Hui, D., dos Santos, R., Chisholm, G., Bansal, S., Souza Crovador, C., & Bruera, E. (2015). Clinical signs of impending death in cancer patients. *The Oncologist, 19*(6), 681–687. DOI: 10.1634/theoncologist.2013-0457

Hui, D., Hannon, B. L., Zimmermann, C., & Bruera, E. (2018). Improving patient and caregiver outcomes in oncology: Team-based, timely, and targeted palliative care. *CA: a Cancer Journal for Clinicians, 68*(5), 356–376. PMID: 30277572

Hui, D., Morgado, M., Vidal, M., Withers, L., Nguyen, Q., Chisholm, G., & Bruera, E. (2013). Dyspnea in hospitalized advanced cancer patients: Subjective and physiologic correlates. *Journal of Palliative Medicine, 16*(3), 274–280. DOI: 10.1089/jpm.2012.0364

Ifrim, R. A., Klugarová, J., Măguri ă, D., Zazu, M., Mazilu, D. C., & Klugar, M. (2022). Communication, an important link between healthcare providers: A best practice implementation project. *JBI Evidence Implementation, 20*(S1), S41–S48. PMID: 36372792

Ighodaro, A., Stefanovics, E., Makanjuola, V., & Rosenheck, R. (2015). An assessment of attitudes towards people with mental illness among medical students and physicians in Ibadan, Nigeria. *Academic Psychiatry, 39*, 280–285. PMID: 24903130

Iida, K., Ryan, A., Payne, S., Hasson, F., & McIlfatrick, S. (2022). Palliative care in Japanese long-term care facilities. *International Journal of Palliative Nursing, 28*(1), 28–37. PMID: 35094533

Iordanou, P., Baltopoulos, G., Giannakopoulou, M., Bellou, P., & Ktenas, E. (2002). Effect of polarized light in the healing process of pressure ulcers. *International Journal of Nursing Practice, 8*(1), 49–55. DOI: 10.1046/j.1440-172x.2002.00338.x PMID: 11831427

Irumba, P., Tugume, D., & Apuulison, D. (2024). Advances in Multidisciplinary Approach for Liver Cancer. *Liver Cancer-Multidisciplinary Approach: Multidisciplinary Approach*, 3.

Irving, J. A., Dobkin, P. L., & Park, J. (2009). Cultivating mindfulness in health care professionals: A review of empirical studies of mindfulness-based stress reduction (MBSR). *Complementary Therapies in Clinical Practice, 15*(2), 61–66. DOI: 10.1016/j.ctcp.2009.01.002

Iyawa, G. E., Herselman, M., & Botha, A. (2016). Digital Health Innovation Ecosystems: From Systematic Literature Review to Conceptual Framework. *Procedia Computer Science, 100*, 244–252. https://doi.org/https://doi.org/10.1016/j.procs.2016.09.149

Iype, T., Rani, P., & Kuriakose, R. (2014). The burden of caregiving for bedridden elderly patients in India. *International Journal of Community Medicine and Public Health, 1*(1), 12–17.

Jack, K., Ridley, C., & Turner, S. (2024). Effective communication with older people. *Nursing Older People, 36*(3). PMID: 31468756

Jaffray, L., Bridgman, H., Stephens, M., & Skinner, T. (2016). Evaluating the effects of mindfulness-based interventions for informal palliative caregivers: A systematic literature review. *Palliative Medicine, 30*(2), 117–131. DOI: 10.1177/0269216315600331

Jamtvedt, G., Dahm, K. T., Christie, A., Moe, R. H., Haavardsholm, E., Holm, I., & Hagen, K. B. (2008). Physical Therapy Interventions for Patients With Osteoarthritis of the Knee: An Overview of Systematic Reviews. *Physical Therapy, 88*(1), 123–136. DOI: 10.2522/ptj.20070043

Jang, H., Lee, K., Kim, S., & Kim, S. (2022). Unmet needs in palliative care for patients with common non-cancer diseases: A cross-sectional study. *BMC Palliative Care, 21*(1). Advance online publication. DOI: 10.1186/s12904-022-01040-0 PMID: 36038840

Janssens, J. P. (2005). Aging of the respiratory system: Impact on pulmonary function tests and adaptation to exertion. *Clinics in Chest Medicine, 26*(3), 469–484. DOI: 10.1016/j.ccm.2005.05.004

Järbrink, K., Ni, G., Sönnergren, H., Schmidtchen, A., Pang, C., Bajpai, R., & Car, J. (2017). The humanistic and economic burden of chronic wounds: A protocol for a systematic review. *Systematic Reviews, 6*(1), 15. DOI: 10.1186/s13643-016-0400-8 PMID: 28118847

Jencks, S. F., Williams, M. V., & Coleman, E. A. (2009). Rehospitalizations among patients in the Medicare fee-for-service program. *The New England Journal of Medicine, 360*(14), 1418–1428. DOI: 10.1056/NEJMsa0803563 PMID: 19339721

Jennings, A. L., Davies, A. N., Higgins, J. P., & Broadley, K. (2001). Opioids for the palliation of breathlessness in terminal illness. *Cochrane Database of Systematic Reviews, 2001*(4), CD002066. Advance online publication. DOI: 10.1002/14651858.CD002066

Jennings, A. L., Davies, A. N., Higgins, J. P., Gibbs, J. S., & Broadley, K. E. (2002). A systematic review of the use of opioids in the management of dyspnea. *Thorax, 57*(11), 939–944. DOI: 10.1136/thorax.57.11.939

Jensen, E., Kristensen, J. K., Bjerglund, R. T., Johnsen, S. P., & Thomsen, J. L. (2022). The pathway and characteristics of patients with non-specific symptoms of cancer: A systematic review. *BMC Cancer*, *22*(1). Advance online publication. DOI: 10.1186/s12885-022-09535-y PMID: 35606715

Jeppesen, S. M., Yderstraede, K. B., Rasmussen, B. S., Hanna, M., & Lund, L. (2016). Extracorporeal shockwave therapy in the treatment of chronic diabetic foot ulcers: A prospective randomised trial. *Journal of Wound Care*, *25*(11), 641–649. DOI: 10.12968/jowc.2016.25.11.641 PMID: 27827284

Jesus, T., Papadimitriou, C., Bright, F., Kayes, N., & Cott, C. (2021). What Person-Centered Rehabilitation Means in Concept and Practice: The Person-Centered Rehabilitation Model for Adult Physical Rehabilitation Derived from a Scoping Review and Thematic Synthesis. *Archives of Physical Medicine and Rehabilitation*, *102*(10), e116. DOI: 10.1016/j.apmr.2021.07.465

Jiang, N., Wu, B., & Li, Y. (2024). Caregiving in Asia: Priority areas for research, policy, and practice to support family caregivers. *Health Care Science*, *3*(6), 374–382. DOI: 10.1002/hcs2.124 PMID: 39735283

Jiao, K., & Chow, A. Y. (2023). The connections of physical and psychosocial symptoms among patients with terminal illnesses: A network analysis. *Palliative Medicine*, *37*(1), 120–130. DOI: 10.1177/02692163221128452

Jodie, F., Anna, K., & Ursula, W. (2025). Effectiveness of music therapy, aromatherapy, and massage therapy on patients in palliative care with end-of-life needs: A systematic review. *Journal of Pain and Symptom Management*, *69*(1), 102–113. DOI: 10.1016/j.jpainsymman.2024.07.024

Johnson, M. J., Bland, J. M., & Currow, D. C. (2017). Breathlessness. In The Oxford Textbook of Palliative Medicine (5th ed., pp. 464-478). Oxford University Press.

Jolley, C. J., & Moxham, J. (2021). The neurophysiology of dyspnea. *Journal of Applied Physiology*, *131*(4), 1283–1293. DOI: 10.1152/japplphysiol.00515.2021

Jones, B., Piet, J., Simonsen, J., & Zachariae, R. (2022). Mindfulness-based interventions and physiological stress markers in cancer caregivers: A randomized pilot trial. *Journal of Psychosocial Oncology*, *40*(2), 237–255. DOI: 10.1080/07347332.2021.1872059

Jones, T., Luth, E. A., Lin, S.-Y., & Brody, A. A. (2021). Advance care planning, palliative care, and end-of-life care interventions for racial and ethnic underrepresented groups: A systematic review. *Journal of Pain and Symptom Management*, *62*(3), e248–e260. PMID: 33984460

Jordan, R. I., Allsop, M. J., ElMokhallalati, Y., Jackson, C. E., Edwards, H. L., Chapman, E. J., & Bennett, M. I. (2020). Duration of palliative care before death in international routine practice: A systematic review and meta-analysis. *BMC Medicine, 18*(1), 368–368. DOI: 10.1186/s12916-020-01829-x

Juckett, G., & Unger, K. (2014). Appropriate use of medical interpreters. *American Family Physician, 90*(7), 476–480. PMID: 25369625

Juergens, M. C., Seekatz, B., Moosdorf, R. G., Petrie, K. J., & Rief, W. (2010). Illness beliefs before cardiac surgery predict disability, quality of life, and depression 3 months later. *Journal of Psychosomatic Research, 68*(6), 553–560. DOI: 10.1016/j.jpsychores.2009.10.004 PMID: 20488272

Just, J., Schmitz, M.-T., Grabenhorst, U., Joist, T., Horn, K., Engel, B., & Weckbecker, K. (2021). Factors influencing length of survival in ambulatory palliative care - a cross sectional study based on secondary data. *BMC Palliative Care, 20*(1). Advance online publication. DOI: 10.1186/s12904-021-00762-x PMID: 34001099

Kabat-Zinn, J. (1990). *Full catastrophe living: Using the wisdom of your body and mind to face stress, pain, and illness*. Delta., DOI: 10.1037/e481272006-001

Kabat-Zinn, J. (1990). *Stress Reduction Clinic. Full catastrophe living : using the wisdom of your body and mind to face stress, pain, and illness. University of Massachusetts Medical Center/Worcester*. Delacorte Press.

Kabat-Zinn, J. (2003). Mindfulness-based interventions in context: Past, present, and future. *Clinical Psychology : a Publication of the Division of Clinical Psychology of the American Psychological Association, 10*(2), 144–156. DOI: 10.1093/clipsy.bpg016

Kaihlanen, A.-M., Ruotsalainen, S., Väisänen, V., Corneliusson, L., Pesonen, T., & Sinervo, T. (2023). Job demand and job resource factors explaining stress and job satisfaction among home care nurses – a mixed-methods sequential explanatory study. *BMC Nursing, 22*(1), 404. DOI: 10.1186/s12912-023-01568-3 PMID: 37891583

Kaiser, A. H., Mao, S., Sundewall, J., Ross, M., Koy, S., Vorn, S., Koeut, P., & Ekman, B. (2025). Assessing the determinants of out-of-pocket health expenditures among Cambodian households in informal employment using survey data. *International Journal for Equity in Health, 24*(1), 33. DOI: 10.1186/s12939-025-02394-6 PMID: 39891289

Kaiser, A. H., Rotigliano, N., Flessa, S., Ekman, B., & Sundewall, J. (2023). Extending universal health coverage to informal workers: A systematic review of health financing schemes in low- and middle-income countries in Southeast Asia. *PLoS One*, *18*(7), e0288269. DOI: 10.1371/journal.pone.0288269 PMID: 37432943

Kako, J., Morita, T., Yamaguchi, T., Kobayashi, M., Sekimoto, A., Kinoshita, H., & Ogawa, A. (2018). Fan therapy is effective in relieving dyspnea in patients with terminally ill cancer: A parallel-arm, randomized controlled trial. *Journal of Pain and Symptom Management*, *56*(4), 493–500. DOI: 10.1016/j.jpainsymman.2018.07.001

Kalaf, E. P., de Souza, P., & Mari, J. J. (2020). Problem-solving therapy versus mindfulness intervention for caregivers of chronic patients: A randomized pilot study. *Clinical Psychology & Psychotherapy*, *27*(2), 187–198.

Kalantari, A. R., Mehrolhassani, M. H., Shati, M., & Dehnavieh, R. (2021). Health service delivery models for elderly people: A systematic review. *Medical Journal of the Islamic Republic of Iran*, *35*, 21. PMID: 34169033

Kalantar-Zadeh, K., Lockwood, M. B., Rhee, C. M., Tantisattamo, E., Andreoli, S., Balducci, A., Laffin, P., Harris, T., Knight, R., Kumaraswami, L., Liakopoulos, V., Lui, S.-F., Kumar, S., Ng, M., Saadi, G., Ulasi, I., Tong, A., & Li, P. K.-T. (2022). Patient-centred approaches for the management of unpleasant symptoms in kidney disease. *Nature Reviews. Nephrology*, *18*(1). Advance online publication. DOI: 10.1038/s41581-021-00518-z PMID: 34980890

Kallas, J., Sterling, M. R., Ajayi, O., Mulroy, E., Kuo, E., Ming, J., Dell, N., & Avgar, A. C. (2023). Making a Bad Situation Worse: Examining the Challenges Facing Rural Home Care Workers. *Journal of Applied Gerontology : The Official Journal of the Southern Gerontological Society*, *42*(4), 768–775. DOI: 10.1177/07334648221134793 PMID: 36510645

Kallis, G. (2025). Exploring the challenges experienced by patients and families using palliative and end-of-life care services: A qualitative focus group study. *Palliative & Supportive Care*.

Kamal Elmasry, A., Elawam, A., Sweed, H., & Fahmy Tolba, M. (2024). Symptoms Burden in Elderly Female Patients Receiving Palliative Care. *EJGG.2024 , 11*(1), 86–97. https://ejgg.journals.ekb.eg/article_350627_e60ab735671bde8a1cf6003fa4beb927.pdf

Kamal, A. H., Maguire, J. M., Wheeler, J. L., Currow, D. C., & Abernethy, A. P. (2012). Dyspnea Review for the Palliative Care Professional: Treatment Goals and Therapeutic Options. *Journal of Palliative Medicine*, *15*(1), 106–114. DOI: 10.1089/jpm.2011.0110

Kamal, A., Currow, D., Bull, J., Ritchie, C., Kutner, J., & Abernethy, A. (2012). The Value of Data Collection to Palliative Care Program Sustainability and Growth (521). *Journal of Pain and Symptom Management, 43*(2), 413–414.

Kane, L., Portman, R. M., Eberhardt, J., Walker, L., Proctor, E.-L., Poulter, H., & O'Neill, C. (2023). Peer supporters' mental health and emotional wellbeing needs: Key factors and opportunities for co-produced training. *Health Expectations, 26*(6), 2387–2395. https://doi.org/https://doi.org/10.1111/hex.13836 PMID: 37565576

Kang, K.-A., Kim, D.-B., Koh, S.-J., Park, M.-H., Park, H. Y., Yoon, D. H., Yoon, S.-J., Lee, S.-J., Choi, J.-E., Han, H.-S., & Chun, J. (2023). Spiritual Care Guide in Hospice Palliative Care. *Journal of Hospice and Palliative Care, 26*(4), 149–159. DOI: 10.14475/jhpc.2023.26.4.149 PMID: 38075589

Kang, K., & Bacci, S. (2022). Photodynamic Therapy. *Biomedicines, 10*, 2701. DOI: 10.3390/biomedicines10112701

Kao, H., Conant, R., Soriano, T., & McCormick, W. (2009). The Past, Present, and Future of House Calls. *Clinics in Geriatric Medicine, 25*(1), 19–34. DOI: 10.1016/j.cger.2008.10.005 PMID: 19217490

Kapoor, Y., & Orr, R. (2016). Effect of therapeutic massage on pain in patients with dementia. *Dementia (London), 16*(1), 119–125. DOI: 10.1177/1471301215583391

Katz, G. M., Arigoni, D., Rice, M. B., & Stall, N. M. (2025). Addressing the Health Impacts of Climate Change in Older Adults. *JAMA Internal Medicine, 185*(4), 362–363. PMID: 39899284

Kawalpreet, K., Rinalben, P., & Ravita, S. (2024). *Managing Anxiety in Palliative Care: Nurses' Non-Pharmacological Intervention.* https://www.theseus.fi/bitstream/handle/10024/886071/Kaur_Parmar_Sharma.pdf?sequence=2

Kawasaki, L., Mushahwar, V. K., Ho, C., Dukelow, S. P., Chan, L. L., & Chan, K. M. (2014). The mechanisms and evidence of efficacy of electrical stimulation for healing of pressure ulcer: A systematic review. *Wound Repair and Regeneration, 22*(2), 161–173. DOI: 10.1111/wrr.12134 PMID: 24372691

Kayonga, C. S., Ristolainen, H., & Lisko, I., Mäki- Petäjä-Leinonen, A., & Tiilikainen, E. (2025). Association Between Social Support and Quality of Life: Cross-Sectional Study Among Older Adults Receiving Home Care Services in Finland. *Home Health Care Management & Practice.* Advance online publication. DOI: 10.1177/10848223251385092

Kelley, A. S., Back, A. L., Arnold, R. M., Goldberg, G. R., Lim, B. B., Litrivis, E., Smith, C. B., & O'Neill, L. B. (2012). Geritalk: Communication skills training for geriatric and palliative medicine fellows. *Journal of the American Geriatrics Society*, *60*(2), 332–337. PMID: 22211768

Kemp, C. (1997). *Terminal illness: A guide to nursing care* (2nd ed.). Lippincott.

Kent, E. E., Rowland, J. H., Northouse, L., Litzelman, K., Chou, W. Y. S., Shelburne, N., Timura, C., O'Mara, A., & Huss, K. (2016). Caring for caregivers and patients: Research and clinical priorities for informal cancer caregiving. *Cancer*, *122*(13), 1987–1995. DOI: 10.1002/cncr.29939

Kernick, L., Glare, P., Hosie, A., Chiu, A., & Kissane, D. W. (2023). Prevalence and management of chronic nonmalignant pain in palliative care populations: A systematic review. *Palliative & Supportive Care*, *22*(4), 1–7. DOI: 10.1017/s1478951523000378 PMID: 37039456

Khaldouni, S., Amane, M., Lamtali, S., Boussaa, S., El Rhanbouri, M., Oussous, A., & Laghouasli, F. (2025). Implementation of Advanced Nursing Practices Through the Adoption of a Patient-Centered Approach. In Amane, M., & Boussaa, S. (Eds.), *Advanced Nursing Practices for Clinical Excellence* (pp. 305–348). IGI Global., DOI: 10.4018/979-8-3693-6730-8.ch014

Khan, H. T., Addo, K. M., & Findlay, H. (2024). Public health challenges and responses to the growing ageing populations. *Public Health Challenges*, *3*(3), e213.

Khan, R., Khan, S., Almohaimeed, H. M., Almars, A. I., & Pari, B. (2025). Utilization, challenges, and training needs of digital health technologies: Perspectives from healthcare professionals. *International Journal of Medical Informatics*, *197*, 105833. https://doi.org/https://doi.org/10.1016/j.ijmedinf.2025.105833 PMID: 39954392

Kibret, A. A., Wolde, H. F., Molla, M. D., Aragie, H., Getnet Adugna, D., Tafesse, E., Melese, E. B., Worku, Y. B., & Belay, D. G. (2022). Factors associated with adherence to guidelines in cancer pain management among adult patients evaluated at oncology unit, in the University of Gondar Comprehensive Specialized Hospital, Northwest Ethiopia. *Frontiers in Pain Research (Lausanne, Switzerland)*, *3*. Advance online publication. DOI: 10.3389/fpain.2022.884253 PMID: 35978991

Kimberg, L. (2019). Trauma and Trauma-Informed Care. *Trauma-Informed Healthcare Approaches: A Guide for Primary Care*, 25-56.

Kim, M.-J., Ahn, K.-H., & Jung, Y. (2002). Distribution of inorganic arsenic species in mine tailings of abandoned mines from Korea. *Chemosphere*, *49*(3), 307–312. https://doi.org/https://doi.org/10.1016/S0045-6535(02)00307-7 PMID: 12363309

Kim, Y., Carver, C. S., Shaffer, K. M., & Cannady, R. S. (2021). Cortisol patterns and psychological distress among spouses of patients with terminal cancer. *Health Psychology*, *40*(8), 530–539. DOI: 10.1037/hea0001124

Kim, Y., & Kim, D.-H. (2024). Interventions for family involvement enhance end-of-life care for hospitalized patients : An integrative review. *BMC Nursing*, *23*(1), 917. DOI: 10.1186/s12912-024-02538-z PMID: 39695593

Kinjo, K., Sairenji, T., Koga, H., Osugi, Y., Yoshida, S., Ichinose, H., Nagai, Y., Imura, H., South-Paul, J. E., Meyer, M., & Honda, Y. (2017). Cost of physician-led home visit care (Zaitaku care) compared with hospital care at the end of life in Japan. *BMC Health Services Research*, *17*(1), 40. DOI: 10.1186/s12913-016-1961-x PMID: 28095906

Klint, Å., Bondesson, E., Rasmussen, B. H., Fürst, C. J., & Schelin, M. E. C. (2019). Dying With Unrelieved Pain—Prescription of Opioids Is Not Enough. *Journal of Pain and Symptom Management*, *58*(5), 784–791.e1. DOI: 10.1016/j.jpainsymman.2019.07.006 PMID: 31319106

Kloth, L. C. (2009). The role of physical therapy in wound management - part one. *The Journal of the American College of Certified Wound Specialists*, *1*(1), 4–5. DOI: 10.1016/j.jcws.2008.08.001 PMID: 24527101

Knaul, a. (2018). Alleviating the access abyss in palliative care and pain relief-an imperative of universal health coverage: The Lancet Commission report. *Lancet*, *391*(10128), 1391–1454. DOI: 10.1016/s0140-6736(17)32513-8

Knaul, F. M., Arreola-Ornelas, H., Kwete, X. J., Bhadelia, A., Rosa, W. E., Touchton, M., Méndez-Carniado, O., Enciso, V. V., Pastrana, T., & Friedman, J. R. (2025). The evolution of serious health-related suffering from 1990 to 2021: An update to The Lancet Commission on global access to palliative care and pain relief. *The Lancet. Global Health*, *13*(3), e422–e436. PMID: 40021301

Koehlmoos, T. P., Anwar, S., & Cravioto, A. (2011). Global health: chronic diseases and other emergent issues in global health. *Infectious Disease Clinics of North America*, *25*(3), 623–638, ix. https://doi.org/DOI: 10.1016/j.idc.2011.05.008

Koel, G., & Houghton, P. E. (2014). Electrostimulation: Current Status, Strength of Evidence Guidelines, and Meta-Analysis. *Advances in Wound Care (New Rochelle, N.Y.)*, *3*(2), 118–126. DOI: 10.1089/wound.2013.0448 PMID: 24761352

Koenig, H. G. (2012). Religion, spirituality, and health: The research and clinical implications. *ISRN Psychiatry*, *2012*, 1–33. DOI: 10.5402/2012/278730

Koper, I., Pasman, H. R. W., Schweitzer, B. P. M., Kuin, A., & Onwuteaka-Philipsen, B. D. (2019). Spiritual care at the end of life in the primary care setting : Experiences from spiritual caregivers - a mixed methods study. *BMC Palliative Care, 18*(1), 98. DOI: 10.1186/s12904-019-0484-8 PMID: 31706355

Kottner, J., Cuddigan, J., Carville, K., Balzer, K., Berlowitz, D., Law, S., & Haesler, E. (2019). Prevention and treatment of pressure ulcers/injuries: The protocol for the second update of the international Clinical Practice Guideline 2019. *Journal of Tissue Viability, 28*(2), 51–58. DOI: 10.1016/j.jtv.2019.01.001 PMID: 30658878

Kovačević, I., Majerić Kogler, V., Krikšić, V., Ilić, B., Friganović, A., Ozimec Vulinec, Š., Pavić, J., Milošević, M., Kovačević, P., & Petek, D. (2022). Non-Medical Factors Associated with the Outcome of Treatment of Chronic Non-Malignant Pain: A Cross-Sectional Study. *International Journal of Environmental Research and Public Health, 19*(5), 2881. DOI: 10.3390/ijerph19052881 PMID: 35270575

Krakauer, E. L. (2025). Palliative Care: Toward a More Responsive Definition. In *Textbook of palliative care* (pp. 115–119). Springer.

Krikorian, A., Maldonado, C., & Pastrana, T. (2020). Patient's Perspectives on the Notion of a Good Death: A Systematic Review of the Literature. *Journal of Pain and Symptom Management, 59*(1), 152–164. DOI: 10.1016/j.jpainsymman.2019.07.033

Krishnaswami, A., Bernacki, G. M., & Bhatt, D. L. (2022). Geriatric and palliative care specialists as valued members of the multidisciplinary heart team. *The American Journal of Medicine, 135*(7), 810–812. PMID: 35134366

Krist, A. H., Tong, S. T., Aycock, R. A., & Longo, D. R. (2017). Engaging Patients in Decision-Making and Behavior Change to Promote Prevention. *Studies in Health Technology and Informatics, 240*, 284–302. PMID: 28972524

Kruger, E. A., Pires, M., Ngann, Y., Sterling, M., & Rubayi, S. (2013). Comprehensive management of pressure ulcers in spinal cord injury: Current concepts and future trends. *The Journal of Spinal Cord Medicine, 36*(6), 572–585. DOI: 10.1179/2045772313y.0000000093 PMID: 24090179

Kuebler, K., Monroe, T., Ricciardi, R., Westlake, C., Sorenson, M., Pederson, J., & Bruera, E. (2024). Integration of palliative care in the management of multiple chronic conditions: An expert consensus paper with policy implications. *Nursing Outlook, 72*(6), 102273.

Kuffler, D. P. (2015). Improving the ability to eliminate wounds and pressure ulcers. *Wound Repair and Regeneration, 23*(3), 312–317. DOI: 10.1111/wrr.12284 PMID: 25801293

Kuipers, S. J., Nieboer, A. P., & Cramm, J. M. (2021). Easier said than done: Healthcare professionals' barriers to the provision of patient-centered primary care to patients with multimorbidity. *International Journal of Environmental Research and Public Health, 18*(11), 6057. PMID: 34199866

Kumari, & Rajapaska. (2025). Global equality, complicated systems and assisted death in palliative care. *International Journal of Palliative Nursing.*

Kumar, S. P., & Jim, A. (2010). Physical therapy in palliative care: from symptom control to quality of life: a critical review. *Indian Journal of Palliative Care, 16*(3), 138–146. DOI: 10.4103/0973-1075.73670

Kumlin, M., Berg, G. V., Kvigne, K., & Hellesø, R. (2020). Elderly patients with complex health problems in the care trajectory: A qualitative case study. *BMC Health Services Research, 20,* 1–10.

Kwak, J., & Salmon, J. (2007). Attitudes and preferences of Korean-American older adults and caregivers on end-of-life care. *Journal of the American Geriatrics Society, 55*(11). Advance online publication. DOI: 10.1111/j.1532-5415.2007.01394.x PMID: 17727642

Labson, M. C. (2015)... *Innovative and Successful Approaches To Improving Care Transitions From Hospital to Home., 33*(2), 88–95.

Lam, T.-C., Chan, S.-K., Choi, C.-W., Tsang, K.-C., Yuen, K.-K., Soong, I., Wong, K.-H., Lui, L., Lo, S.-H., & Tong, M. (2021). Integrative palliative care service model improved end-of-life care and overall survival of advanced cancer patients in Hong Kong: A review of ten-year territory-wide cohort. *Journal of Palliative Medicine, 24*(9), 1314–1320. PMID: 33507834

Landers, S. H. (2006). Home care: A key to the future of family medicine? *Annals of Family Medicine, 4*(4), 366–368. DOI: 10.1370/afm.550 PMID: 16868241

Landers, S., Madigan, E., Leff, B., Rosati, R. J., McCann, B. A., Hornbake, R., MacMillan, R., Jones, K., Bowles, K., Dowding, D., Lee, T., Moorhead, T., Rodriguez, S., & Breese, E. (2016). The Future of Home Health Care: A Strategic Framework for Optimizing Value. *Home Health Care Management & Practice, 28*(4), 262–278. DOI: 10.1177/1084822316666368 PMID: 27746670

Larking, A. M., Duport, S., Clinton, M., Hardy, M., & Andrews, K. (2010). Randomized control of extracorporeal shock wave therapy versus placebo for chronic decubitus ulceration. *Clinical Rehabilitation, 24*(3), 222–229. DOI: 10.1177/0269215509346083 PMID: 20156981

LaRocca-Pitts, M. (2015). Four FACTs spiritual assessment tool. *Journal of Health Care Chaplaincy*, *21*(2), 51–59. PMID: 25793421

Larsen, L. T. (2022). Not merely the absence of disease: A genealogy of the WHO's positive health definition. *History of the Human Sciences*, *35*(1), 111–131.

Latimer, S., Chaboyer, W., Thalib, L., McInnes, E., Bucknall, T., & Gillespie, B. M. (2019). Pressure injury prevalence and predictors among older adults in the first 36 hours of hospitalisation. *Journal of Clinical Nursing*, *28*(21-22), 4119–4127. DOI: 10.1111/jocn.14967 PMID: 31216388

Lauffenburger, J. C., Robinson, J. G., Oramasionwu, C., & Brookhart, M. A. (2019). Racial/ethnic and gender disparities in the use of high-risk medications among Medicare beneficiaries. *Journal of the American Geriatrics Society*, *67*(11), 2296–2302. DOI: 10.1111/jgs.16071

Lazzaroni, L., Bellotti, F., & Berta, R. (2024). An embedded end-to-end voice assistant. *Engineering Applications of Artificial Intelligence*, *136*, 108998.

Leao, D. L. L., Cremers, H.-P., van Veghel, D., Pavlova, M., & Groot, W. (2023). The Impact of Value-Based Payment Models for Networks of Care and Transmural Care: A Systematic Literature Review. *Applied Health Economics and Health Policy*, *21*(3), 441–466. DOI: 10.1007/s40258-023-00790-z PMID: 36723777

Lee, V., Lam, T., Jing, H., Liu, F., Zhang, Y., Huang, J., & Lee, A. (2019). Integrative palliative cancer care in Hong Kong: An overview and an example from the East. *Clinical Oncology*, *31*(8), 589–594. PMID: 31230834

Lee, Y. J., Kim, S.-H., Yoo, S. H., Kim, A.-S., Lin, C.-P., Martina, D., Mori, M., & Suh, S.-Y. (2024). Advance Care Planning in Palliative Care in Asia: Barriers and Implications. *Journal of Hospice and Palliative Care*, *27*(4), 107. PMID: 39691175

Leff, B., & Burton, J. R. (2001). The future history of home care and physician house calls in the United States. *The Journals of Gerontology. Series A, Biological Sciences and Medical Sciences*, *56*(10), M603–M608. DOI: 10.1093/gerona/56.10.m603 PMID: 11584032

Leff, B., Burton, L., Mader, S. L., Naughton, B., Burl, J., Inouye, S. K., Greenough, W. B.III, Guido, S., Langston, C., & Frick, K. D. (2005). Hospital at home: Feasibility and outcomes of a program to provide hospital-level care at home for acutely ill older patients. *Annals of Internal Medicine*, *143*(11), 798–808. PMID: 16330791

Lei, H., Zhong, K., Chen, Z., Li, P., Chen, J., Li, H., & Zhou, J. (2025). Global Burden of Pressure Ulcer and Contributing Factors from 1990 to 2021: A Systematic Analysis with Forecasts to 2035. *Advances in Wound Care (New Rochelle, N.Y.)*. Advance online publication. DOI: 10.1089/wound.2025.0021 PMID: 40272818

Lei, L., Lu, Y., Gan, Q., Hu, Z., & Luo, Y. (2022). Awareness and perceptions of palliative care among the elderly: A qualitative study. *Journal of Palliative Care*, *37*(2), 204–212. PMID: 35195464

Leininger, M. (2002). Culture care theory: A major contribution to advance transcultural nursing knowledge and practices. *Journal of Transcultural Nursing*, *13*(3), 189–192.

Lei, Y.-Y., Ya, S. R. T., Zheng, Y.-R., & Cui, X.-S. (2023). Effectiveness of nurse-led multidisciplinary interventions in primary health care: A systematic review and meta-analysis. *International Journal of Nursing Practice*, *29*(6), e13133. DOI: 10.1111/ijn.13133 PMID: 36658754

Lengacher, C. A., Reich, R., & Paterson, C.. (2019). Biobehavioral mechanisms of mindfulness-based interventions for cancer caregivers: A systematic review. *Supportive Care in Cancer*, *27*(11), 4209–4222. DOI: 10.1007/s00520-019-04873-7

Lepherd, L. (2015). Spirituality: Everyone has it, but what is it? *International Journal of Nursing Practice*, *21*(5), 566–574. PMID: 24666816

Leppert, W., & Nosek, K. (2019). Comparison of the Quality of Life of Cancer Patients with Pain Treated with Oral Controlled-Release Morphine and Oxycodone and Transdermal Buprenorphine and Fentanyl. *Current Pharmaceutical Design*, *25*(30), 3216–3224. DOI: 10.2174/1381612825666190717091230 PMID: 31333114

Leslye Rojas-Concha, L., Bang Hansen, M., & Groenvold, M. (2024). Symptoms and problems reported by patients with non-cancer diseases through open-ended questions in specialist palliative care: A national register-based study. *Supportive Care in Cancer*, *32*(2). Advance online publication. DOI: 10.1007/s00520-024-08345-1 PMID: 38305835

Leung, A. C.-t., Liu, C.-p., Chow, N. W.-s., & Chi, I. (2004). Cost-benefit analysis of a case management project for the community-dwelling frail elderly in Hong Kong. *Journal of Applied Gerontology*, *23*(1), 70–85.

Li, W. W. (2021). Death Acceptance in Vietnamese Cancer Patients: A Phenomenological Study. *journal of Transcultural Nursing*.

Li, D. M., Parikh, S., & Costa, A. (2025). A critical look into artificial intelligence and healthcare disparities. *Frontiers in Artificial Intelligence*, *8*, 1545869.

Ligibel, J. A., Bohlke, K., May, A. M., Clinton, S. K., Demark-Wahnefried, W., Gilchrist, S. C., & Alfano, C. M. (2022). Exercise, Diet, and Weight Management During Cancer Treatment: ASCO Guideline. *Journal of Clinical Oncology, 40*(22), 2491–2507. DOI: 10.1200/jco.22.00687

Li, K., Cardoso, C., Moctezuma-Ramirez, A., Elgalad, A., & Perin, E. (2023). Heart Rate Variability Measurement through a Smart Wearable Device: Another Breakthrough for Personal Health Monitoring? *International Journal of Environmental Research and Public Health, 20*(24), 7146. DOI: 10.3390/ijerph20247146

Li, L., Yang, Y., Yang, Z., Zheng, M., Luo, G., He, W., & Yin, R. (2022). Effects of ALA-PDT on the macrophages in wound healing and its related mechanisms in vivo and in vitro. *Photodiagnosis and Photodynamic Therapy, 38*, 102816. DOI: 10.1016/j.pdpdt.2022.102816 PMID: 35378277

Lillie, A. K., Read, S., Mallen, C., Croft, P., & McBeth, J. (2013). Musculoskeletal pain in older adults at the end-of-life: A systematic search and critical review of the literature with priorities for future research. *BMC Palliative Care, 12*(1), 27–27. DOI: 10.1186/1472-684X-12-27

Lindauer, A., & Harvath, T. A. (2014). Pre-death grief in the context of dementia caregiving: A concept analysis. *Journal of Advanced Nursing, 70*(10), 2196–2207. DOI: 10.1111/jan.12411

Liu, M. F., Ho, M.-H., Montayre, J., Wang, Y.-W., & Lin, C.-C. (2021). Palliative care development in the Asia pacific region: A review of assessment indicators. *Journal of Pain and Symptom Management, 62*(5), 1008–1014. PMID: 33933621

Liu, X., Wang, S., Chang, K., & Chen, J. (2021). Mindfulness training modifies intrinsic brain networks associated with emotional regulation: A meta-analytic review of fMRI studies. *Neuroscience and Biobehavioral Reviews, 131*, 1211–1223. DOI: 10.1016/j.neubiorev.2021.11.019

Liu, Y., Zavareh, A. T., & Zoghi, B. (2024). Enhancing Well-Being and Alleviating Stress via Wearable-Driven Emotion Recognition and EQ Intentional Practice with Deep Reinforcement Learning. *IEEE Sensors Letters.*

Livingston, G., Kelly, L., Lewis-Holmes, E., Baio, G., Morris, S., Patel, N., & Cooper, C. (2014). Non-pharmacological interventions for agitation in dementia: Systematic review of randomised controlled trials. *The British Journal of Psychiatry, 205*(6), 436–442. DOI: 10.1192/bjp.bp.113.141119

Li, W. W. (2021). A Cross-Cultural Study of Filial Piety and Palliative Care Knowledge: Moderating Effect of Culture and Universality of Filial Piety. *Frontiers in Psychology*, •••, 787724.

Li, Z., Zhang, Z., Ren, Y., Wang, Y., Fang, J., Yue, H., Ma, S., & Guan, F. (2021). Aging and age-related diseases: From mechanisms to therapeutic strategies. *Biogerontology*, *22*(2), 165–187. DOI: 10.1007/s10522-021-09910-5

Loh, K. P., Soto-Perez-de-Celis, E., Hsu, T., de Glas, N. A., Battisti, N. M. L., Baldini, C., Rodrigues, M., Lichtman, S. M., & Wildiers, H. (2018). What every oncologist should know about geriatric assessment for older patients with cancer: Young international society of geriatric oncology position paper. *Journal of Oncology Practice / American Society of Clinical Oncology*, *14*(2), 85–94. PMID: 29436306

Løhre, E. T., Jakobsen, G., Solheim, T. S., Klepstad, P., & Thronæs, M. (2023). Breakthrough and Episodic Cancer Pain from a Palliative Care Perspective. *Current Oncology (Toronto, Ont.)*, *30*(12), 10249–10259. DOI: 10.3390/curroncol30120746 PMID: 38132380

Lok, C. W. (2016). Palliative care in chronic obstructive pulmonary disease. *Journal of Thoracic Disease*, *8*(10), E1117–E1121. DOI: 10.21037/jtd.2016.09.43

Long, H., Huang, W., Zheng, P., Li, J., Tao, S., Tang, S., & Zhang, L. (2016). The effectiveness and safety of palliative oxygen therapy for dyspnea in patients with advanced cancer: A meta-analysis. *Oncotarget*, *7*(43), 70862–70871. DOI: 10.18632/oncotarget.12234

Long, N. H. (2018). Death Acceptance in Vietnamese Cancer Patients: A Phenomenological Study. *Journal of Transcultural Nursing*.

Loosen, S. H., Schwartz, J., Grewe, S., Krieg, S., Krieg, A., Luedde, T., Batzler, Y.-N., Kostev, K., Neukirchen, M., & Roderburg, C. (2023). Drug landscape in patients receiving general outpatient palliative care in Germany: Results from a retrospective analysis of 10,464 patients. *BMC Palliative Care*, *22*(1), 118. PMID: 37596590

López, D. M., Rico-Olarte, C., Blobel, B., & Hullin, C. (2022). Challenges and solutions for transforming health ecosystems in low-and middle-income countries through artificial intelligence. *Frontiers in Medicine*, *9*, 958097.

Luckett, T., Phillips, J., Agar, M., Virdun, C., Green, A., & Davidson, P. M. (2014). Elements of effective palliative care models: A rapid review. *BMC Health Services Research*, *14*, 1–22. PMID: 24670065

Lupiáñez-Pérez, I., Gómez-González, A. J., Marfil-Gómez, R. M., Morales-Asencio, J. M., García-Mayor, S., León-Campos, Á., & Morilla-Herrera, J. C. (2021). Tissue temperature, flux and oxygen of sacral and trochanteric area under pressure of healthy subjects: A quasi-experimental study. *Journal of Tissue Viability*, *30*(2), 207–215. DOI: 10.1016/j.jtv.2021.01.006 PMID: 33487523

Lu, Y., Gu, Y., & Yu, W. (2018). Hospice and palliative care in China: Development and challenges. *Asia-Pacific Journal of Oncology Nursing*, *5*(1), 26–32. PMID: 29379830

Machado, R. S., Viana, S., & Sbruzzi, G. (2017). Low-level laser therapy in the treatment of pressure ulcers: Systematic review. *Lasers in Medical Science*, *32*(4), 937–944. DOI: 10.1007/s10103-017-2150-9 PMID: 28116536

Mahajan, A., Heydari, K., & Powell, D. (2025). Wearable AI to enhance patient safety and clinical decision-making. *npj. Digital Medicine*, *8*(1), 176.

Mahdiabadi, F. R., Mirzaei, S., Entezari, A., & Nasiriani, K. (2023). The effect of implementing the COMFORT communication model on communication skills of nursing students. *International Journal of Palliative Nursing*, *29*(9), 412–420. PMID: 37757811

Maita, K. C., Maniaci, M. J., Haider, C. R., Avila, F. R., Torres-Guzman, R. A., Borna, S., Lunde, J. J., Coffey, J. D., Demaerschalk, B. M., & Forte, A. J. (2024). The Impact of Digital Health Solutions on Bridging the Health Care Gap in Rural Areas: A Scoping Review. *The Permanente Journal*, *28*(3), 130–143. DOI: 10.7812/TPP/23.134 PMID: 39135461

Maj, A., Kusiak, A., Garbacz, K., Cichońska, D., & Świetlik, D. (2025). Photodynamic therapy in non-surgical treatment of periodontitis. *Scientific Reports*, *15*(1), 5903. DOI: 10.1038/s41598-025-89563-3 PMID: 39966437

Majedi, H., Dehghani, S. S., Soleyman-Jahi, S., Tafakhori, A., Emami, S. A., Mireskandari, M., & Hosseini, S. M. (2019). (in press). Assessment of Factors Predicting Inadequate Pain Management in Chronic Pain Patients. *Anesthesiology and Pain Medicine, In Press*. Advance online publication. DOI: 10.5812/aapm.97229 PMID: 32280619

Maltoni, M. C., Donati, C. M., Rossi, R., & Morganti, A. G. (2023). Timely Palliative Care Could Be Another Benefit for Cancer Patients with Non-Malignant Pain. *Cancers (Basel)*, *15*(9), 2588. DOI: 10.3390/cancers15092588 PMID: 37174054

Manfredini, a. (2016). Exercise in Patients on Dialysis: A Multicenter, Randomized Clinical Trial. *Journal of the American Society of Nephrology*, *28*(4), 1259–1268. DOI: 10.1681/asn.2016030378

Marengoni, A., Angleman, S., Melis, R., Mangialasche, F., Karp, A., Garmen, A., Meinow, B., & Fratiglioni, L. (2011). Aging with multimorbidity: A systematic review of the literature. *Ageing Research Reviews*, *10*(4), 430–439. DOI: 10.1016/j.arr.2011.03.003

Maresova, P. (2024). Cost-effectiveness of home-based palliative care. *Systematic Reviews*.

Marmot, M. (2005). Social determinants of health inequalities. *Lancet*, *365*(9464), 1099–1104. DOI: 10.1016/S0140-6736(05)71146-6 PMID: 15781105

Martins Pereira, S., Hernández-Marrero, P., Pasman, H. R., Capelas, M. L., Larkin, P., & Francke, A. L. (2021). Nursing education on palliative care across Europe: Results and recommendations from the EAPC Taskforce on preparation for practice in palliative care nursing across the EU based on an online-survey and country reports. *Palliative Medicine*, *35*(1), 130–141. PMID: 32912033

Maslach, C., & Leiter, M. P. (2016). Understanding the burnout experience: Recent research and its implications for psychiatry. *World Psychiatry; Official Journal of the World Psychiatric Association (WPA)*, *15*(2), 103–111. DOI: 10.1002/wps.20311

Masoumi, N., Hosseinzadeh, M., VanSon, C., & Ghezeljeh, T. N. (2021). Home healthcare in Iran: A hybrid concept analysis. *Iranian Journal of Nursing and Midwifery Research*, *26*(3), 196–203. DOI: 10.4103/ijnmr.IJNMR_198_20 PMID: 34277369

Mat, S., Ng, C. T., Tan, P. J., Ramli, N., Fadzli, F., Rozalli, F. I., Tan, M. P. (2017). Effect of Modified Otago Exercises on Postural Balance, Fear of Falling, and Fall Risk in Older Fallers With Knee Osteoarthritis and Impaired Gait and Balance: A Secondary Analysis. *PM&R*, *10*(3), 254-262. doi:DOI: 10.1016/j.pmrj.2017.08.405

Matchim, W. K., & Chaipetch, O., & Yaowarat. (2012). Thai Buddhist families' perspective of a peaceful death in ICUs. *Nursing in Critical Care*.

Mattingly, T. J., Silverman, E., & Lavenberg, J. (2022). Inclusion of informal caregiver costs in cost-of-illness studies: A systematic review. *Value in Health*, *25*(3), 394–402.

Maugans, T. A. (1996). The spiritual history. *Archives of Family Medicine*, *5*(1), 11–16. PMID: 8542049

McCABE, C., Begley, C., Collier, S., & McCANN, S. (2007). Methodological issues related to assessing and measuring quality of life in patients with cancer : Implications for patient care. *European Journal of Cancer Care, 0*(0), 070611034311001-??? DOI: 10.1111/j.1365-2354.2007.00809.x

McCarthy, B., O'Donovan, M., & Trace, A. (2021). A new therapeutic communication model "TAGEET" to help nurses engage therapeutically with patients suspected of or confirmed with COVID-19. *Journal of Clinical Nursing*, *30*(7-8), 1184–1191. PMID: 33350012

McInnes, E., Jammali-Blasi, A., Bell-Syer, S. E., Dumville, J. C., Middleton, V., & Cullum, N. (2015). Support surfaces for pressure ulcer prevention. *Cochrane Database of Systematic Reviews*, *2015*(9), Cd001735. DOI: 10.1002/14651858.CD001735.pub5 PMID: 26333288

McLaney, E., Morassaei, S., Hughes, L., Davies, R., Campbell, M., & Di Prospero, L. (2022). A framework for interprofessional team collaboration in a hospital setting: Advancing team competencies and behaviours. *Healthcare Management Forum*, *35*(2), 112–117. DOI: 10.1177/08404704211063584

McLaughlin, D., Hasson, F., Reid, J., Brazil, K., Rutherford, L., Stone, C., & Ballentine, J. (2022). Evaluating a partnership model of hospice enabled dementia care: A three-phased monitoring, focus group and interview study. *Palliative Medicine*, *36*(9), 1351–1363. DOI: 10.1177/02692163221116763

McQuay, H. (2010). Drug Treatment of Chronic Pain. In Stannard, C. F., Kalso, E., & Ballantyne, J. (Eds.), *Evidence-Based Chronic Pain Management.*, DOI: 10.1002/9781444314380.ch31

Meitar, D., & Karnieli-Miller, O. (2022). Twelve tips to manage a breaking bad news process: Using SPw-ICE-S–A revised version of the SPIKES protocol. *Medical Teacher*, *44*(10), 1087–1091. PMID: 34057007

Mercadante, S., Adile, C., Tirelli, W., Ferrera, P., Penco, I., & Casuccio, A. (2020). Barriers and Adherence to Pain Management in Advanced Cancer Patients. *Pain Practice*, *21*(4). Advance online publication. DOI: 10.1111/papr.12965 PMID: 33200548

Mercadante, S., Gregoretti, C., & Cortegiani, A. (2018). Palliative care in intensive care units: Why, where, what, who, when, how. *BMC Anesthesiology*, *18*, 1–6. PMID: 30111299

Mercier, C., & Filion, J. (2006). La qualité de la vie : Perspectives théoriques et empiriques. *Sante Mentale au Quebec, 12*(1), 135–143. DOI: 10.7202/030380ar PMID: 16946975

Meredith, S., Feldman, P., Frey, D., Giammarco, L., Hall, K., Arnold, K., Brown, N. J., & Ray, W. A. (2002). Improving medication use in newly admitted home healthcare patients: A randomized controlled trial. *Journal of the American Geriatrics Society, 50*(9), 1484–1491. PMID: 12383144

Mezzalira, E., Canzan, F., Marini, G., Longhini, J., Leardini, C., Saiani, L., & Ambrosi, E. (2024). Introduction of novel complex integrated care models supported by digital health interventions in European primary settings: A scoping review. *Health Policy and Technology, 13*(4), 100896. https://doi.org/https://doi.org/10.1016/j.hlpt.2024.100896

Michel, J.-P., & Cha, H. B. (2015). Filling the geriatric education gap around the world. *Journal of the American Medical Directors Association, 16*(12), 1010–1013. PMID: 26410106

Michels, G., Schallenburger, M., Neukirchen, M., John, S., Janssens, U., Raake, P., Schütt, K., Bauersachs, J., Barchfeld, T., Schucher, B., Delis, S., Karpf-Wissel, R., Kochanek, M., von Bonin, S., Erley, C. M., Kuhlmann, S. D., Müllges, W., Gahn, G., Heppner, H. J., & Wiese, C. H. R. (2023). Recommendations on palliative care aspects in intensive care medicine. *Critical Care, 27*(1). Advance online publication. DOI: 10.1186/s13054-023-04622-3 PMID: 37723595

Miller, R. K., Morgan-Gouveia, M. D., & DeCherrie, L. V. (2022). Medical Training in Home Care Medicine: The Time is Now. *Journal of General Internal Medicine, 37*(9), 2302–2305. DOI: 10.1007/s11606-022-07514-4 PMID: 35710677

Mills, J., Kim, S.-H., Chan, H. Y., Ho, M.-H., Montayre, J., Liu, M. F., & Lin, C.-C. (2021). Palliative care education in the Asia Pacific: Challenges and progress towards palliative care development. *Progress in Palliative Care, 29*(5), 251–254.

Miranda, R., Bunn, F., Lynch, J., Van Den Block, L., & Goodman, C. (2019). Palliative care for people with dementia living at home : A systematic review of interventions. *Palliative Medicine, 33*(7), 726–742. DOI: 10.1177/0269216319847092 PMID: 31057088

Miroslav S. (2020). Mindfulness in Palliative Care - the Healing Effect of the Present Moment. Mindfulness/všímavost v paliativní péči - léčivý efekt přítomného okamžiku. *Klinicka onkologie: casopis Ceske a Slovenske onkologicke spolecnosti, 33*(Supplementum - 2), 138–140.

Mitchell, R. J., Wijekulasuriya, S., du Preez, J., Lystad, R., Chauhan, A., Harrison, R., Curtis, K., & Braithwaite, J. (2024). Population-level quality indicators of end-of-life-care in an aged care setting: Rapid systematic review. *Archives of Gerontology and Geriatrics, 116*, 105130. PMID: 37535984

Miura, H. (2015). Historical changes in home care service and its future challenges. *JMA Journal, 58*(1–2), 1–5. PMID: 26557453

Mohammed, M. (2024). Exercise intervention in frailty, challenges, and recommendations. In *Difficulties and challenges in geriatric health management* (p. 30). IGI Global., DOI: 10.4018/979-8-3693-0675-8.ch007

Mohammed, M. (2025). Rehabilitation and assistive robotics for the elderly and physically challenged. In *Modern technologies in healthcare* (1st ed., p. 20). CRC Press., DOI: 10.1201/9781003481959

Mohammed, M., & Li, J. (2022). Stroke-Related Sarcopenia among Two Different Developing Countries with Diverse Ethnic Backgrounds (Cross-National Study in Egypt and China). *Health Care, 10*(11), 2336. DOI: 10.3390/healthcare10112336

Mohammed, M., & Li, J. (2023). Knowledge mapping and visualization of current sarcopenia and cancer research: A bibliometric analysis. *Beni-Suef University Journal of Basic and Applied Sciences, 12*(1), 51. DOI: 10.1186/s43088-023-00386-5

Mohammed, M., Mehani, S., Aziz, A. A., Mohamed, M. F., & El Nahas, N. (2023). Efficacy of threshold inspiratory muscle trainer versus diaphragmatic plus pursed lip breathing in occupational COPD. *Beni-Suef University Journal of Basic and Applied Sciences, 12*(1), 73. DOI: 10.1186/s43088-023-00409-1

Mo, L., Geng, Y., Chang, Y. K., Philip, J., Collins, A., & Hui, D. (2021). Referral criteria to specialist palliative care for patients with dementia: A systematic review. *Journal of the American Geriatrics Society, 69*(6), 1659–1669. PMID: 33655535

Molero Jurado, M. D. M., Pérez-Fuentes, M. C., Barragán Martín, A. B., Soriano Sánchez, J. G., Oropesa Ruiz, N. F., Sisto, M., & Gázquez Linares, J. J. (2020). Mindfulness in family caregivers of persons with dementia: Systematic review and meta-analysis. *Healthcare (Basel), 8*(3), 193. DOI: 10.3390/healthcare8030193

Montagnini, M., Javier, N. M., & Mitchinson, A. (2020). The Role of Rehabilitation in Patients Receiving Hospice and Palliative Care. *Rehabilitation Oncology, 38*(1), 9–21. DOI: 10.1097/01.reo.0000000000000196

Montgomery, A., & Lynn, J. (2014). The MediCaring™ Model: Best plan for frail elders in the longevity era. *The Public Policy and Aging Report, 24*(3), 112–117.

Montori, V. M., Ruissen, M. M., Hargraves, I. G., Brito, J. P., & Kunneman, M. (2023). Shared decision-making as a method of care. *BMJ Evidence-Based Medicine, 28*(4), 213–217. DOI: 10.1136/bmjebm-2022-112068 PMID: 36460328

Morgan, O. J., Hillstrom, H. J., Ellis, S. J., Golightly, Y. M., Russell, R., Hannan, M. T., & Hillstrom, R. (2019). Osteoarthritis in England: Incidence Trends From National Health Service Hospital Episode Statistics. *ACR Open Rheumatology, 1*(8), 493–498. DOI: 10.1002/acr2.11071

Mori, M. (2023). Communication in Cancer Care in Asia: A Narrative Review. *JCO Global Oncology.*

Mori, M. (2025). Definition and recommendations of advance care planning: A Delphi study in five Asian sectors. *Palliative Medicine.*

Muecke, R., Paul, M., Conrad, C., Stoll, C., Muenstedt, K., Micke, O., & Huebner, J. (2016). Complementary and Alternative Medicine in Palliative Care: A Comparison of Data From Surveys Among Patients and Professionals. *Integrative Cancer Therapies, 15*(1), 10–16. DOI: 10.1177/1534735415596423

Mukamel, D. B., Ladd, H., Nuccio, E., Zinn, J. S., Sorkin, D. H., & Ettner, S. L. (2022). Home Health Care Quality, Its Costs and Implications for Home Health Value-Based Purchasing. *Medical Care Research and Review : MCRR, 79*(1), 90–101. DOI: 10.1177/1077558720974528 PMID: 33233999

Mulaga, A. N., Kamndaya, M. S., & Masangwi, S. J. (2022). Decomposing socioeconomic inequality in catastrophic out-of-pocket health expenditures in Malawi. *PLOS Global Public Health, 2*(2), e0000182. DOI: 10.1371/journal.pgph.0000182 PMID: 36962147

Murphree, D. H., Wilson, P. M., Asai, S. W., Quest, D. J., Lin, Y., Mukherjee, P., & Storlie, C. B. (2021). Improving the delivery of palliative care through predictive modeling and healthcare informatics. *Journal of the American Medical Informatics Association : JAMIA, 28*(6), 1065–1073.

Murray, C. J., & Lopez, A. D. (1997). Alternative projections of mortality and disability by cause 1990–2020: Global Burden of Disease Study. *Lancet, 349*(9064), 1498–1504. PMID: 9167458

Naderi, N. B., Rafiei, S. Z., Pourramzani, A., Mirpour, S. H., Biazar, G., Atrkarroushan, Z., Mortazavi, M., & Ahmadi, M. (2022). *Physicians.* Skills in Breaking Bad News to Patients With Cancer Using SPIKES Protocol.

Nahavandi, D., Alizadehsani, R., Khosravi, A., & Acharya, U. R. (2022). Application of artificial intelligence in wearable devices: Opportunities and challenges. *Computer Methods and Programs in Biomedicine, 213*, 106541.

Narayan, S. M., Chung, M. K., Adedinsewo, D., Brant, L. C. C., Davis, L. L., Duncker, D., Hall, J. L., Han, J. K., Lam, C. S. P., Lewis, E., Loscalzo, J., Márquez, M. F., Rahimzadeh, V., Rodriguez, F., Sanders, P., Svennberg, E., Stein, K., Turakhia, M., Yancy, C., & Armoundas, A. A. (2025). Access to digital health technologies: Personalized framework and global perspectives. *Nature Reviews. Cardiology*. Advance online publication. DOI: 10.1038/s41569-025-01184-5 PMID: 40670723

National Clinical Guideline. C. (2014). National Institute for Health and Clinical Excellence: Guidance *Osteoarthritis: Care and Management in Adults*. London: National Institute for Health and Care Excellence (UK)

National Pressure Injury Advisory Panel. E. P. U. A. P. a. P. P. P. I. A. (2025). Prevention and Treatment of Pressure Ulcers/Injuries: Quick Reference Guide. *The International Guideline: Fourth Edition.*

Navigante, A., Cresta Morgado, P., Daud, M. L., Dos Santos Regis, H., Kolberg, M., Marazzi, C., & De Simone, G. (2022). Physical exercise and fatigue in advanced gastrointestinal cancer during chemotherapy. *BMJ Supportive &amp. Palliative Care, 13*(2), 218–227. DOI: 10.1136/bmjspcare-2021-003516

Naylor, M. D., Brooten, D. A., Campbell, R. L., Maislin, G., McCauley, K. M., & Schwartz, J. S. (2004). Transitional care of older adults hospitalized with heart failure: A randomized, controlled trial. *Journal of the American Geriatrics Society, 52*(5), 675–684. PMID: 15086645

Ne, L. S., Ne, L. S., & Ne, L. S. (2023). *The Honorable Jessica Rosenworcel Chairwoman Federal Communications Commission Washington, DC 20554 The Honorable Brendan Carr Commissioner Federal Communications Commission Washington, DC 20554 The Honorable Geoffrey Starks Commissioner Federal Communi. 14*, 1–6.

Nguyen, V., Khanh, Q. T., Hocaoglu, M., Huyen, H. T. M., Thinh, D. H. Q., & Krakauer, E. L. (2023). Integrated hospital-and home-based palliative care for cancer patients in Vietnam: People-centered outcomes. *Journal of pain and symptom management, 66*(3), 175–182. e173.

NHPCO facts and figures on hospice care. 2014. Web site. http://www.nhpco. org/sites/default/files/public/Statistics_Research/2012_Facts_Fig ures.pdf. Accessed April 15, 2015. (2014). *National Hospice and Palliative Care Organization*. doi:-DOI: 10.1097/01.naj.0000454840.97361.f2

Nichola, G., Gwyther, L., Tiso, T., & Harding, R. (2013). Traditional Healers' Views of the Required Processes for a ''Good Death'' Among Xhosa Patients Pre- and Post-Death. *Journal of Pain Symptoms and Management.*

Nissen, R. D., Viftrup, D. T., & Hvidt, N. C. (2021). The process of spiritual care. *Frontiers in Psychology, 12*, 674453. PMID: 34557128

Nkhoma, K. B., Bates, M. J., van Breevoort, D., Chifamba, D. D., Evans, C. J., Kwaitana, D., Mensah, A. B. B., Mnenula, M. C., Mupaza, L., & Opare-Lokko, E. B. A. (2025). Integrating palliative care into primary care for older people with multimorbid serious illness: A multinational qualitative cross-sectional study in Sub-Saharan Africa. *BMJ Public Health, 3*(1). PMID: 40134537

Nukunu, F., Ahwireng, S. O., Gandaa, M., Donkor, W., & Odoi, P. (2024). Legal and Ethical Issues in Geriatric Care in Ghana. *JL Pol'y & Globalization, 140*, 20.

O'Lone, E., Connors, M., Masson, P., Wu, S., Kelly, P. J., Gillespie, D., & Webster, A. C. (2016). Cognition in People With End-Stage Kidney Disease Treated With Hemodialysis: A Systematic Review and Meta-analysis. *American Journal of Kidney Diseases, 67*(6), 925–935. DOI: 10.1053/j.ajkd.2015.12.028

Obermeyer, Z., Powers, B., Vogeli, C., & Mullainathan, S. (2019). Dissecting racial bias in an algorithm used to manage the health of populations. *Science, 366*(6464), 447–453. DOI: 10.1126/science.aax2342 PMID: 31649194

OECD. (2021). *OECD ageing population projections*. OECD Publishing.

OECD. (2023). *Time for Better Care at the End of Life*. OECD., DOI: 10.1787/722b927a-

Ogundunmade, B. G., John, D. O., & Chigbo, N. N. (2024). Ensuring quality of life in palliative care physiotherapy in developing countries. *Frontiers in Rehabilitation Sciences, 5*, 1331885–1331885. DOI: 10.3389/fresc.2024.1331885

Ohinata, H., Aoyama, M., & Miyashita, M. (2022). Complexity in the context of palliative care: A systematic review. *Annals of Palliative Medicine, 11*(10), 3231–3246. DOI: 10.21037/apm-22-623 PMID: 36226646

Ohr, S. (2017). Cultural and religious beliefs and values, and their impact on preferences for end-of-life care among four ethnic groups of community-dwelling older persons. *Journal of Clinical Nursing*, •••, 1681–1689.

Oldervoll, L. M., Loge, J. H., Paltiel, H., Asp, M. B., Vidvei, U., Wiken, A. N., Hjermstad, M. J., & Kaasa, S. (2006). The Effect of a Physical Exercise Program in Palliative Care : A Phase II Study. *Journal of Pain and Symptom Management, 31*(5), 421–430. DOI: 10.1016/j.jpainsymman.2005.10.004 PMID: 16716872

Olyaie, M., Rad, F. S., Elahifar, M. A., Garkaz, A., & Mahsa, G. (2013). High-frequency and noncontact low-frequency ultrasound therapy for venous leg ulcer treatment: A randomized, controlled study. *Ostomy/Wound Management, 59*(8), 14–20. PMID: 23934374

Omoyeni, E., & Gwyther, L. (2018). Assessing the palliative care needs of elderly patients seen at The University College Hospital, Ibadan, Nigeria (TH321A). *Journal of Pain and Symptom Management, 55*(2), 571–572.

Onuh, G. (2025, October 1). AI in healthcare risks could exclude 5 billion people: Here's what we can do about it. World Economic Forum. Retrieved November 10, 2025, from https://www.weforum.org/stories/2025/10/ai-in-healthcare-risks-could-exclude-5-billion-people-here-s-what-we-can-do-about-it/

Open MedScience. (2024, December 6). Healthcare reimagined: How virtual assistants are revolutionising patient care. Open MedScience. Retrieved June 6, 2025, from https://openmedscience.com/healthcare-reimagined-how-virtual-assistants-are-revolutionising-patient-care/

Othman, E. H. (2025). Death and Dying Through the Lens of Jordanian Muslim Patients and Caregivers. *Omega*, •••, 228–242.

Ozgok Kangal, M. K., & Kopitnik, N. L. (2025). Physiology, Wound Healing. In *StatPearls*. Treasure Island (FL) ineligible companies. Disclosure: Nancy Kopitnik declares no relevant financial relationships with ineligible companies.: StatPearls Publishing Copyright © 2025, StatPearls Publishing LLC.

Paal, P., Brandstötter, C., Lorenzl, S., Larkin, P., & Elsner, F. (2019). Postgraduate palliative care education for all healthcare providers in Europe: Results from an EAPC survey. *Palliative & Supportive Care, 17*(5), 495–506. PMID: 30683163

Paiva, C. E., Bonilla-Sierra, P., Tripodoro, V. A., Rodríguez-Nunez, A., De Simone, G., Rodriguez, L. H., de Oliveira Vidal, E. I., Ríos, M. R., Crispim, D. H., & Pérez-Cruz, P. (2023). How to advance palliative care research in South America? Findings from a delphi study. *Journal of Pain and Symptom Management, 65*(3), 193–202. PMID: 36455800

Palmieri, B., Vadalà, M., & Laurino, C. (2020). Electromedical devices in wound healing management: A narrative review. *Journal of Wound Care*, *29*(7), 408–418. DOI: 10.12968/jowc.2020.29.7.408 PMID: 32654604

Pandya, S., Hamal, M., Abuya, T., Kintu, R., Mwanga, D., Warren, C. E., & Agarwal, S. (2022). Understanding Factors That Support Community Health Worker Motivation, Job Satisfaction, and Performance in Three Ugandan Districts: Opportunities for Strengthening Uganda's Community Health Worker Program. *International Journal of Health Policy and Management*, *11*(12), 2886–2894. DOI: 10.34172/ijhpm.2022.6219 PMID: 35461208

Panel., E. P. U. A. P. a. N. P. U. A. (2009). Prevention and treatment of pressure ulcers: quick reference guide. *Washington DC: National Pressure Ulcer Advisory Panel, 2009.*

Panel, N. P. U. A. (2014). *National Pressure Ulcer Advisory Panel, European Pressure Ulcer Advisory Panel and Pan Pacific Pressure Injury*. Cambridge Media.

Papp, M. E., Henriques, M., Biguet, G., Wändell, P. E., & Nygren-Bonnier, M. (2018). Experiences of hatha yogic exercises among patients with obstructive pulmonary diseases: A qualitative study. *Journal of Bodywork and Movement Therapies*, *22*(4), 896–903. DOI: 10.1016/j.jbmt.2017.11.001

Park, M., & Giap, T.-T.-T. (2020). Patient and family engagement as a potential approach for improving patient safety: A systematic review. *Journal of Advanced Nursing*, *76*(1), 62–80. https://doi.org/https://doi.org/10.1111/jan.14227 PMID: 31588602

Patel, K. V., Guralnik, J. M., Phelan, E. A., Gell, N. M., Wallace, R. B., Sullivan, M. D., & Turk, D. C. (2018). Symptom Burden Among Community-Dwelling Older Adults in the United States. *Journal of the American Geriatrics Society*. Advance online publication. DOI: 10.1111/jgs.15673 PMID: 30548453

Pauline, I., David, A., & Daniel, T. (2024). Challenges in Geriatrics Palliative Care: A Global Concern. In *Difficulties and Challenges in Geriatric Health Management* (pp. 83–97). IGI Global.

Peddle-McIntyre, C. J., Singh, F., Thomas, R., Newton, R. U., Galvão, D. A., & Cavalheri, V. (2019). Exercise training for advanced lung cancer. *Cochrane Database of Systematic Reviews*, *2*(2), CD012685–CD012685. DOI: 10.1002/14651858.CD012685.pub2

Pelleg, A. R., Schiller, G., Goldhirsch, S. L., Fernandez, H. M., & Lindenberger, E. C. (2021). Geriatrics and palliative medicine leadership is needed now more than ever: What are the training gaps? *Journal of the American Geriatrics Society*, *69*(4), 1063–1070. PMID: 33580716

Peralta, T., Castel-Branco, M. M., Reis-Pina, P., Figueiredo, I. V., & Dourado, M. (2022). Prescription trends at the end of life in a palliative care unit: Observational study. *BMC Palliative Care*, *21*(1), 65. PMID: 35505394

Percival, S. L., Francolini, I., & Donelli, G. (2015). Low-level laser therapy as an antimicrobial and antibiofilm technology and its relevance to wound healing. *Future Microbiology*, *10*(2), 255–272. DOI: 10.2217/fmb.14.109 PMID: 25689537

Pergolizzi, J.Jr, LeQuang, J. A. K., Wagner, M., & Varrassi, G. (2024). Challenges in Palliative Care in Latin America: A Narrative Review. *Cureus*, *16*(5). PMID: 38899235

Perreault, L. (2018). Les directives anticipées des personnes atteintes d'une démence de type Alzheimer : Comment faire pour bien faire? *BioéthiqueOnline*, *5*. Advance online publication. DOI: 10.7202/1044261ar

Peters, L., Cant, R., Payne, S., O'Connor, M., McDermott, F., Hood, K., & Morphet, J. (2013). How death anxiety impacts nurses' caring for patients at the end of life: A review of literature. *The Open Nursing Journal*, *7*, 14–21. DOI: 10.2174/1874434601307010014

Peterson, D. S., & Martin, P. E. (2010). Effects of age and walking speed on coactivation and cost of walking in healthy adults. *Gait &amp. Posture*, *31*(3), 355–359. DOI: 10.1016/j.gaitpost.2009.12.005

Petrie, J. R., Guzik, T. J., & Touyz, R. M. (2018). Diabetes, hypertension, and cardiovascular disease: Clinical insights and vascular mechanisms. *The Canadian Journal of Cardiology*, *34*(5), 575–584.

Phillips, J. L., & Currow, D. (2019). Challenges and future directions of palliative care. *Textbook of palliative care*, 111–130.

Physiopedia. (2025). *Psychological basis of pain*. Physiopedia. https://www.physio-pedia.com/index.php?title=Psychological_basis_of_pain&redirect=no

Pinquart, M., & Sörensen, S. (2003). Differences between caregivers and noncaregivers in psychological health and physical health: A meta-analysis. *Psychology and Aging*, *18*(2), 250–267. DOI: 10.1037/0882-7974.18.2.250

Pinsky, M. R., Bedoya, A., Bihorac, A., Celi, L., Churpek, M., Economou-Zavlanos, N. J., & Clermont, G. (2024). Use of artificial intelligence in critical care: Opportunities and obstacles. *Critical Care*, *28*(1), 113.

Polak, A., Franek, A., Blaszczak, E., Nawrat-Szoltysik, A., Taradaj, J., Wiercigroch, L., & Juras, G. (2014). A prospective, randomized, controlled, clinical study to evaluate the efficacy of high-frequency ultrasound in the treatment of Stage II and Stage III pressure ulcers in geriatric patients. *Ostomy/Wound Management*, *60*(8), 16–28. PMID: 25105475

Polak, A., Kloth, L. C., Blaszczak, E., Taradaj, J., Nawrat-Szoltysik, A., Ickowicz, T., & Kucio, C. (2017). The Efficacy of Pressure Ulcer Treatment With Cathodal and Cathodal-Anodal High-Voltage Monophasic Pulsed Current: A Prospective, Randomized, Controlled Clinical Trial. *Physical Therapy*, *97*(8), 777–789. DOI: 10.1093/ptj/pzx052 PMID: 28789467

Polak, A., Taradaj, J., Nawrat-Szoltysik, A., Stania, M., Dolibog, P., Blaszczak, E., & Kucio, C. (2016). Reduction of pressure ulcer size with high-voltage pulsed current and high-frequency ultrasound: A randomised trial. *Journal of Wound Care*, *25*(12), 742–754. DOI: 10.12968/jowc.2016.25.12.742 PMID: 27974012

Pollak, K. I., Arnold, R. M., Jeffreys, A. S., Alexander, S. C., Olsen, M. K., Abernethy, A. P., Sugg Skinner, C., Rodriguez, K. L., & Tulsky, J. A. (2007). Oncologist communication about emotion during visits with patients with advanced cancer. *Journal of Clinical Oncology*, *25*(36), 5748–5752. PMID: 18089870

Price, E. G., Beach, M. C., Gary, T. L., Robinson, K. A., Gozu, A., Palacio, A., Smarth, C., Jenckes, M., Feuerstein, C., Bass, E. B., Powe, N. R., & Cooper, L. A. (2005). A systematic review of the methodological rigor of studies evaluating cultural competence training of health professionals. *Academic Medicine*, *80*(6), 578–586. DOI: 10.1097/00001888-200506000-00013 PMID: 15917363

Prince, M. J. (2015). The burden of disease in older people and implications for health policy and practice. *Lancet*, •••, 549–562.

Puchalski, & Donnel. (2005). Religious and spiritual beliefs in end of life care: how major religions view death and dying. 114-121.

Purnell, L. (2000). A description of the Purnell model for cultural competence. *Journal of Transcultural Nursing*, *11*(1), 40–46.

Puspawati, N., Shimizu, Y., & Ishimaru, M. (2017). The effectiveness of fan therapy in reducing dyspnea in patients with chronic obstructive pulmonary disease: A systematic review. *JBI Database of Systematic Reviews and Implementation Reports, 15*(8), 2026–2053. DOI: 10.11124/JBISRIR-2016-003282

Putt, K., Faville, K. A., Lewis, D., McAllister, K., Pietro, M., & Radwan, A. (2017). Role of physical therapy intervention in patients with life-threatening illnesses: A systematic review. *The American Journal of Hospice & Palliative Care, 34*(2), 186–196.

Pyszora, A., Budzyński, J., Wójcik, A., Prokop, A., & Krajnik, M. (2017). Physiotherapy programme reduces fatigue in patients with advanced cancer receiving palliative care: randomized controlled trial. *Supportive care in cancer: official journal of the Multinational Association of Supportive Care in Cancer, 25*(9), 2899-2908. doi:DOI: 10.1007/s00520-017-3742-4

Qamar, S., Sarfraz, M., Ishtiaq, H., Akbar, A., Khattak, M. I., Raja, S. K., & Khan, M. (2025). The Complexity of Aging: Managing Multimorbidity in Geriatrics. *Cureus*. Advance online publication. DOI: 10.7759/cureus.87615 PMID: 40786252

Qaseem, A. (2008). *Evidence-Based Interventions to Improve the Palliative Care of Pain, Dyspnea, and Depression at the End of Life: A Clinical Practice Guideline from the American College of Physicians*. American College of Physicians.

Qiu, W. Q., Dean, M., Liu, T., George, L., Gann, M., Cohen, J., & Bruce, M. L. (2010). Physical and Mental Health of Homebound Older Adults: An Overlooked Population. *Journal of the American Geriatrics Society, 58*(12), 2423–2428. https://doi.org/https://doi.org/10.1111/j.1532-5415.2010.03161.x PMID: 21070195

Quah, E. L. Y., Chua, K. Z. Y., Lua, J. K., Wan, D. W. J., Chong, C. S., Lim, Y. X., & Krishna, L. (2023). A Systematic Review of Stakeholder Perspectives of Dignity and Assisted Dying. *Journal of Pain and Symptom Management, 65*(2), e123–e136. DOI: 10.1016/j.jpainsymman.2022.10.004 PMID: 36244639

Quigley, D. D., & McCleskey, S. G. (2021). Improving Care Experiences for Patients and Caregivers at End of Life: A Systematic Review. *The American Journal of Hospice & Palliative Care, 38*(1), 84–93. DOI: 10.1177/1049909120931468

Radbruch, a. (2020). Redefining Palliative Care-A New Consensus-Based Definition. *Journal of Pain and Symptom Management, 60*(4), 754–764. DOI: 10.1016/j.jpainsymman.2020.04.027

Radbruch, L., De Lima, L., Knaul, F., Wenk, R., Ali, Z., Bhatnaghar, S., Blanchard, C., Bruera, E., Buitrago, R., & Burla, C. (2020). Redefining palliative care—A new consensus-based definition. *Journal of Pain and Symptom Management, 60*(4), 754–764. PMID: 32387576

Radhoe, S. P., Clephas, P. R., Mokri, H., & Brugts, J. J. (2023). The CardioMEMS Heart Failure System for chronic heart failure–a European perspective. *Expert Review of Medical Devices, 20*(5), 349–356.

Rad, J. (2025). Health inequities: A persistent global challenge from past to future. *International Journal for Equity in Health, 24*(1). Advance online publication. DOI: 10.1186/s12939-025-02526-y PMID: 40410748

Raeder, K., Jachan, D. E., Müller-Werdan, U., & Lahmann, N. A. (2020). Prevalence and risk factors of chronic wounds in nursing homes in Germany: A Cross-Sectional Study. *International Wound Journal, 17*(5), 1128–1134. DOI: 10.1111/iwj.13486 PMID: 32815303

Raimann, a. (2016). The Effect of Increased Frequency of Hemodialysis on Volume-Related Outcomes: A Secondary Analysis of the Frequent Hemodialysis Network Trials. *Blood Purification, 41*(4), 277–286. DOI: 10.1159/000441966

Rajendran, S. B., Challen, K., Wright, K. L., & Hardy, J. G. (2021). Electrical Stimulation to Enhance Wound Healing. *Journal of Functional Biomaterials, 12*(2). Advance online publication. DOI: 10.3390/jfb12020040 PMID: 34205317

Ramachandran, A. K., Das, S., Joseph, A., Shenoy, G. G., Alex, A. T., & Mudgal, J. (2021). Neurodegenerative Pathways in Alzheimer's Disease: A Review. *Current Neuropharmacology, 19*(5), 679–692. DOI: 10.2174/1570159X18666200807130637

Ramm, M., Chung, M. L., Schnabel, K., Schnabel, A., Jedamzik, J., Hesse, M., Hach, M., Radbruch, L., Mücke, M., & Conrad, R. (2024). Pain in palliative cancer patients – Analysis of the German National Palliative Care Registry. *Journal of Pain and Symptom Management.* Advance online publication. DOI: 10.1016/j.jpainsymman.2024.10.030 PMID: 39505055

Rawlinson, F., Gwyther, L., Kiyange, F., Luyirika, E., Meiring, M., & Downing, J. (2014). The current situation in education and training of health-care professionals across Africa to optimise the delivery of palliative care for cancer patients. *ecancermedicalscience, 8*, 492.

Reckrey, J. M., Ornstein, K. A., Wajnberg, A., Kopke, M. V., & DeCherrie, L. V. (2017). Teaching Home-Based Primary Care. *Home Healthcare Now*, *35*(10). https://journals.lww.com/homehealthcarenurseonline/fulltext/2017/11000/teaching_home_based_primary_care.6.aspx PMID: 29095335

Regnard, C., & Dean, M. (2022). *A guide to symptom relief in palliative care*. CRC Press.

Reinhard, S. C., Given, B., Petlick, N. H., & Bemis, A. (2008). Supporting Family Caregivers in Providing Care. In Hughes, R. G. (Ed.), *Patient Safety and Quality: An Evidence-Based Handbook for Nurses*. Agency for Healthcare Research and Quality.

Ren, Z., Xu, Y., Sun, J., Han, Y., An, L., & Liu, J. (2023). Chronic diseases and multimorbidity patterns, their recent onset, and risk of new-onset Parkinson's disease and related functional degeneration in older adults: A prospective cohort study. *EClinicalMedicine*, •••, 65.

Rhee, J. C., Done, N., & Anderson, G. F. (2015). Considering long-term care insurance for middle-income countries: Comparing South Korea with Japan and Germany. *Health Policy (Amsterdam)*, *119*(10), 1319–1329. https://doi.org/https://doi.org/10.1016/j.healthpol.2015.06.001 PMID: 26117093

Ricks-Aherne, E. S. (2020). Practice Considerations for Trauma-Informed Care at End of Life. *Journal of Social Work in End-of-Life & Palliative Care*, •••, 313–329.

Ringdal, G. I. (2002). Health-related quality of life (HRQOL) in family members of cancer victims: Results from a longitudinal intervention study in Norway and Sweden. *Palliative Medicine*.

Robinson, M. R., Al-Kindi, S. G., & Oliveira, G. H. (2017). Trends in palliative care use in elderly men and women with severe heart failure in the United States. *JAMA Cardiology*, *2*(3), 344–344. PMID: 27926774

Robledo, L. M. G., Cano-GutiéRrez, C., & Garcia, E. V. (2022). Healthcare for older people in Central and South America. *Age and Ageing*, *51*(5), afac017. PMID: 35604089

Rochon, P. A., & Gurwitz, J. H. (2017). The prescribing cascade revisited. *Lancet*, *389*(10081), 1778–1780. DOI: 10.1016/S0140-6736(17)31188-1

Rodgers-Melnick, S. N., Rivard, R. L., Block, S., & Dusek, J. A. (2023). Effectiveness of music therapy within community hospitals: An EMMPIRE retrospective study. *Pain Reports (Baltimore, Md.)*, *8*(3), e1074. DOI: 10.1097/pr9.0000000000001074

Roeland, E. J., Triplett, D. P., Matsuno, R. K., Boero, I. J., Hwang, L., Yeung, H. N., Mell, L., & Murphy, J. D. (2016). Patterns of palliative care consultation among elderly patients with cancer. *Journal of the National Comprehensive Cancer Network : JNCCN, 14*(4), 439–445. PMID: 27059192

Roller-Wirnsberger, R., Thurner, B., Pucher, C., Lindner, S., & Wirnsberger, G. H. (2020). The clinical and therapeutic challenge of treating older patients in clinical practice. *British Journal of Clinical Pharmacology*, *86*(10), 1904–1911.

Romanò, M., Oldani, S., Reina, V., Sofia, M., & Castiglioni, C. (2022). Palliative Care for Patients with End-Stage, Non-Oncologic Diseases—A Retrospective Study in Three Public Palliative Care Departments in Northern Italy. *Health Care*, *10*(6), 1031. DOI: 10.3390/healthcare10061031 PMID: 35742082

Ronanki, R. (2024). *Revolutionizing Health Care with AI: A New Era of Efficiency, Trust, and Care Excellence*. NEJM AI Sponsored.

Rossi, I. (2010). Culture palliative : Pour anticiper et accueillir la mort. *Revue internationale de soins palliatifs, 25*(1), 37-43. DOI: 10.3917/inka.101.0037

Roubaud-Baudron, C., & Guerville, F. (2022). Multimorbidity. *Lessons from the ICU*, 111–122. https://doi.org/DOI: 10.1007/978-3-030-94133-8_8

Rousseau, C. (2022). Safe enough? Rethinking the concept of cultural safety in healthcare and training. *The British Journal of Psychiatry*, •••, 587–588.

Sadiq, F. U., Yu-Lyu, Y., Hung-En, L., Eka, P. M. A., Sneha, P., & Shih, Y.-H. (2025). The benefits, barriers, and specific needs of palliative care for adults with cancer in sub-Saharan Africa: A systematic review. *Global Health Action*, *18*(1), 2485742. DOI: 10.1080/16549716.2025.2485742 PMID: 40208058

Sakamoto, R. (2025). Aging in Southeast Asia and Japan: Challenges and opportunities. *Geriatrics & Gerontology International*, •••, 837–854.

Sakurai, Y. (2025). A Comparative Analysis of End-of-Life Care for Older Adults in East Asia, the US and Europe: With a Particular Focus on Family Involvement, Advance Directives and ACP. *Yokohama International Society and Social Science Research*, *29*(3), 107–124.

Salikhanov, I.. (2023). Economic evaluation of hospice and palliative care interventions. *Systematic Reviews*.

Salikhanov, I., Katapodi, M. C., Kunirova, G., & Crape, B. L. (2023). Improving palliative care outcomes in remote and rural areas of LMICs through family caregivers : Lessons from Kazakhstan. *Frontiers in Public Health, 11*, 1186107. DOI: 10.3389/fpubh.2023.1186107 PMID: 37601198

Samba, E. I., Mensah, G. B., Frimpong, P. O., Addy, A., & Otoo, J. (2023). The State of Gerontological and Geriatric Studies in Sub-Saharan Africa and Ghanaian Studies: Literature Review. *International Journal for Multidisciplinary Research*

Samia, L. W., Ellenbecker, C. H., Friedman, D. H., & Dick, K. (2012). Home care nurses' experience of job stress and considerations for the work environment. *Home Health Care Services Quarterly, 31*(3), 243–265. DOI: 10.1080/01621424.2012.703903 PMID: 22974083

Sampson, E. L., Candy, B., Davis, S., Gola, A. B., Harrington, J., King, M., Kupeli, N., Leavey, G., Moore, K., Nazareth, I., Omar, R. Z., Vickerstaff, V., & Jones, L. (2018). Living and dying with advanced dementia : A prospective cohort study of symptoms, service use and care at the end of life. *Palliative Medicine, 32*(3), 668–681. DOI: 10.1177/0269216317726443 PMID: 28922625

Sani, D. K., Yunusa, U., Kombo, S. A., Ibrahim, A., Sani, H. M., Umar, S. S., & Ladan, M. A. (2024). Home-based care models for patients with terminal illnesses in low and middle-income countries: A systematic review of randomized and quasi-experimental studies. *Archives of Gerontology and Geriatrics, 127*, 105580. DOI: 10.1016/j.archger.2024.105580 PMID: 39029345

Saracino, R. M., Bai, M., Blatt, L., Solomon, L., & McCorkle, R. (2018). Geriatric palliative care: Meeting the needs of a growing population. *Geriatric Nursing, 39*(2), 225–229. PMID: 29042070

Sarfraz, A., & Siddiqui, S. (2023). Cultural adaptation of a mindfulness-based intervention for young adults: An application of heuristic framework. *Pakistan Journal of Social Research, 5*(2), 40–53. DOI: 10.52567/pjsr.v5i02.1107

Sarhill, N. (2001). The terminally ill Muslim: Death and dying from the Muslim perspective. *American Journal of Hospice and Palliative Medicine®.*

Savva, G. M., Zaccai, J., Matthews, F. E., Davidson, J. E., McKeith, I., & Brayne, C. (2009). Prevalence, correlates and course of behavioural and psychological symptoms of dementia in the population. *The British Journal of Psychiatry, 194*(3), 212–219. DOI: 10.1192/bjp.bp.108.049619

Schefold, J. C. (2025). The impact of religion on changes in end-of-life practices in European intensive care units: A comparative analysis over 16 years. *Intensive Care Medicine*.

Schoenherr, L. A., Bischoff, K. E., Marks, A. K., O'Riordan, D. L., & Pantilat, S. Z. (2019). Trends in Hospital-Based Specialty Palliative Care in the United States From 2013 to 2017. *JAMA Network Open*, *2*(12), e1917043–e1917043. DOI: 10.1001/jamanetworkopen.2019.17043

Schulz, R., Eden, J., & Adults, C. on F. C. for O., Services, B. on H. C., Division, H. and M., & National Academies of Sciences, E. (2016). Family Caregiving Roles and Impacts. In *Families Caring for an Aging America*. National Academies Press (US). https://www.ncbi.nlm.nih.gov/books/NBK396398/

Schulz, R., Beach, S. R., Czaja, S. J., Martire, L. M., & Monin, J. K. (2020). Family Caregiving for Older Adults. *Annual Review of Psychology*, *71*, 635–659. DOI: 10.1146/annurev-psych-010419-050754

Schulz, R., & Czaja, S. J. (2018). Family Caregiving : A Vision for the Future. *The American Journal of Geriatric Psychiatry: Official Journal of the American Association for Geriatric Psychiatry*, *26*(3), 358–363. DOI: 10.1016/j.jagp.2017.06.023 PMID: 28774786

Schulz, R., & Sherwood, P. R. (2008). Physical and mental health effects of family caregiving. *The American Journal of Nursing*, *108*(9, Suppl), 23–27. DOI: 10.1097/01.NAJ.0000336406.45248.4c

Seckinger, J., Dschietzig, W., Leimenstoll, G., Rob, P. M., Kuhlmann, M. K., Pommer, W., & Schwenger, V. (2016). Morbidity, mortality and quality of life in the ageing haemodialysis population: Results from the ELDERLY study. *Clinical Kidney Journal*, *9*(6), 839–848. DOI: 10.1093/ckj/sfw087

Seise, C. (2021). Dying a Good Death: Indonesian Rituals and Negotiations About the End of Life. *International Journal of Islam in Asia*, 168-190.

Seo, M. S., Shim, J. Y., Choi, Y. S., Kim, D. Y., Hwang, I. G., Baek, S. K., Shin, J. Y., Lee, J., & Lee, C. G. (2017). Physician's Attitude toward Treating Breakthrough Cancer Pain in Korea. *Han'guk Hosup'isu Wanhwa Uiryo Hakhoe Chi = The Korean Journal of Hospice and Palliative Care*, *20*(1), 18–25. DOI: 10.14475/kjhpc.2017.20.1.18

Sepúlveda, C., Marlin, A., Yoshida, T., & Ullrich, A. (2002). Palliative Care. *Journal of Pain and Symptom Management*, *24*(2), 91–96. DOI: 10.1016/S0885-3924(02)00440-2 PMID: 12231124

Sepúlveda, C., Marlin, A., Yoshida, T., & Ullrich, A. (2002). Palliative care: The World Health Organization's global perspective. *Journal of Pain and Symptom Management, 24*(2), 91–96. PMID: 12231124

Sethuraman, S. C., Kompally, P., Mohanty, S. P., & Choppali, U. (2020). MyWear: A smart wear for continuous body vital monitoring and emergency alert. *arXiv preprint arXiv:2010.08866.*

Sewpersad, S. (2024). Ageing in South Africa: Trends and Determinants. *Geriatrics & Gerontology International.*

Sganga, F., Salerno, A., Frizza, A., Turriziani, A., Barillaroa, C., & Bernabei, R. (2022). The role of geriatricians in hospital palliative care units for elderly patients affected by end stage diseases. *International Journal of Palliative Nursing, 28*(5), 202–207. DOI: 10.12968/ijpn.2022.28.5.202

Shabnam, J., Timm, H. U., Nielsen, D. S., & Raunkiaer, M. (2022). Palliative care utilization among non-western migrants in Europe: A systematic review. *Journal of Immigrant and Minority Health*, •••, 1–19. PMID: 34709528

Shahriari, M., Nia, D. H., Kalij, F., & Hashemi, M. S. (2024). Challenges of home care: A qualitative study. *BMC Nursing, 23*(1), 215. DOI: 10.1186/s12912-024-01878-0 PMID: 38549100

Shajari, S., Kuruvinashetti, K., Komeili, A., & Sundararaj, U. (2023). The emergence of AI-based wearable sensors for digital health technology: A review. *Sensors (Basel), 23*(23), 9498.

Shalaby, R. A. H., & Agyapong, V. I. O. (2020). Peer Support in Mental Health: Literature Review. *JMIR Mental Health, 7*(6), e15572. DOI: 10.2196/15572 PMID: 32357127

Shalev, D. (2020). End-of-Life Care in Individuals With Serious Mental Illness. *Psychosomatics*, •••, 428–435.

Shapiro, S. L., Carlson, L. E., Astin, J. A., & Freedman, B. (2006). Mechanisms of mindfulness. *Journal of Clinical Psychology, 62*(3), 373–386. DOI: 10.1002/jclp.20237

Sharma, G., & Goodwin, J. (2006). Effect of aging on respiratory system physiology and immunology. *Clinical Interventions in Aging, 1*(3), 253–260. DOI: 10.2147/ciia.2006.1.3.253

Shaw, J., Rudzicz, F., Jamieson, T., & Goldfarb, A. (2019). Artificial intelligence and the implementation challenge. *Journal of Medical Internet Research, 21*(7), e13659.

Sheik, A. (1998). Death and dying-a Muslim perspective. *Journal of the Royal Society of Medicine*.

Shennan, C., Payne, S., & Fenlon, D. (2011). What is the evidence for the use of mindfulness-based interventions in cancer care? A review. *Psycho-Oncology*, *20*(7), 681–697. DOI: 10.1002/pon.1819

Shoemake, A. (1994). Solutions to the Home Healthcare Nursing Shortage. *Home Healthcare Now*, *12*(4). https://journals.lww.com/homehealthcarenurseonline/fulltext/1994/07000/solutions_to_the_home_healthcare_nursing_shortage.6.aspx PMID: 7960869

Sholjakova, M., Durnev, V., Kartalov, A., & Kuzmanovska, B. (2018). Pain relief as an integral part of the palliative care. *Open Access Macedonian Journal of Medical Sciences*, *6*(4), 739–741. DOI: 10.3889/oamjms.2018.163 PMID: 29731950

Sibai, A. M., Semaan, A., Tabbara, J., & Rizk, A. (2017). Ageing and health in the Arab region: Challenges, opportunities and the way forward. *Population Horizons*, *14*(2), 73–84. DOI: 10.1515/pophzn-2017-0007

Silva, A. M. D., Silva, G. M., Martins, J. C., Bavaresco, T., & Echevarría-Guanilo, M. E. (2025). Photobiomodulation and photodynamic therapy in the treatment of pressure injuries: A scoping review. *Revista Latino-Americana de Enfermagem*, *33*, e4488. DOI: 10.1590/1518-8345.7495.4488 PMID: 39969041

Simon, P. M., Schwartzstein, R. M., Weiss, J. W., Fencl, V., Teghtsoonian, M., & Weinberger, S. E. (1990). Distinguishable types of dyspnea in patients with shortness of breath. *The American Review of Respiratory Disease*, *142*(5), 1009–1014. DOI: 10.1164/ajrccm/142.5.1009

Simon, S. T., Köskeroglu, P., Gaertner, J., & Voltz, R. (2016). Benzodiazepines for the relief of breathlessness in advanced malignant and non-malignant diseases in adults. *Cochrane Database of Systematic Reviews*, *2016*(10), CD007354. Advance online publication. DOI: 10.1002/14651858.CD007354.pub3

Sindhukumari, S. U., & Varkey Thomas, K. (2023). Analyzing the Influence of Socioeconomic Status on Public Healthcare Access: An Interdisciplinary Framework. *EuroMid Journal of Business and Tech-Innovation (EJBTI)*, 33–48. https://doi.org/ DOI: 10.51325/ejbti.v2i2.176

Singer, P. A. (1999). Quality end-of-life care. Patients' perspectives. *Journal of the American Medical Association*.

Skalla, K. A. (2006). Spiritual assessment of patients with cancer: the moral authority, vocational, aesthetic, social, and transcendent model. *Number 4/July 2006, 33*(4), 745–751.

Skevington, S. M., Lotfy, M., & O'Connell, K. A.WHOQOL Group. (2004). The World Health Organization's WHOQOL-BREF quality of life assessment : Psychometric properties and results of the international field trial. A report from the WHOQOL group. *Quality of Life Research: An International Journal of Quality of Life Aspects of Treatment, Care and Rehabilitation, 13*(2), 299–310. DOI: 10.1023/B: QURE.0000018486.91360.00 PMID: 15085902

Skou, S. T., Mair, F. S., Fortin, M., Guthrie, B., Nunes, B. P., Miranda, J. J., Boyd, C. M., Pati, S., Mtenga, S., & Smith, S. M. (2022). Multimorbidity. *Nature Reviews. Disease Primers, 8*(1), 1–22. DOI: 10.1038/s41572-022-00376-4 PMID: 35835758

Sleeman, K. E., De Brito, M., Etkind, S., Nkhoma, K., Guo, P., Higginson, I. J., Gomes, B., & Harding, R. (2019). The escalating global burden of serious health-related suffering: Projections to 2060 by world regions, age groups, and health conditions. *The Lancet. Global Health, 7*(7), e883–e892. PMID: 31129125

Smeekes, O. S., De Boer, T. R., Van Der Mei, R. D., Buurman, B. M., & Willems, H. C. (2024). Receiving home care forms and the risk for emergency department visits in community-dwelling Dutch older adults, a retrospective cohort study using national data. *BMC Public Health, 24*(1), 1792.

Snyder, R., Galiano, R., Mayer, P., Rogers, L. C., & Alvarez, O. (2018). Diabetic foot ulcer treatment with focused shockwave therapy: Two multicentre, prospective, controlled, double-blinded, randomised phase III clinical trials. *Journal of Wound Care, 27*(12), 822–836. DOI: 10.12968/jowc.2018.27.12.822 PMID: 30557108

Soares, L. G. L., Japiassu, A. M., Gomes, L. C., Pereira, R., Peçanha, C., & Goldgaber, T. (2018). Prevalence and intensity of dyspnea, pain, and agitation among people dying with late stage dementia compared with people dying with advanced cancer: A single-center preliminary study in Brazil. *Annals of Palliative Medicine, 7*(4), 437–443. DOI: 10.21037/apm.2018.05.06

Soban, L. M., Kim, L., Yuan, A. H., & Miltner, R. S. (2017). Organisational strategies to implement hospital pressure ulcer prevention programmes: Findings from a national survey. *Journal of Nursing Management, 25*(6), 457–467. DOI: 10.1111/jonm.12416 PMID: 27487972

Son, Y.-J., Lee, Y., & Lee, H.-J. (2020). Effectiveness of Mobile Phone-Based Interventions for Improving Health Outcomes in Patients with Chronic Heart Failure: A Systematic Review and Meta-Analysis. *International Journal of Environmental Research and Public Health, 17*(5). Advance online publication. DOI: 10.3390/ijerph17051749 PMID: 32156074

Sopel, M., Kuberka, I., Szczuka, I., Taradaj, J., Rosińczuk, J., & Dymarek, R. (2024). Can Shockwave Treatment Elicit a Molecular Response to Enhance Clinical Outcomes in Pressure Ulcers? The SHOck Waves in wouNds Project. *Biomedicines, 12*(2). Advance online publication. DOI: 10.3390/biomedicines12020359 PMID: 38397961

Sörensen, S. M. (2002). How effective are interventions with caregivers? an updated meta-analysis. *The Gerontologist.*

Spathis, A., Booth, S., & Moffat, C. (2017). The breathing, thinking, functioning clinical model: A proposal to facilitate evidence-based breathlessness management in chronic respiratory disease. *NPJ Primary Care Respiratory Medicine, 27*, 27. DOI: 10.1038/s41533-017-0024-z

Sribunlue, P., Boondet, K., Charoenpol, F., & Pairojkul, S. (2024). Factors Predicting the Difficulty of Pain Management in Patients Receiving First Palliative Care Consultation. *The Journal of Thailand Nursing and Midwifery Council, 39*(03), 313–327. DOI: 10.60099/jtnmc.v39i03.267495

Stamm, B. H. (2010). The concise ProQOL manual, *2nd edition.* Pocatello, ID: ProQOL.org.

Steffens, D. C., & Zdanys, K. F. (2022). *The American Psychiatric Association Publishing Textbook of Geriatric Psychiatry.* American Psychiatric Pub.

Stewart, S. (1998). Effects of a home-based intervention among patients with congestive heart failure discharged from acute hospital care. *Archives of Internal Medicine.*

Stow, D., Spiers, G., Matthews, F. E., & Hanratty, B. (2019). What is the evidence that people with frailty have needs for palliative care at the end of life? A systematic review and narrative synthesis. *Palliative Medicine, 33*(4), 399–414. PMID: 30775957

Strang, P. (2022). Palliative oncology and palliative care. *Molecular Oncology, 16*(19). Advance online publication. DOI: 10.1002/1878-0261.13278 PMID: 35762045

Stringuetta Belik, F., & Oliveira, E Silva, Viviana R., Braga, Gabriel P., Bazan, R., Perez Vogt, B., Costa Teixeira Caramori, J., . . . da Silva Franco, Roberto J. (2018). Influence of Intradialytic Aerobic Training in Cerebral Blood Flow and Cognitive Function in Patients with Chronic Kidney Disease: A Pilot Randomized Controlled Trial. *Nephron, 140*(1), 9–17. DOI: 10.1159/000490005

Strömgren, A. S., Sjogren, P., Goldschmidt, D., Petersen, M. A., Pedersen, L., & Groenvold, M. (2006). Symptom priority and course of symptomatology in specialized palliative care. *Journal of Pain and Symptom Management, 31*(3), 199–206. DOI: 10.1016/j.jpainsymman.2005.07.007 PMID: 16563314

Stucki, G., Bickenbach, J., Gutenbrunner, C., & Melvin, J. (2018). Rehabilitation: The health strategy of the 21st century. *Journal of Rehabilitation Medicine, 50*(4), 309–316. DOI: 10.2340/16501977-2200

Suija, K., Mason, S. R., Elsner, F., & Paal, P. (2024). Palliative care training in medical undergraduate education: A survey among the faculty. *BMC Palliative Care, 23*(1), 19. PMID: 38233862

Suleman, M. (2023). The balancing of virtues—Muslim perspectives on palliative and end of life care: Empirical research analysing the perspectives of service users and providers. *Bioethics*, •••, 57–68.

Sungur, H., van den Muijsenbergh, M. E., van Weert, J. C., & Schouten, B. C. (2022). Caring for older culturally and linguistically diverse patients with Cancer: Healthcare Providers' perceived barriers to communication. *Journal of Geriatric Oncology, 13*(6), 862–870. PMID: 35589543

Sun, H., Li, Q., & Zhang, W. (2022). Comparing mindfulness-based intervention with group supportive therapy for caregiver stress: A randomized controlled study. *Palliative & Supportive Care, 20*(5), 620–629.

Sun, X., & Li, X. (2023). Editorial: Aging and chronic disease: public health challenge and education reform. *Frontiers in Public Health, 11*, 1175898. DOI: 10.3389/fpubh.2023.1175898

Sutin, A. R., Stephan, Y., & Terracciano, A. (2018). Psychological Distress, Self-Beliefs, and Risk of Cognitive Impairment and Dementia. *Journal of Alzheimer's Disease, 65*(3), 1041–1050. DOI: 10.3233/JAD-180119

Svendsen, S. J., Grov, E. K., & Staats, K. (2024). Patients' experiences with shared decision-making in home-based palliative care – navigation through major life decisions. *BMC Palliative Care, 23*(1), 101. DOI: 10.1186/s12904-024-01434-2 PMID: 38627710

Taha, M. M., El-Nagar, M. M., Elrefaey, B. H., Elkholy, R. M., Ali, O. I., Alkhamees, N., & Felaya, E. E. E. (2022). Effect of Polarized Light Therapy (Bioptron) on Wound Healing and Microbiota in Diabetic Foot Ulcer: A Randomized Controlled Trial. *Photobiomodulation, Photomedicine, and Laser Surgery, 40*(12), 792–799. DOI: 10.1089/photob.2021.0175 PMID: 36315226

Takechi, H., Tsuzuki, A., Matsumoto, K., Fukui, A., Kawakita, H., Yoshino, H., & Kanada, Y. (2022). Differences in the frequency of subjective geriatric complaints along with aging and their associations with physical function, multimorbidity, and mood: A cross-sectional study. *PLoS One*, *17*(2), e0263889. PMID: 35148335

Takemura, N., Cheung, D. S. T., Fong, D. Y. T., Hui, D., Lee, A. W. M., Lam, T.-C., & Lin, C.-C. (2024). Tai Chi and Aerobic Exercise on Cancer-Related Dyspnea in Advanced Lung Cancer Patients: A Randomized Clinical Trial. *Journal of Pain and Symptom Management*, *68*(2), 171–179. DOI: 10.1016/j.jpainsymman.2024.04.025

Tanaka, S., Imaizumi, T., Morohashi, A., Kobayashi, K., Takagi, D., Hattori, K., Yoshito, N., Takeuchi, S., Tsuchikawa, Y., Inoue, T., Nagaya, M., Nishida, Y., Morimoto, R., Kondo, T., Hiraiwa, H., Kazama, S., Okumura, T., & Murohara, T. (2025). Prognostic value of symptom burden as a simple patient-reported outcome measure in older patients with heart failure. *Scientific Reports*, *15*(1). Advance online publication. DOI: 10.1038/s41598-025-06615-4 PMID: 40594461

Taradaj, J., Shay, B., Dymarek, R., Sopel, M., Walewicz, K., Beeckman, D., & Rosińczuk, J. (2018). Effect of laser therapy on expression of angio- and fibrogenic factors, and cytokine concentrations during the healing process of human pressure ulcers. *International Journal of Medical Sciences*, *15*(11), 1105–1112. DOI: 10.7150/ijms.25651 PMID: 30123047

Taran, S. (2011). An examination of the factors contributing to poor communication outside the physician-patient sphere. *McGill Journal of Medicine : MJM : an International Forum for the Advancement of Medical Sciences by Students*, *13*(1), 86. PMID: 22363186

Taren, A. A., Creswell, J. D., & Gianaros, P. J. (2022). Neural mechanisms of mindfulness in stress reduction: Insights for caregivers of terminally ill patients. *Biological Psychiatry: Cognitive Neuroscience and Neuroimaging*, 7(4), 396–405. DOI: 10.1016/j.bpsc.2021.04.006

Tark, A., Estrada, L. V., Tresgallo, M. E., Quigley, D. D., Stone, P. W., & Agarwal, M. (2020). Palliative care and infection management at end of life in nursing homes : A descriptive survey. *Palliative Medicine*, *34*(5), 580–588. DOI: 10.1177/0269216320902672 PMID: 32153248

Teal, C. R., & Street, R. L. (2009). Critical elements of culturally competent communication in the medical encounter: A review and model. *Social Science & Medicine*, *68*(3), 533–543. PMID: 19019520

Team-Based Models for End-of-Life Care: An Evidence-Based Analysis. (2014). *Ont Health Technol Assess Ser,* *14*(20), 1-49.

Tefferi, a. (2015). In Support of a Patient-Driven Initiative and Petition to Lower the High Price of Cancer Drugs. *Mayo Clinic Proceedings*, *90*(8), 996–1000. DOI: 10.1016/j.mayocp.2015.06.001

Teut, M., Roesner, E. J., Ortiz, M., Reese, F., Binting, S., Roll, S., Fischer, H. F., Michalsen, A., Willich, S. N., & Brinkhaus, B. (2013). Mindful walking in psychologically distressed individuals: A randomized controlled trial. *Evidence-Based Complementary and Alternative Medicine : eCAM*, *489856*. Advance online publication. DOI: 10.1155/2013/489856

Thiele, D., Rodseth, R., Friedland, R., Berger, F., Mathew, C., Maslo, C., & Nee, J. (2025). Machine Learning Models for the Early Real-Time Prediction of Deterioration in Intensive Care Units—A Novel Approach to the Early Identification of High-Risk Patients. *Journal of Clinical Medicine*, *14*(2), 350.

Thiel, M., Mattison, D., Goudie, E., Licata, S., Brewster, J., & Montagnini, M. (2021). Social work training in palliative care: Addressing the gap. *The American Journal of Hospice & Palliative Care*, *38*(8), 893–898. PMID: 32969240

Thomas, E. (2010). 185Pain in older people. In P. Croft, F. M. Blyth, & D. van der Windt (Eds.), *Chronic Pain Epidemiology: From Aetiology to Public Health* (pp. 0): Oxford University Press.

Thomas, S. A., Browning, C. J., Charchar, F. J., Klein, B., Ory, M. G., Bowden-Jones, H., & Chamberlain, S. R. (2023). Transforming global approaches to chronic disease prevention and management across the lifespan: Integrating genomics, behavior change, and digital health solutions. *Frontiers in Public Health*, *11*, 1248254. DOI: 10.3389/fpubh.2023.1248254 PMID: 37905238

Ting, R., Edmonds, P., Higginson, I. J., & Sleeman, K. E. (2020). The use of a handheld fan as a breathlessness intervention in palliative care: A randomized controlled trial. *Journal of Pain and Symptom Management*, *60*(5), 861–868. DOI: 10.1016/j.jpainsymman.2020.06.014

Tjernberg, J. (2020). Older persons' thoughts about death and dying and their experiences of care in end-of-life: A qualitative study. *BMC Nursing*.

Tolep, K., & Kelsen, S. G. (1993). Effect of aging on respiratory skeletal muscles. *Clinics in Chest Medicine*, *14*(3), 363–378.

Topol, E. J. (2019). High-performance medicine : The convergence of human and artificial intelligence. *Nature Medicine*, *25*(1), 44–56. DOI: 10.1038/s41591-018-0300-7 PMID: 30617339

Torrey, E. F. (2025). Epilogue 2025: How to Fix the Mental Illness Treatment System.

Tripodoro, V. A. (2025). First-Ever Global Ranking of Palliative Care: 2025 World Map Under the New WHO Framework. *Journal of Pain and Symptom Management.*

Tsai, Y. J., Lin, C. H., Yen, Y. H., Wu, C. C., Carvajal, C., Molte, N. F., & Hsieh, C. H. (2023). Risk factors for pressure ulcer recurrence following surgical reconstruction: A cross-sectional retrospective analysis. *Frontiers in Surgery, 10,* 970681. DOI: 10.3389/fsurg.2023.970681 PMID: 36936658

Turner, G., & Clegg, A. (2014). Best practice guidelines for the management of frailty : A British Geriatrics Society, Age UK and Royal College of General Practitioners report. *Age and Ageing, 43*(6), 744–747. DOI: 10.1093/ageing/afu138 PMID: 25336440

U.S. Department of Health & Human Services. (2013). *Health Insurance Portability and Accountability Act of 1996 (HIPAA).* https://www.hhs.gov/hipaa/for-professionals/privacy/index.html

Ukpo, S. D., Imohiosen, C. E., Owot, J. A., & Ajuluchukwu, P. (2024). The impact of religious and spiritual counseling on mental health outcomes in geriatric care. *International Journal of Multidisciplinary Research and Growth Evaluation, 5*(6), 1538–1547.

Umar, Z., Tahir, Z., & Nizami, A. (2023). Impact of severe mental illnesses on health-related quality of life among patients attending the Institute of Psychiatry, Rawalpindi from 2019 to 2021 : A cross-sectional study. *PLoS One, 18*(8), e0289080. DOI: 10.1371/journal.pone.0289080 PMID: 37535604

UNICEF. (2019). *Mental Health and Psychosocial Technical Note*

United Nations (UN). (2022). *Ageing* [Internet]. Retrieved June 4, 2025, from https://www.un.org/en/global-issues/ageing

United Nations. (2019). *World Population Prospects, The 2019 Revision - Volume I : Comprehensive Tables.* UN. DOI: 10.18356/15994a82-en

United Nations. (2023). Second Committee approves 14 draft resolutions, including texts on agriculture development, biological diversity, combating sand and dust storms. UN Press. https://press.un.org/en/2023/gaef3587.doc.htm Retrieved June 13, 2025.

Upasen, R. (2022). Death Acceptance Process in Thai Buddhist Patients With Life-Limiting Cancer: A Grounded Theory. *Global Qualitative Nursing Research.*

Vaiphei, S. D. (2025). *Understanding End-of-Life Care*. Google Books. https://books.google.com/books?hl=en&lr=&id=Q8RIEQAAQBAJ&oi=fnd&pg=PA1&dq=Ignoring+the+emotional+or+psychological+component+of+the+terminally+ill+patient%E2%80%99s+symptoms

Vaiphei, S. D. (2021). The psychological aspect of pain and symptom management in clinical practices: Scoping review. *Journal of Clinical Medicine of Kazakhstan, 18*(6). https://cyberleninka.ru/article/n/the-psychological-aspect-of-pain-and-symptom-management-in-clinical-practices-scoping-review

Van Dam, N. T., van Vugt, M. K., Vago, D. R., Schmalzl, L., Saron, C. D., Olendzki, A., Meissner, T., Lazar, S. W., Kerr, C. E., Gorchov, J., & Fox, K. C. R. (2018). Mind the hype: A critical evaluation and prescriptive agenda for research on mindfulness and meditation. *Perspectives on Psychological Science, 13*(1), 36–61. DOI: 10.1177/1745691617709589

van den Brink, J. L., Moorman, P. W., de Boer, M. F., Hop, W. C. J., Pruyn, J. F. A., Verwoerd, C. D. A., & van Bemmel, J. H. (2007). Impact on quality of life of a telemedicine system supporting head and neck cancer patients : A controlled trial during the postoperative period at home. *Journal of the American Medical Informatics Association : JAMIA, 14*(2), 198–205. DOI: 10.1197/jamia.M2199 PMID: 17213498

van der Stap, L., de Heij, A. H., van der Heide, A., Reyners, A. K. L., & van der Linden, Y. M. (2022). Barriers and facilitators to multidimensional symptom management in palliative care: A focus group study among patient representatives and clinicians. *Palliative & Supportive Care, 21*(4), 1–12. DOI: 10.1017/s147895152200133x PMID: 36177886

Van Driel, T., Hilderink, P., Hanssen, D., De Boer, P., Rosmalen, J., & Oude Voshaar, R. (2018). Assessment of somatization and medically unexplained symptoms in later life. *Assessment, 25*(3), 374–393. PMID: 28745072

Van Hecke, N., Claes, C., Vanderplasschen, W., De Maeyer, J., De Witte, N., & Vandevelde, S. (2018). Conceptualisation and Measurement of Quality of Life Based on Schalock and Verdugo's Model : A Cross-Disciplinary Review of the Literature. *Social Indicators Research, 137*(1), 335–351. DOI: 10.1007/s11205-017-1596-2

Vanholder, R., Davenport, A., Hannedouche, T., Kooman, J., Kribben, A., Lameire, N., Lonnemann, G., Magner, P., Mendelssohn, D., Saggi, S. J., Shaffer, R. N., Moe, S. M., Van Biesen, W., van der Sande, F., Mehrotra, R., & Nephrology, on behalf of the D. A. G. of the A. S. of. (2012). Reimbursement of Dialysis: A Comparison of Seven Countries. *Journal of the American Society of Nephrology, 23*(8). https://journals.lww.com/jasn/fulltext/2012/08000/reimbursement_of_dialysis__a_comparison_of_seven.7.aspx

Vargas-Escobar, L. M., Sánchez-Cárdenas, M. A., Guerrero-Benítez, A. C., Suarez-Prieto, V. K., Moreno-García, J. R., Cañón Piñeros, Á. M., Rodríguez-Campos, L. F., & León-Delgado, M. X. (2022). Barriers to access to palliative care in Colombia: A social mapping approach involving stakeholder participation. *INQUIRY: The Journal of Health Care Organization, Provision, and Financing*, *59*, 00469580221133217. PMID: 36317765

Vedel, I., De Stampa, M., Bergman, H., Ankri, J., Cassou, B., Mauriat, C., Blanchard, F., Bagaragaza, E., & Lapointe, L. (2009). A novel model of integrated care for the elderly: COPA, Coordination of Professional Care for the Elderly. *Aging Clinical and Experimental Research*, *21*, 414–423. PMID: 20154510

Veronese, N., Custodero, C., Demurtas, J., Smith, L., Barbagallo, M., Maggi, S., Cella, A., Vanacore, N., Aprile, P. L., & Ferrucci, L. (2022). Comprehensive geriatric assessment in older people: An umbrella review of health outcomes. *Age and Ageing*, *51*(5), afac104. PMID: 35524746

Vetter, V. J. (2022). Palliative care screening tools in the gynecologic oncology population: A narrative review. *Annals of Palliative Medicine*, *11*(10), 3263–3272. DOI: 10.21037/apm-22-728 PMID: 36226647

Vick, J. B., & Wolff, J. L. (2021). A scoping review of person and family engagement in the context of multiple chronic conditions. *Health Services Research, 56 Suppl 1*(Suppl 1), 990–1005. https://doi.org/DOI: 10.1111/1475-6773.13857

Visiting Nurses Association of America (V.N.A.A.). (n.d.). https://www.vnaa.org/

Vo, M. T. H., & Fong, B. Y. F. (2025). Long-Term Care Initiatives in Southeast Asian Countries with Emerging Ageing Population and the Sustainability of Health and Social Care Systems. In *The Handbook of Public Health in the Asia-Pacific* (pp. 1–32). Springer.

von Leupoldt, A., Sommer, T., Kegat, S., Baumann, H. J., Klose, H., Dahme, B., & Büchel, C. (2008). The unpleasantness of perceived dyspnea is processed in the anterior insula and amygdala. *American Journal of Respiratory and Critical Care Medicine*, *177*(9), 1026–1032. DOI: 10.1164/rccm.200712-1821OC

Von Roenn, J. H. (2013). Advance Care Planning : Ensuring That the Patient's Voice Is Heard. *Journal of Clinical Oncology, 31*(6), 663–664. DOI: 10.1200/JCO.2012.46.8181 PMID: 23284035

Voumard, R., Rubli Truchard, E., Benaroyo, L., Borasio, G., Büla, C., & Jox, R. (2018). Geriatric palliative care: A view of its concept, challenges and strategies. *BMC Geriatrics, 18*, 1–6. PMID: 30236063

W.H.O. (2025). *News Release*. Retrieved from W.H.O.

Wachterman, M. W., & Sommers, B. D. (2021). Dying poor in the US—Disparities in end-of-life care. *Journal of the American Medical Association, 325*(5), 423–424. PMID: 33528526

Wagenschieber, E., & Blunck, D. (2024). Impact of reimbursement systems on patient care - a systematic review of systematic reviews. *Health Economics Review, 14*(1), 22. DOI: 10.1186/s13561-024-00487-6 PMID: 38492098

Wang, C., Huang, S., Zhu, T., Sun, X., Zou, Y., & Wang, Y. (2014). [Efficacy of photodynamic antimicrobial therapy for wound flora and wound healing of pressure sore with pathogen infection]. *Zhonghua Yi Xue Za Zhi, 94*(31), 2455–2459. PMID: 25400056

Wang, M., & Ding, X. (2025). Integrated palliative care improves the quality of life of advanced cancer patients. *BMC Palliative Care, 24*(1), 162. DOI: 10.1186/s12904-025-01800-8 PMID: 40483417

Wang, Y., Zhang, X., Huang, Y., & Ma, X. (2024). Palliative care for cancer patients in asia: Challenges and countermeasures. *Oncology Reviews, 17*, 11866. PMID: 38293617

Warden, V., Hurley, A., & Volicer, L. (2003). Development and Psychometric Evaluation of the Pain Assessment in Advanced Dementia (PAINAD) Scale. *Journal of the American Medical Directors Association, 4*(1), 9–15. DOI: 10.1016/s1525-8610(04)70258-3

Warth, M., Kessler, J., Koenig, J., Wormit, A. F., Hillecke, T. K., & Bardenheuer, H. J. (2014). Music therapy to promote psychological and physiological relaxation in palliative care patients: Protocol of a randomized controlled trial. *BMC Palliative Care, 13*(1), 60. DOI: 10.1186/1472-684x-13-60

Watson, L., Qi, S., Link, C., DeIure, A., Afzal, A., & Barbera, L. (2023). Patient-Reported Symptom Complexity and Acute Care Utilization Among Patients With Cancer: A Population-Based Study Using a Novel Symptom Complexity Algorithm and Observational Data. *Journal of the National Comprehensive Cancer Network : JNCCN, 21*(2), 173–180. DOI: 10.6004/jnccn.2022.7087 PMID: 36791760

Wenger, N. S. (2001). Quality indicators for end-of-life care in vulnerable elders. *Annals of Internal Medicine*, •••, 677–685.

Wenrich, M. D. (2003). Dying patients' need for emotional support and personalized care from physicians: Perspectives of patients with terminal illness, families, and health care providers. *Journal of Pain and Symptom Management*, •••, 236–246.

Whitebird, R. R., Kreitzer, M. J., Crain, A. L., Lewis, B. A., Hanson, L. R., & Enstad, C. J. (2013). Mindfulness-based stress reduction for family caregivers: A randomized controlled trial. *The Gerontologist, 53*(4), 676–686. DOI: 10.1093/geront/gns126

WHO. (1993). Study protocol for the World Health Organization project to develop a Quality of Life assessment instrument (WHOQOL). *Quality of Life Research: An International Journal of Quality of Life Aspects of Treatment, Care and Rehabilitation, 2*(2), 153–159. PMID: 8518769

WHO. (1997). *WHOQOL Measuring Quality of Life*. World Health Organization. https://iris.who.int/handle/10665/63482

WHO. (2002). *National cancer control programmes: policies and managerial guidelines*. World Health Organization.

WHO. (2014). *Renforcement des soins palliatifs en tant qu'élément du traitement intégré à toutes les étapes de la vie.*

WHO. (2021). Assessing the development of palliative care worldwide: a set of actionable indicators. Available at: https://www.who.int/publications/i/item/9789240033351: World Health Organization.

WHO. (2022). World Health Organization *Palliative care fact sheet.* doi:DOI: 10.1097/grh.0000000000000052

WHO. (2023a). Policy brief on integrating rehabilitation into palliative care services. Copenhagen: Licence: CC BY NC-SA 3.0 IGO. *World Health Organization Regional Office for Europe.*

WHO. (2023b). World Health Organisation Palliative Care (2020). Available online at: https://www. who.int/news-room/fact-sheets/detail/palliative-care (assessed October 25, 2023). *World Health Organisation*. doi:DOI: 10.1016/s0266-6138(14)00213-7

WHO. W. H. O. (2020). *Palliative Care*. WHO. Retrieved 23/04/2025 from https://www.who.int/news-room/fact-sheets/detail/palliative-care

WHPCA. W. P. C. A. (2020). *Global Atlas of Palliative Care* (2nd Edition ed.).

Wiencek, C., & Coyne, P. (2014). Palliative care delivery models. Seminars in oncology nursing, Wittenberg, E., Ferrell, B., Goldsmith, J., & Ruel, N. H. (2016). Family Caregiver Communication Tool: A New Measure for Tailoring Communication with Cancer Caregivers: For submission to Psycho Oncology. *Psycho-Oncology*, *26*(8), 1222.

Wilaras, A. (2024). Cognitive behavioural interventions for palliative care in adult patients: A scoping review. *Progress in Palliative Care*, *32*(6), 1–43. DOI: 10.1080/09699260.2024.2408127

Willadsen, T. G., Siersma, V., Nicolaisdottir, D. R., Jarbol, D., Guassora, A. D., Reventlow, S., & Køster-Rasmussen, R. (2021). Symptom burden in multimorbidity: A population-based combined questionnaire and registry study from Denmark. *BMJ Open*, *11*(4), e041877. DOI: 10.1136/bmjopen-2020-041877 PMID: 33849847

Wilson, I. B., & Cleary, P. D. (1995). Linking clinical variables with health-related quality of life. A conceptual model of patient outcomes. *Journal of the American Medical Association*, *273*(1), 59–65. PMID: 7996652

Wittenberg, E., Reb, A., & Kanter, E. (2018). Communicating with patients and families around difficult topics in cancer care using the COMFORT communication curriculum. Seminars in oncology nursing, Wolf, C., & Wedding, U. (2025). Geriatric Oncology Highlights from the European Society for Medical Oncology Annual Meeting 2024. *Oncology Research and Treatment*.

Wittenberg, E., Goldsmith, J. V., Ragan, S. L., & Parnell, T. A. (2019). *Communication in Palliative Nursing: The COMFORT Model*. Oxford University Press., DOI: 10.1093/med/9780190061326.001.0001

Wittenberg, E., Kravits, K., Goldsmith, J., Ferrell, B., & Fujinami, R. (2017). Validation of a model of family caregiver communication types and related caregiver outcomes. *Palliative & Supportive Care*, *15*(1), 3–11. PMID: 27032294

Wong, L. P. (2015). Associations between religiosity and death attitudes: Different between christians and buddhists? *Psychology of Religion and Spirituality*.

World Health Organization. (1996). *WHOQOL-BREF: Introduction, administration, scoring, and generic version of the assessment*. WHO.

World Health Organization. (2020). *Decade of healthy ageing: Baseline report*. World Health Organization. https://www.who.int/publications/i/item/9789240017900

World Health Organization. (2024, October 1). *Ageing and health* [Fact sheet]. Retrieved June 3, 2025, from https://www.who.int/news-room/fact-sheets/detail/ageing-and-health

Wu, Y., Tao, Z., Qiao, Y., Chai, Y., Liu, Q., Lu, Q., Zhou, H., Li, S., Mao, J., Jiang, M., & Pu, J. (2022). Prevalence and characteristics of somatic symptom disorder in the elderly in a community-based population: A large-scale cross-sectional study in China. *BMC Psychiatry*, *22*(1). Advance online publication. DOI: 10.1186/s12888-022-03907-1 PMID: 35413865

Xie, W., & Butcher, R. (2023). *Artificial Intelligence Decision Support Tools for End-of-Life Care Planning Conversations : CADTH Horizon Scan*. Canadian Agency for Drugs and Technologies in Health. https://www.ncbi.nlm.nih.gov/books/NBK599854/

Yaghi, G., & Chahine, B. (2023). Potentially inappropriate medications use in a psychiatric elderly care hospital: A cross-sectional study using Beers criteria. *Health Science Reports*, *6*(5), e1247. PMID: 37234198

Yan, A. F., Chen, Z., Wang, Y., Campbell, J. A., Xue, Q.-L., Williams, M. Y., Weinhardt, L. S., & Egede, L. E. (2022). Effectiveness of Social Needs Screening and Interventions in Clinical Settings on Utilization, Cost, and Clinical Outcomes: A Systematic Review. *Health Equity*, *6*(1), 454–475. DOI: 10.1089/heq.2022.0010 PMID: 35801145

Yang, Y., Liang, X., Liu, Q., & Liu, J. (2025). Navigating limited resources: Experiences of caregivers for elderly terminal cancer patients in a region with limited palliative care services. *Supportive Care in Cancer*, *33*(3), 207. PMID: 39971822

Yao, H., Jingyue, W., Rui, Z., Hou, Y., & Hui, Y. (2025). E-CARE as core competencies for palliative social workers: A systematic review. *BMC Palliative Care*, *24*(1). Advance online publication. DOI: 10.1186/s12904-025-01735-0 PMID: 40490802

Yao, M., Zhou, X.-y., Xu, Z.-j., Lehman, R., Haroon, S., Jackson, D., & Cheng, K. K. (2021). The impact of training healthcare professionals' communication skills on the clinical care of diabetes and hypertension: A systematic review and meta-analysis. *BMC Family Practice*, *22*, 1–23. PMID: 34261454

Yao, R., Zhang, W., Evans, R., Cao, G., Rui, T., & Shen, L. (2022). Inequities in Health Care Services Caused by the Adoption of Digital Health Technologies: Scoping Review. *Journal of Medical Internet Research, 24*(3), e34144. DOI: 10.2196/34144 PMID: 35311682

Yeung, W.-J. J., & Thang, L. L. (2018). Long-Term care for older adults in ASEAN plus three: The roles of family, community, and the state in addressing unmet eldercare needs. *Journal of Aging and Health, 30*(10), 1499–1515. PMID: 30239253

Yorke, J., Moosavi, S. H., Shuldham, C., & Jones, P. W. (2010). Quantification of dyspnea using descriptors: Development and initial testing of the Dyspnea-12. *Thorax, 65*(1), 21–26. DOI: 10.1136/thx.2009.118521

Zanin, A. (2023). End-of-life decisions and practices as viewed by health professionals in pediatric critical care: A European survey study.

Zarit, S. H., Reever, K. E., & Bach-Peterson, J. (1980). Relatives of the impaired elderly: Correlates of feelings of burden. *The Gerontologist, 20*(6), 649–655. DOI: 10.1093/geront/20.6.649

Zeidan, F., Johnson, S. K., Diamond, B. J., David, Z., & Goolkasian, P. (2010). Mindfulness meditation improves cognition: Evidence of brief mental training. *Consciousness and Cognition, 19*(2), 597–605. DOI: 10.1016/j.concog.2010.03.014

Zernicke, K. A., Campbell, T. S., Speca, M., & Carlson, L. E. (2020). Autonomic and inflammatory correlates of caregiver stress and the potential role of mindfulness-based interventions. *Brain, Behavior, and Immunity, 89*, 275–284. DOI: 10.1016/j.bbi.2020.06.005

Zertuche-Maldonado, T., Figueroa, S. A. V., Cantisani, A. F., Lim, F., & Silva, M. F. (2020). Management of palliative care in Latin America. *Journal of Alternative Medical Research, 12*(1), 63–75.

Zhang, D., Lee, E. K. P., Mak, E. C. W., Ho, C. Y., & Wong, S. Y. S. (2021). Mindfulness-based interventions: An overall review. *British Medical Bulletin, 138*(1), 41–57. DOI: 10.1093/bmb/ldab005

Zhang, L., Zeng, Y., Wang, L., & Fang, Y. (2020). Urban-Rural Differences in Long-Term Care Service Status and Needs Among Home-Based Elderly People in China. *International Journal of Environmental Research and Public Health, 17*(5). Advance online publication. DOI: 10.3390/ijerph17051701 PMID: 32150946

Zhang, N., Li, Q., Chen, S., Wu, Y., Xin, B., Wan, Q., Shi, P., He, Y., Yang, S., & Jiang, W. (2024). Effectiveness of nurse-led electronic health interventions on illness management in patients with chronic heart failure: A systematic review and meta-analysis. *International Journal of Nursing Studies, 150*, 104630. DOI: 10.1016/j.ijnurstu.2023.104630 PMID: 38029453

Zhang, Q. H., Sun, Z. R., Yue, J. H., Ren, X., Qiu, L. B., Lv, X. L., & Du, W. (2013). Traditional Chinese medicine for pressure ulcer: A meta-analysis. *International Wound Journal, 10*(2), 221–231. DOI: 10.1111/j.1742-481X.2012.00969.x PMID: 22512889

Zhang, Q., Sun, Z., & Yue, J. (2015). Massage therapy for preventing pressure ulcers. *Cochrane Database of Systematic Reviews, 2015*(6), Cd010518. DOI: 10.1002/14651858.CD010518.pub2 PMID: 26081072

Zhang, X., Zhang, X., Li, Y., Chen, T., Wang, Y., Siow, L., Wang, Y., Ming, W.-K., Sun, X., & Wu, Y. (2022). Factors affecting acceptance of palliative care in mainland China: A national cross-sectional study. *The Lancet. Oncology, 23*, S3.

Zhang, Y.-h., Yang, Z.-k., Wang, J.-w., Xiong, Z.-y., Liao, J.-l., Hao, L., & Dong, J. (2018). Cognitive Changes in Peritoneal Dialysis Patients: A Multicenter Prospective Cohort Study. *American Journal of Kidney Diseases, 72*(5), 691–700. DOI: 10.1053/j.ajkd.2018.04.020

Zhang, Y., Leuk, J. S. P., & Teo, W. P. (2023). Domains, Feasibility, Effectiveness, Cost, and Acceptability of Telehealth in Aging Care: Scoping Review of Systematic Reviews. *JMIR Aging, 6*, 1–16. DOI: 10.2196/40460 PMID: 37071459

Zhao, W., Kelly, R. M., Rogerson, M. J., & Waycott, J. (2024, May). Older adults imagining future technologies in participatory design workshops: Supporting continuity in the pursuit of meaningful activities. In *Proceedings of the 2024 CHI Conference on Human Factors in Computing Systems* (pp. 1-18).

Zhao, X., Tong, S., & Yang, Y. (2022). The Correlation Between Quality of Life and Positive Psychological Resources in Cancer Patients : A Meta-Analysis. *Frontiers in Psychology, 13*, 883157. DOI: 10.3389/fpsyg.2022.883157 PMID: 35783766

Zhao, Y., Wang, J., Zhu, X., Zhang, X., Zhang, Y., Zhang, W., & Dong, Y. (2023). Multimorbidity and polypharmacy in hospitalized older patients: A cross-sectional study. *BMC Geriatrics, 23*(1), 423. DOI: 10.1186/s12877-023-04109-4 PMID: 37434147

Zhou, L., Li, W., Wu, T., Fan, Z., Ismaili, L., Komolafe, T. E., & Zhang, S. (2024). Adaptive weighted stacking model with optimal weights selection for mortality risk prediction in sepsis patients. *Applied Intelligence*, *54*(22), 11892–11913.

Zhou, L., Wu, R., Wang, S., Komolafe, T. E., Guo, J., Fan, Z., & Zhang, Z. (2025). An explicable machine learning approach for predicting 30-day septic mortality for ICU patients. *International Journal of Information and Communication Technology*, *26*(9), 1–22.

Zhu, T. (2023). Preferences and Attitudes Towards Life-Sustaining Treatments of Older Chinese Patients and Their Family Caregivers. *Clinical Interventions in Aging*, •••, 467–475.

About the Contributors

Adil Alharthi, MD consultant Internist KFAFH Jeddah interested in General medicine, Geriatrics, Multimorbidity, Palliative Care

Marwa Mohammed Eleawa is an Assistant Professor at faculty of allied medical science,department of physiotherapy,applied science private university,Amman,Jordan . She obtained a PhD in rehabilitation medicine and physical therapy at Nanjing Medical University, China, in 2022. Dr. Mohammed has published numerous peer-reviewed research and review articles in internationally acclaimed journals. Her areas of expertise include cardiopulmonary rehabilitation, geriatric robotics, AI in rehabilitation, cancer research, exercise physiology,neurorehabilitation, sarcopenia, frailty, and cachexia. She serves as a peer reviewer for several journals, including IGI Global, Frontiers in Neurology, Journal of Advanced Research, and Journal of Cachexia, Sarcopenia, and Muscle. Additionally, she supervises master's theses at Faculty of physical therapy, Beni-Suef University,Egypt

***

Adegbola O Adeniji is an Otorhinolaryngologist- head and neck surgeon. He had his University degree from the University of Ilorin, Nigeria and his Otolaryngology fellowship from the West African college of surgeons. He currently practices as a Consultant in the Ear, nose and Throat department of the Federal Medical center, Owo. He is a visiting consultant to the University of Medical sciences Teaching Hospital, Ondo. His areas of research interest include Endoscopic sinus and skull base surgery, Head and neck oncology, Neurootology and skull base surgery to mention a few. He is a member of Otolaryngological society of Nigeria(ORLSON), American Accademy of Otolaryngology Head and Neck Surgeons (AAOHNS).

His research interests are in Head and Neck tumours, Heareing loss and Cochlear implants.

Wafaa Ramadan Ahmed is an Assistant Professor of Medical-Surgical Nursing at Faculty of Nursing, Assiut University, Egypt, and currently working at the Nursing Science Program, School of Health and Medical Sciences, Libyan International Medical University (LIMU), Libya. She has over 15 years of experience in nursing education and researches, with a focus on chronic disease management, patient education, and evidence-based Nursing practice. Dr. Ahmed has published nearly 20 research papers in reputable international journals, supervised postgraduate theses, and led curriculum development initiatives. She is actively involved in academic leadership, serving as Training and Development Supervisor, Interprofessional Learning Education (IPE) Supervisor, and member of ERASMUS+ EU projects. Dr. Ahmed is a reviewer for Rehabilitation Nursing Journal and Frontiers in Medicine, contributing to the advancement of high-quality scientific scholarship in healthcare.

Akintunde Oluseye David is a researcher and scholar with a strong background in History and International Relations. Oluseye had his Bachelor's degree in History and International Relations, and later completed his Master's degree in International Relations. Oluseye's academic interests include public health, peace and conflicts, cultural history, global diplomacy and international policy analysis. With a dedication to academic growth, Oluseye is poised to impact both the academic community and policy making environments.

Tosin Yinka Akintunde is a Senior Research and Data Analyst with the Government of Alberta. He holds a PhD and MSc in Sociology from Hohai University, China, and a BSc in Demography and Social Statistics from Obafemi Awolowo University, Nigeria. Tosin's research spans public health, child and adolescent development, trauma, and social determinants of violence, with a growing focus on cross-cultural analysis. He has held academic and research roles at the University of Alberta and Hohai University, and received prestigious awards including the Chinese Government Scholarship and Hohai University First-Class Scholarship. Tosin has authored over 50 peer-reviewed publications across journals such as Public Health, Journal of Aggression, Maltreatment & Trauma, child and adolesce social work, and Adversity and Resilience Science. His work reflects a commitment to advancing evidence-based insights into psychosocial vulnerabilities of those exposed to childhood adversity and violence.

Joseph Obiri Asante is a lecturer and researcher at the School of Pharmacy, Jiangsu Food and Pharmaceutical Science College, with expertise in palliative care, geriatric pharmacotherapy, and quality-of-life research. He holds a PhD in Social

Medicine and Health Management, as well as advanced degrees in Education, Medicine, and Pharmacy. His scholarly work focuses on the intersections of clinical pharmacology, geriatric care, and health outcomes, with a particular emphasis on symptom management in terminal illness, ethical decision-making in healthcare, and patient- and caregiver-centered approaches in end-of-life care. Dr. Asante has authored and co-authored numerous peer-reviewed publications addressing quality-of-life assessment, medical ethics, and pharmacological interventions in advanced disease, contributing significantly to the fields of palliative medicine and health systems research. As an academic, Dr. Asante is committed to training the next generation of healthcare professionals, integrating evidence-based clinical practice with compassionate care models. His ongoing research projects explore innovative frameworks for the management of distressing symptoms such as non-hypoxic dyspnea, aiming to improve patient comfort, dignity, and family support in terminal care.

Samia Boussaa is currently Professor in ISPITS (Institut Supérieur des Professions Infirmières et des Techniques de Santé) of Rabat (Morocco). She obtained her PhD, in Ecology and Epidemiology, at Cadi Ayyad University (Morocco) and at Strasbourg University (France) in 2008. Her research is focused on Medical Entomology, Vector Borne Disease and especially on Epidemiology of leishmaniasis in Morocco.

Stanley Isangha is an Assistant Lecturer at The Department of Social Work and Social Administration, The University of Hong Kong, where he coordinates the BSOCSC Counseling programme Capstone Project. His teaching emphasizes multiculturalism, trauma, and youth support. His research focuses on Mental health, Child Protection, Violence, Family Violence and Men's Health, particularly Intimate Partner Violence against men, aiming to promote effective interventions for community well-being.

Ashba Javed is a driven and enthusiastic student pursuing her Master's degree from Aligarh Muslim University in psychology. With a passion for learning and a keen interest in making a meaningful impact, Ashba is dedicated to exceling in her field of study. As a proactive and engaged learner, she is eager to contribute to the academic community and make a positive difference. Her academic pursuits and enthusiasm for growth make her a promising talent in her field.

Arshy Kamal is a dedicated researcher in the field of Clinical Psychology, pursuing her research at JNMCH College, Aligarh Muslim University (AMU). A qualified NET and GATE scholar, Arshy has demonstrated exceptional academic prowess and a strong commitment to her field. Her research contributions include publications in peer-reviewed papers and chapters, showcasing her expertise and potential to make a significant impact in Clinical Psychology. As a driven and accomplished researcher, Arshy Kamal is poised to make valuable contributions to the field and inspire future generations.

Arshy Kamal is currently a Research Scholar at a reputed Medical Psychiatric College, where their work focuses on the psychological dimensions of health and illness. They have successfully qualified the National Eligibility Test (NET) and the Graduate Aptitude Test in Engineering (GATE), reflecting their strong academic foundation. With two research publications in peer-reviewed journals, Arshy Kamal is actively contributing to the advancement of psychiatric and psychological research. Their scholarly interests span mental health interventions, psychosocial factors in medical care, and integrative approaches to psychiatry. They aim to bridge clinical practice with psychological theory, fostering holistic perspectives in patient care and research.

Ayesha Khan is a distinguished guest faculty member with a PhD in psychology. They have made significant contributions to research, actively publishing in peer-reviewed journals, and are deeply involved in teaching and mentoring students. Dr. Ayesha Khan has also played a key role in curriculum development and syllabus modifications, ensuring that academic programs remain current and aligned with emerging trends in the field. Their work bridges rigorous research with effective teaching, fostering an enriched learning environment for students and advancing scholarly knowledge in psychology.

Blessing Funmi Komolafe is a Lecturer at the College of International Education, Shanghai University of Medicine & Health Sciences. She previously worked in the Department of Science Education at Adekunle Ajasin University, Nigeria. Her research focuses on pre-service physics teacher training, curriculum development, pedagogy, medical education, and AI-based teaching methods. She earned her Ph.D. in Curriculum and Pedagogy from Zhejiang Normal University, China, in 2021. Dr. Komolafe has published extensively in international journals and serves as a reviewer for peer-reviewed journals, as well as an Article Editor for Sage Open and a Book Editor for Taylor & Francis.

Temitope Emmanuel Komolafe received his Ph.D. in Biomedical Engineering from the University of Science and Technology of China, Hefei, in 2021. He then worked as a postdoctoral researcher at the School of Biomedical Engineering, ShanghaiTech University, from 2021 to 2023. He is currently an Assistant Professor at the Collaborative Research Centre, Shanghai University of Medicine and Health Sciences. His research interests include intelligent medicine, medical image processing, and precision medical rehabilitation robotic devices. Dr. Komolafe has published extensively in peer-reviewed journals and serves as a Review Editor for Data Mining and Management (Frontiers in Big Data) and as a Book Editor for Taylor & Francis.

Hassan Hussein Musa is a world-renowned scientist in Molecular Genetics and Immunology. His rich academic history involves postgraduate studies at renowned world establishments like Yangzhou University in China, the Institute of Genetic Engineering and Biotechnology in Iran, the USA's University of Pennsylvania School of Medicine, the University of Nottingham in the UK, and the Chinese Academy of Sciences. Professor Musa's exceptional research has drawn him numerous prestigious awards and recognition, including the CAS President International Fellowship Initiative in China, TWAS-UNESCO Associateship in Italy, and competitive grants from the Chinese Postdoctoral Science Foundation. He conducted his PhD through the Chinese Scholarship Council and postdoctoral research at Yangzhou University. His professional awards and achievements are Fellowship in the Chinese Academy of Science and membership in Sudanese National Academy of Science. Professor Musa is also a member of several top-level international scientific societies, i.e., the American Association of Immunologists, the African/European/American Societies of Human Genetics, and the International Society for Stem Cell Research. Directing cutting-edge multidisciplinary research programs in Genetics, Genomics, Immunology, and Stem Cells, Professor Musa has authored a renowned set of over 200 peer-reviewed articles, book chapters, and conference proceedings. He has supervised 8 PhD and 22 MSc students to successful completion of their degrees, testifying to his firm academic growth and capacity building obligation to the future generation of scientists. Through his excellent global training, large volume of research contributions, and dedication to the education of science, Professor Musa has become an elite global expert in molecular genetics and immunology with significant contributions to the advancement of science and future scientists.

Idriss Hussein Musa is a distinguished Senior Specialist in General Surgery with over a decade of experience, renowned for his clinical expertise and dedication to advancing surgical care and medical education. His career spans significant contributions at both national and international levels. Currently, Dr. Idriss serves as a Senior Specialist in General Surgery at Wad Madani Teaching Hospital. Concurrently, he shapes the future of medicine as a faculty member in the School of Medical Sciences at Darfur University College, Sudan. His international credentials include a clinical attachment in Hepatobiliary Surgery at Sultan Qaboos University Hospital in Oman and a prestigious License in General Surgery from the Oman Medical Specialization Board (2024). Prior to his current roles, Dr. Idriss gained extensive experience across various private and public hospitals in Sudan. A key position was his tenure as a General Surgery Specialist at Bashair University Hospital in Khartoum, where he demonstrated strong leadership by guiding a surgical team and overseeing referral clinics, outpatient services, and elective operations.

Taha Hussein Musa is a distinguished Sudanese epidemiologist and biostatistician whose career seamlessly integrates advanced academic research with impactful fieldwork in public health and infectious diseases. With a professional dedication to addressing health challenges in vulnerable communities across Sudan and globally, Dr. Musa has emerged as a leading voice in epidemiology and community health. His academic journey is characterized by excellence and international recognition. He earned his PhD in Epidemiology and Health Statistics from Southeast University in China, complemented by a Master's in Professional Public Health from the same institution. His foundational studies in Environmental Science and Natural Resources were completed at the University of Gezira, Sudan. His academic achievements were further highlighted through multiple prestigious scholarships from the Chinese Scholarship Council. Currently serving as an Assistant Professor, Dr. Musa lectures on critical subjects including Biostatistics, Epidemiology, Hospital Management, and Research Methods. He is also a co-founder of the Organization of African Academic Doctors (OAAD), underscoring his commitment to fostering research capacity and talent development across Africa. Dr. Musa's extensive professional experience includes significant roles in renowned humanitarian organizations such as Médecins Sans Frontières (MSF), Oxfam GB, and UNHCR. In these capacities, he has managed public health programs, led food security initiatives, and delivered essential health services in challenging environments, including refugee and internally displaced persons (IDPs) settings in Sudan. As a prolific researcher, Dr. Musa serves as a leading staff member at the Biomedical Research Institute, Darfur University College. With over 160 publications and 1,243 citations, his work focuses on infectious diseases, public health, and epidemiological studies. He also contributes as an editor for several peer-reviewed journals published by Elsevier, Springer, Wiley, and Frontiers. Driven by a passion for disease prevention and health promotion, Dr. Musa effectively collaborates with global partners and local communities. His unique blend of academic rigor, field experience, and dedication to mentoring future researchers solidifies his status as a distinguished figure in public health and epidemiology.

Madiha Rahman is a dedicated special Educator and Researcher with a Ph.D in Psychology, holding certification from the Rehabilitation Council of India (RCI) with extensive experience working with children with diverse needs, including Autism Spectrum Disorder, ADHD, and Learning disabilities, she combines evidence-based interventions with compassionate care to support holistic development . Her work bridges academic research and practical application m ensuring that children with special needs receive individualized support that nurtures their abilities and enhances inclusion .Passionate about advancing special education, Dr. Madiha Rehman continues to contribute through teaching, researchDr Madiha Rahman is a dedicated special Educator and Researcher with a Ph.D in Psychology, holding certification from the Rehabilitation Council of India (RCI) with extensive experience working with children with diverse needs, including Autism Spectrum Disorder, ADHD, and Learning disabilities, she combines evidence-based interventions with compassionate care to support holistic development . Her work bridges academic research and practical application, ensuring that children with special needs receive individualized support that nurtures their abilities and enhances inclusion .Passionate about advancing special education, Dr. Madiha Rehman continues to contribute through teaching, research, and advocacy for children with developmental and Learning challenges.

Madiha Rehman is a distinguished psychologist and special educator, having earned her doctoral degree from Aligarh Muslim University (AMU). Her research contributions include publications in reputable platforms, showcasing her expertise in psychology. As an RCI Registered Special Educator, she is committed to providing specialized support and education, making a positive impact in the lives of individuals with special needs.

Syed Zafar Sultan Rizvi is a noted academician, researcher, and psychologist, currently serving as an Assistant Professor in the Department of Psychology at Mohammad Ali Jauhar University, Rampur (India). His work reflects a deep commitment to advancing psychological education, research, and mental health awareness. Dr. Rizvi completed his Ph.D. in Psychology from Aligarh Muslim University (AMU), one of India's premier centers of higher learning. His doctoral research, titled "Academic Performance as Related to Procrastination, Stress and Anxiety among University Students," explored the interconnection between psychological stressors and academic outcomes — a theme that continues to shape his research and teaching philosophy. He also holds a Master's degree in Social Psychology from AMU. With expertise covering Social Psychology, Cognitive Psychology, Neuropsychology, Biological Psychology, Clinical and Counselling Psychology, and Educational Psychology, Dr. Rizvi brings an interdisciplinary perspective to both teaching and research. His scholarly contributions include seven research papers, a book chapter in "COVID-19: Biopsychosocial Perspectives," participation in fourteen workshops, and presentations at five international conferences. Dr. Rizvi's teaching approach emphasizes critical inquiry, reflective learning, and the integration of theory with practice. He is known for motivating students to explore the human mind scientifically while nurturing empathy and ethical sensitivity — qualities essential for the next generation of mental health professionals. Technically adept, he utilizes tools such as SPSS, Minitab, and Python for data analysis and research, combining traditional psychological insights with modern computational methods. His primary research interests include student mental health, stress management, procrastination, emotional regulation, and cognitive resilience. Through his academic leadership and compassionate engagement with learners, Dr. Syed Zafar Sultan Rizvi continues to make a meaningful contribution to the field of psychology, shaping both minds and hearts in pursuit of holistic education and well-being.

Syed Zafar Sultan Rizvi is an accomplished academic and researcher, currently serving as an Assistant Professor with over three years of teaching experience in psychology. They hold a PhD and have authored more than 10 publications, including a Scopus-indexed book chapter. Actively involved in academic governance, Dr Syed Zafar Sultan Rizvi has contributed to Boards of Studies, NEP initiatives, and NAAC-related work. They have participated in over 20 national and international workshops and seminars and have shared their expertise in interviews on psychological topics published in leading media outlets, including Times of India, The Pioneer, Hindustan Times, News18, and Economic Times. Their work bridges research, teaching, and practical applications in the field of psychology.

Afreen Waseem is an Assistant Professor at GITAM University, holding a PhD in Psychology. She has published numerous research papers in peer-reviewed journals and is actively engaged in both teaching and research. Earlier, she worked as a Teaching Assistant at Aligarh Muslim University and completed internships at Dr. Ram Manohar Lohia Hospital (PGIMER) and as a School Counselor at Jamia Millia Islamia. Her academic and professional journey reflects a strong commitment to advancing psychological research while fostering practical learning and student development.

Liang Zhou is currently with the Department of Radiology, Jiading District Central Hospital Affiliated Shanghai University of Medicine & Health Sciences, Shanghai. His research interests include big data analysis and decision support.

Index

A

C

D

E

F

G

H

M

N

O

P

Q

R

S

T

W

www.ingramcontent.com/pod-product-compliance
Lightning Source LLC
LaVergne TN
LVHW062322300926
849161LV00007B/1537